P9-DGI-978

BIO-AGE

Ten Steps to a Younger You

Brad J. King and
Dr. Michael A. Schmidt

Macmillan Canada
Toronto

First published in Canada in 2001 by
Macmillan Canada, an imprint of CDG Books Canada

Copyright © Brad J. King 2001
Copyright © Dr. Michael A. Schmidt: Chapter 7 ("Fatty Acids"), Chapter 18 ("Mind Over Aging")

Chapters by the following contributors have been printed with their permission:
Dr. Fereydoon Batmanghelidj, Stephen Cherniske, Dr. Edward J. Conley, Dr. Daniel Crisafi,
Sam Graci, Dr. Donald Henderson, Dr. Kenneth Seaton, and Dr. Michael A. Zeligs.

Kenneth Seaton's chapter "The Aging Process: How to Slow it or Reverse it with Albumin"
is reprinted with permission from the author and from the Winter 2000 issue of *The Inter-national Journal of Anti-Aging Medicine*. Copyright 2000 by Intertec Publishing, a PRIMEDIA
Company. All rights reserved.

All rights reserved. The use of any part of this publication reproduced, transmitted in
any form or by any means, electronic, mechanical, recording or otherwise, or stored in a
retrieval system, without the prior consent of the publisher, is an infringement of the
copyright law. In the case of photocopying or other reprographic copying of the material,
a licence must be obtained from the Canadian Copyright Licensing Agency (CANCOPY)
before proceeding.

Canadian Cataloguing in Publication Data

King, Brad (Brad J.)
    Bio-age: ten steps to a younger you
Includes bibliographical references and index.
ISBN 1-55335-004-9

1. Aging—Prevention. I. Schmidt, Michael A., 1958–. II. Title
RA776.75.K56 2001   613   C2001-930071-9

This book is available at special discounts for bulk purchases by your group or organiza-tion for sales promotions, premiums, fundraising and seminars. For details, contact:
CDG Books Canada Inc., 99 Yorkville Avenue, Suite 400, Toronto, ON, M5R 3K5.
Tel: 416-963-8830. Toll Free: 1-877-963-8830. Fax: 416-923-4821. Web site: cdgbooks.com.

1 2 3 4 5 FP 05 04 03 02 01

Cover design by CS Richardson; text design by Heidy Lawrance Associates; photo credits:
cover photo by SuperStock; Dozier Photography (Michael Schmidt); Scope Photography,
Victoria, B.C. (Brad King)

Authors and Publisher have used their best efforts in preparing this book. CDG Books
Canada, the sponsor, and the authors make no representations or warranties with respect
to the accuracy or completeness of the contents of this book and specifically disclaim any
implied warranties of merchantability or fitness for a particular purpose. There are no
warranties that extend beyond the descriptions contained in this paragraph. No warranty
may be created or extended by sales representatives or written sales materials. The accu-racy and completeness of the information provided herein and the opinions stated herein
are not guaranteed or warranted to produce any specific results, and the advice and strate-gies contained herein may not be suitable for every individual. Neither CDG Books Canada,
the sponsor, nor the authors shall be liable for any loss of profit or any other commercial
damages including but not limited to special, incidental, consequential or other damages.

Bio-Age contains information summarized from medical literature, interviews with experts
and the authors' own clinical experience. Readers should recognize that interpretations of
scientific studies vary among scientists. The information in this book should not be construed
as medical advice, nor should it replace the advice of a licensed health care professional.

Macmillan Canada
An imprint of CDG Books Canada Inc.
Toronto
Printed in Canada

Contents

Acknowledgments

I owe a great debt to many people who have played an important role in shaping my destiny today and influencing the writing of this and other books. My late mother, Elva, who showed me what unconditional love is all about. My late father, Alan, who without realizing it pushed me to always strive for higher ground in life. My soul mother, Peggy Groom, who was sent from above to teach me the ways of the heart. You are truly a gift from the Universe, Peggy. To my beautiful Renee, for being so patient and understanding with my time commitments on this project, and for gifting me with your incredible love. To one of my closest friends and mentors, Sam Graci, who has always amazed me with his ability to magnetize those around him. You have inspired me to be the researcher, lecturer and health advocate I am today. To my great friend and mentor, Dr. Michael Schmidt, who it was an absolute honor to have as my co-author on this project. To Beth Potter, truly one of the best publicity agents and supporters I could ever have asked for. To Amy Black, assistant editor at CDG Books, you were great to work with and extremely professional in your conduct. To Stewart Brown, for his continued support of my research. To one of my greatest supporters and best friends, Fred Hagadorn, who has always amazed me by his ability to communicate. To Deane Parkes, the most underrated marketing genius in the health industry today. And last but not least to my sisters, Debbie, Lisa and Chris, I love you all very, very much.

It's time to become inspired by the miracle of life, and stand up and create a life worth living.

Health, happiness and longevity to you all.

—Brad J. King

I would like to first thank every mystic, poet, storyteller, musician, child, lover and humorist that has inspired humans to enter into greater passion, wisdom and meaning throughout their lives. I would also like to thank the patients who have taught me greater wisdom and compassion.

I thank all of my teachers; those who have helped me see with new eyes at each step of my journey as an explorer in life's mystery.

And I would like to thank the group at NASA Ames Research Center from whom I continue to learn so much. Included is Ralph Pelligra, M.D., Chief Medical Officer. He continues to share his insights as a scientist with his kindness and compassion as a man. He is always generous and willing to offer friendship. To Pat Cowings, Ph.D., and Bill Toscano, Ph.D., both at NASA.

To Wade Henrichs, M.D., Torrey Lystra, and Dr. Paul Westby: your strength and support are appreciated beyond words. To Ira Fritz, Ph.D., for your intelligent kindness.

I wish to thank my sons, Caleb and Julian. They have inspired me to be more fully who I am as a human being and as an explorer. To Julie, who has offered her generous heart to the process of partnership for 22 years.

Finally, I wish to thank Brad King. Brad lives the spirit of openness, kindness and respect. His enthusiasm for life is contagious, spreading to all who cross his good-natured path.

—Michael A. Schmidt

Introduction

When we set out to write a book on biological aging, the last thing we wanted to do was create yet another "anti-aging" book. Let's face it, we all know we are eventually going to age; this is one of the inevitabilities of life. But what many of us may not yet fully understand is that we can have a profound influence on exactly how aging affects us in the most crucial way of all—on a biological level. It was through this realization that the concept of *Bio-Age* was developed.

With *Bio-Age*, we knew exactly what we wanted to accomplish: a thoughtful book that explored the key points of aging with an eye to practical solutions. We reviewed the subjects we felt were best supported by scientific research and then sought out a number of experts in these selected areas. We asked these scientists to probe deeply into the complexities of their subject and tease out the most relevant points in a way that was accessible, friendly and useful. In many cases, these contributors have spent much of their scientific careers exploring how to improve human function. In addition to their scientific expertise and clinical experience, we were attracted to their integrity as individuals who, in the course of their work, have striven to help others and benefit society.

HEALTHY LONGEVITY

As you will see, many of the presumed inevitabilities of the aging process can be slowed or even halted in certain cases, but the goals in any longevity program should reflect *quality* instead of just *quantity*. We propose that the biological forces driving us toward our maturing years can be met with a rich appreciation unmatched by our experiences of youth. Our philosophy of aging is that if we so choose, we can meet the physical changes of adulthood with a wisdom that will offset the changes so commonly encountered by aging adults. We believe that by using the strategies put forth in *Bio-Age*, you can look forward to enjoying increased vitality and vigor in your later years of life.

When we talk about "healthy longevity" we are really describing the totality of the experience of day-to-day life. This goes well beyond a healthy diet, exercise and sleep. For it also involves attention to our most intimate relationships, the expression of our innermost feelings and desires and the attitudes we adopt in approaching life's challenges. Our approach in *Bio-Age* has been influenced by the evidence that our hormonal changes and nutritional needs in the aging process may signal the rise and fall of our vitality. We explore these in great, practical depth. But we are equally impressed by the ways in which forgiveness, acceptance and love affect nearly every aspect of body chemistry, immunity and well-being. These also receive their due attention in the *Bio-Age* plan, corroborating what many advanced health professionals realize: that to truly talk about health we need to fully appreciate the role of the mind, body and spirit.

Think about how you keep a car running at its best for many years—this involves much more than just putting in quality high-octane fuel to keep its engine purring. The human body is very much like that car, so when we refer to a healthy lifestyle, we are not referring only to just eating the right foods. Instead, we are talking about a multi-faceted approach to well-being and longevity, which incorporates proper eating, exercise, supplementation, stress reduction and an effective mind-set. This is exactly what *Bio-Age* is all about.

DEBUNKING AGING MYTHS

In their best-selling book, *Successful Aging*, John Rowe, M.D., and Robert Kahn, Ph.D., both members of the MacArthur Foundation Research Network, which funded the most extensive, comprehensive study on aging in America, thoroughly debunk the myth that debilitation and decrepitude are the inevitable results of aging. The authors state that after 65 years of age, what counts in the process of aging, more than a tendency toward inherited diseases, is the way you live your life. In other words, your genes will definitely load the gun, but your lifestyle is responsible for pulling the trigger!

Copious research on biological aging has proven beyond any doubt that two people possessing the same genetic code (twins) will age differently depending on their lifestyles. This is evidence that you can change your habits to enjoy true healthy longevity. Many such findings further show that the damage caused by an unhealthy lifestyle is cumulative. The more the body is neglected, the greater its chances of breaking down.

THE *BIO-AGE* PLAN

We have structured this book in three parts: in Part I, we outline some of the crucial factors and aspects of our biochemistry; in Part II, we have assembled the contributions of some of the best scientific minds on various topics related to aging; and in Part III we offer you 10 steps you can adopt to achieve a young and vital Bio-Age.

Most people who follow the lifestyle program advocated in *Bio-Age* notice a difference almost immediately. By adopting the various recommendations throughout *Bio-Age* you will begin to fill in the pieces of your biological puzzle. The end result will be worth the effort. It's time to think of your body as a work of art in progress. After all, you're about to complete a masterpiece.

Part I

The Basics of Bio-Age

There are many theories of aging. Throughout this book, we have focused on the ones that we feel best explain the main causes of aging. The combined wisdom of these theories, in addition to others, served as the foundation of the *Bio-Age* program. This is a compilation of our choices:

THE NEUROENDOCRINE THEORY

Anti-aging scientists realize that biological aging is caused by a combination of many factors that disrupt the equilibrium of our bodies' systems. This is often referred to as homeostasis. Homeostasis is the regulator that keeps the body's systems in balance. It is governed by the constant internal physiological conditions that take place on a moment by moment basis. This internal milieu is very much affected by its external environment, such as light exposure, temperature, nutrition and thoughts, to name just a few. You can't have an optimum running engine without taking care of the external components.

Approximately 30 years ago, Vladimir Dilman, the late Russian aging researcher from the Soviet Academy of Science, developed the neuroendocrine theory of aging, which states that as we age, our endocrine (hormonal) system begins to run awry. In a sense we lose the communication of our cellular generals. Dr. Dilman believed that if we could reestablish the homeostasis of our body, then we could possibly tap into the fountain of youth.

His theory makes sense since hormones are the main controllers of overall biochemical balance. Perhaps hormones are the missing keys. Our hormones are controlled by the hypothalamic-pituitary axis in our brains. This axis, located in the center of the brain, regulates the secretion of growth hormone, the activity of the adrenal glands, which are responsible for controlling the body's stress and the activity of the sex and thyroid glands. This axis forms a kind of neuroendocrine "clock" of aging, which governs our biochemical functions.

This hormonal theory of aging is very important to our Bio-Age philosophy because without proper hormonal communication, the body can no longer deliver clear anti-aging messages. Researchers call these messages "longevity signals" and they are in a sense a continual dialogue between the brain and the body (more on this in Chapter 8 in Part II). We all know the saying, "You are only as old as you think you are." In this case, however, you are only as old as the messages being relayed back to your brain.

THE FREE RADICAL THEORY OF AGING

The free radical theory of aging originated nearly 40 years ago with Dr. Denham Harman, a researcher from the University of Nebraska Medical Center. Free radicals are unstable molecules that can damage cell structures and lead to cell death. It is the free radicals that are made constantly by cell processes such as energy production, as well as exposure to smoke, pollutants and solar radiation, that cause the cumulative damage to our structures. Ninety-five percent of the free radical production takes place in the muscles' energy centers, the mitochondria (where fat is burned), so it becomes very important to protect these energy centers from undue damage.

As any biochemist will tell you, oxygen is a paradoxical substance. While oxygen is necessary for life, it can also take life away, slowly eroding us from the inside out. Let's look at this concept a little more closely. The oxygen we extract from the air and breathe is by far the most important nutrient for life. The actual oxygen molecule itself is relatively inactive. Through the normal energy process, electrons that surround the oxygen molecule become detached. It is through this extraction of electrons from oxygen that drives the biological functions of our bodies. The downside becomes the reactivity of these detached electrons or, as they are commonly referred to, oxygen free radicals. Free radicals are constantly in search of a partner electron to pair up with, even if it means stealing that electron from a neighboring molecule. It is this process that is responsible for the destructive chain reaction we see with free radicals.

Antioxidants: A Powerful Anti-Aging Force

Antioxidants are substances that slow down or stop the damage caused from oxygen free radicals. Antioxidants are produced by the body as a network of antioxidant enzymes and are also present in many foods. They allow our cells to function properly by protecting us from the harmful effects of free radicals by donating their own electrons to the destructive free radical, ultimately reducing it to a passive state. There are four main antioxidant enzymes produced from within the body: Superoxide dismutase (SOD), glutathione peroxidase, catalase and glutathione reductase. These specialized enzymes must be produced from within the body by using various vitamins, minerals and amino acids to form their unique structures. In other words, you can't just go to a vitamin store and buy these important allies. They all function together to help slow the damage of excess free radicals, but when it comes to slowing premature aging, SOD and glutathione peroxidase are the clear champions. SOD cannot function without the minerals zinc, copper and manganese, while glutathione peroxidase requires selenium and the amino acid cysteine to function. All of these nutrients must be obtained through the diet.

Free radicals are with us constantly. Scientists have identified 1100 varieties of these cellular attackers to date. Recent research confirms that various antioxidants work together, each supporting the other in stopping cell-damaging free radicals in their tracks. As we will discuss, there are five pivotal antioxidants that form what is referred to as the network antioxidants: vitamin C, vitamin E, lipoic acid, CoQ10 and glutathione. Research shows that these antioxidants work in combination to help stop the excess damage from free radicals.

As you'll see in our discussion of recommended antioxidants in Part III, we have incorporated the important findings of the free radical theory of aging into our *Bio-Age* regime, giving you the most recent and effective tools to combat the cell damage caused by free radicals.

THE TELOMERE THEORY OF AGING

Our bodies are constantly replacing cells that are damaged or dead. New cells are made when an existing cell divides. This is also referred to as the anabolic process, better known as anabolism, which governs the repair and rejuvenation processes of the body. If these processes of cell replacement always produced new healthy cells as often as needed, aging would not occur. However, as we age the rate of cell replacement and the quality of the new cells decline. When you put cells into a test tube and grow them, they divide only a certain number of times. The number of times normal human cells will divide is approximately 50–60 times = 110–120 years. When we are young and highly anabolic, this process of cellular renewal is very efficient, but as we get older, it begins to decline to the point where it eventually ceases. This is known as the Hayflick limit, named for the scientist, Leonard Hayflick, Ph.D., who discovered it. Once a cell stops dividing, it ages and becomes a senescent cell that hangs around and causes havoc to nearby healthy ones. Dr. Judith Campisi, from the Lawrence Berkeley National Laboratory in California, is one of the pioneers in the research of cellular senescence. Through her extensive research in molecular biology, Dr. Campisi has shown that a senescent cell emits harmful proteins to neighboring cells, eventually leading to malfunction. Studies have suggested that age is related to our cells' division potential.

How Telomerase Helps Your Cells

The latest scientific evidence indicates that there is a "clock" or "counter" in each cell that is governed by the piece of DNA, which is located at the end of each bar-shaped chromosome in the nucleus of our cells. Many researchers believe that this so-called clock of aging can either be turned on (causing us to age biologically) or turned off (allowing the cells to multiply almost indefinitely). This terminal piece of DNA is known as the telomere. This end section of DNA protects the rest of the molecule from being damaged. During cell division, DNA replicates or makes a new copy of itself.

Scientists at the University of Texas Southwestern Medical Center were able to extend the life span of normal human cells by adding the active component of an enzyme (telomerase, the off switch) responsible for elongating telomeres in the cells. The scientists introduced telomerase into normal human cells to see if the cells' life spans could be prolonged. The cells with telomerase extended the length of their telomeres, dividing for 20 additional generations past the time they normally would have. The cells also grew and divided in a normal manner, producing cells with the normal number of chromosomes.

"This research raises the possibility that we could take a patient's own cells, rejuvenate them, then modify the cells as needed and give them back to the patient to treat a variety of genetic and other diseases," notes Dr. Woodring Wright, professor of cell biology at the University of Texas. "The potential long-term applications are simply staggering. I think this finally nails down the fundamental cause of cell aging, and provides a direct means of altering the clock of cell aging for therapeutic effect."

There is another side of the coin, however, when it comes to possible telomerase future therapy. Cells that divide indefinitely are also referred to as cancer cells. If scientists were to prove that telomerase therapy could definitely lead to normal healthy cells, then it would be a future option worth considering. Even though the telomere theory of aging is an interesting one, we are not presenting it in *Bio-Age* for you to sit back, do nothing, and wait for such therapies to become a reality.

The cold, hard truth is that if you do not take the necessary steps today to ward off cumulative cellular damage (especially to your genetic information—your DNA), then you will not be given the luxury of taking advantage of this possible science of tomorrow. You must partake in the science of today in order to benefit from anti-aging therapies on the horizon. We are merely pointing out the possibility of the science of tomorrow.

Dolly, the famous sheep clone, was cloned from an udder cell of a 6-year-old sheep. The question is whether Dolly's older parent cell would make her age faster. The answer so far is maybe.

According to Scottish scientists, Dolly, now 2 years old, has the telomeres of a 6 to 8–year-old animal. The shortened telomeres reflected the age of the original cells, as well as their time in culture. It remains to be seen whether this will affect the longevity of cloned animals. Veterinarians report that Dolly has given birth to two healthy litters of normal lambs.

THE CALORIE RESTRICTION THEORY OF AGING

Another theory of aging stems from the calorie-reduction study by Dr. Richard Weindruch and Dr. Roy Walford. Walford, a respected gerontologist and coauthor of the "Weindruch-Walford Paper" at the University of California in Los Angeles, had for the past 13 years restricted his own food intake to about two thirds of what he used to eat.

Calorie restriction has proven to be an effective method to extend the life span in every single species ever tested, from one-celled organisms to rhesus monkeys. It stands to reason that if it works so well all across the animal kingdom, it should also work in humans. About 90% of the 300 animals studied remained biologically younger longer on a calorie-restricted diet.

Calorie-restricted diets for mice and rats extended biological youth or prevented most major diseases like cancer, kidney disease, cataracts, hypertension, renal disease, diabetes and lupus, to name a few. The decrease of certain immune responses began at age 2 compared to age 1 in normal mice and rats. Calorie restriction that started in middle-aged mice extended their maximum life span by 10–20% and blocked cancer development. To prove his point, Dr. Walford got involved in a human experiment. In 1991, Dr. Walford signed on as a team doctor for the highly publicized experiment known as Biosphere 2. He lived together with seven other biospherians in a self-sustaining greenhouse in the Arizona desert. They lived on a 1500-calorie diet comprising mostly vegetables, beans, grains and fruit.

This diet was close to the diet Dr. Walford had already been following for four years. Thus he was able to help the other participants with their diet transition. His findings during the two years they spent in the biosphere were that many of the physiological measurements that usually get worse with age—such as high cholesterol levels, high blood pressure and glucose metabolism—actually decreased among the biospherians. It is important to state that calorie restriction without nutrient increases does not work. In order to see results in any of the studies, the diets of the animals were kept calorically sparse while nutrient dense. The message for all of you *Bio-Age* readers is not to eat everything your hearts desire. Instead, cut down on portions of food while keeping the nutrient density as high as possible. Don't worry, you'll learn how in Part III.

The Benefits of Caloric Restriction

So why would a reduction in calories and an increase in nutrients be a benefit when it comes to one's Bio-Age anyway? According to Dr. Barry Sears, the best-selling author of *The Zone* series of books, the main benefits from caloric restriction occur on three separate levels:

1. The more calories you consume, the more free radicals you produce due to the extra energy the body uses to metabolize all the extra food.
2. It reduces excess blood glucose levels in the body, which, as you will discover in Part II, will stop the "cooking effect" in your internal and external structures.
3. It reduces excess insulin levels. In Chapter 5 we will discuss the premature aging effects of an overproduction of insulin.

We want to make it clear that we do not support a drastically reduced caloric intake, especially if it is not accompanied by an increase in essential nutrients. But suppose a calorie-restricted diet does add years to your life. Is it worth it to you to spend the rest of your life hungry to gain a few years? Who would be willing to be on a limited diet of 1500 calories a day? Who would want to live with a nagging feeling of hunger? As you will see throughout *Bio-Age*, there are many other ways to affect aging on a cellular level.

1

How Young Do You Want to Be?

We have known for many years now that it doesn't really matter how many candles are on your cake. The truth is you are the only one who can make a difference in how you age on the most fundamental level of all, the cellular level. Chronological aging only refers to the linear aging of the body. The real magic lies in your biological age, or your Bio-Age for short, which refers to *the way you look, feel and perform.* Everything you do in your life—every meal you eat, every thought you think, every exercise you do or don't do— all of these lifestyle factors have an impact on your Bio-Age. Therefore, the quality of your life, and how long you live, is mostly up to you. This is the whole premise behind *Bio-Age.* So the question is no longer "How old are you?" but instead, "How young do you want to be?"

Chronological Age Doesn't Count!

Realizing this is the first crucial step toward achieving healthy longevity, but it's a dramatically different way of conceptualizing the aging process than what we're used to. Just think about how many times you've been asked "How old are you?" If you're under 30 and like most of us, you'd probably come back with a reply almost as quickly as the question was asked. But after the age of 30 something oddly protective seems to happen; we seem to hold back somewhat on the reply. "Why is age so important anyway?" we'd like to respond, but begrudgingly we eventually answer the question, and sometimes we even disclose our real age, the chronological one, that is. Why is it that chronological age seems to be such an off-limits topic after a certain birthday? Because for most people, many things have already begun to run awry both physiologically and sometimes psychologically. Let's face it, after age 30 we feel and sometimes look older, and most of us don't like these changes.

MEASURING YOUR BIO-AGE

But is there any other way of measuring age besides counting the number of candles on our birthday cakes? The answer is a surprising and astounding yes! Over the last decade or so, many scientists have come up with the inescapable conclusion that the actual biological age (that is, the cellular age) of an individual should no longer be measured in chronological years. Instead, science now has ways of measuring the biological age, and the good news is that many of the biological measurements can be performed without the aid of a laboratory. One can even start with a simple mirror, as long as you can take a really discerning look at yourself and report back what you see. Remember that mirrors don't lie.

As a society, we are constantly preoccupied with our physical appearances. How could we not be? Images of physical perfection are everywhere we look—on billboards, in magazines, on TV and now even on buses. Everywhere we are faced with the Hollywood concept of beauty—chiseled faces, thick hair, lean and incredibly attractive people, all with one thing in common: youth. The appeal of youth is now nearly universal, and we will reach out to anything that promises to make us look and feel younger. We constantly paint, coif, cleanse, moisturize and perfume ourselves. We long to be admired and accepted. The fact is, like it or not, we are judged by our appearance, even though underneath the nearly 20,000 square centimeters of skin that covers our frames we are all much the same.

As we age, it becomes more and more difficult to uphold the Hollywood standard. We look in the mirror and notice that we are not exactly what we used to be; our hair is beginning to gray and lose its shine, we see a wrinkle here and there and it is becoming increasingly difficult to lose that extra roll. Our weight may be the same, but in many cases it has shifted south.

Inner Health Is the Key

So many of us get caught up in this pursuit of outer beauty that we often forget and neglect our inner health. How could we ignore the truth, that our inner health is the ultimate key to our outer beauty? Everything we choose to consume in the way of food, supplements and even our thoughts has a profound influence on how our genes control our bodies. If we decide to fill our bodies and our minds with the proper fuels, then we can expect excellent results from our efforts. But if we choose to ignore what we really need and continue to place the wrong fuels in our bodies and minds, then we can most certainly expect trouble down the line.

REMEMBER WHEN YOU WERE YOUNG?

Remember when you were really young? Do you remember what you felt like? If you're like most of us, you probably took your excess energy for granted. Looking, feeling and performing great were things that just happened; you didn't have to think twice about them. Your natural energy was always there. The reason everything worked so well was because your body invested a lot of time and energy on repairs. It was as if you had a full-time mechanic on the premises.

If you take time to watch a child, you will soon understand the miracle of life—life in the truest sense of the word! A child lives every moment to the fullest. Children contain the essential mechanics of life that keep them in a constant repair mode. Children are highly anabolic, meaning that they are in a constant state of rebuilding and renewing their bodies. A child is the most incredible self-repairing organism of all.

Our bodies are in a constant mode of regeneration, or at least they should be! The cells that comprise our organs, the bones that frame them, the muscles that hold up the frame and the skin that covers the structures are all being renewed at an astonishing rate when we are young and vital. When we are healthy, we can rebuild and replace our structures at the rate of almost 200 million cells a minute, which equates to nearly 300 billion repaired, replaced and replenished cells per day. In a sense, we wake up as a different person each morning!

THE ANABOLIC STATE

The human body is constantly shifting through various metabolic states during the day and night. It is through these various states that biological aging makes its biggest impact. The anabolic state of health is where the cells are constantly renewing and rebuilding themselves. In the anabolic state, all of the body's systems are in a constant mode of regeneration.

The process of renewal is controlled by our *anabolic metabolism*, the rate at which our 100 trillion cells rebuild, replenish and repair themselves. In a sense, anabolic metabolism is our repair budget. The more anabolic we are, the more we can afford the repair bills. When we are young and healthy, our repair budget is extremely high. We regenerate ourselves on the cellular level at incredible speed and efficiency. As we get older and neglect to make the healthy choices our bodies need us to make, we start to break down. This is when we move into the catabolic state.

THE CATABOLIC STATE

The catabolic state, or catabolism, in science refers to any destructive process in which complex substances are converted into more simple compounds with a release of energy. A more simple description of catabolism in anti-aging science is when your repair mechanisms start to run awry. The catabolic process depletes the body systems, especially the bones and muscles. Thus health and vitality begin to degenerate regardless of age. Many anti-aging researchers now believe that premature aging really begins the day that catabolic metabolism exceeds anabolic metabolism. In other words, when your body breaks down faster than it can rebuild itself is when you begin to die.

Premature Aging Starts Early

Moving from childhood into adolescence can be the start of premature aging—the beginning of the transition from a highly anabolic state to a catabolic one. The reason for the rapid breakdown of the teenage body is directly related to the way teenagers live their lives. In today's society, after age 11 a child's mortality rate doubles every eight years.

Teenagers today are under constant stress and peer pressure. Their diets and social life consist of junk food meals. TV and video games after school and on weekends consume their extra time. Many teens have lost interest in exercise and other physical activities. A Canadian study conducted in 2000 revealed that 29% of boys were overweight, almost twice as many as the 1981 rate, which was 15%. Among girls, the rate rose to 24% from 15% in the same period. The enormous stress and responsibility associated with issues such as sexually transmitted diseases and teenage abortions have increased. With more and more teens contending with factors like these, the teen body moves ever closer to a predominantly catabolic state and begins to break down prematurely.

Many girls in the U.S. are entering puberty earlier than normal, according to a recent study reported in the journal *Pediatrics*. Marcia Herman-Giddens's report, entitled "Secondary Sexual Characteristics and Menses in Young Girls Seen in Office Practice," states that 48% of African American girls and 15% of Caucasian girls have begun some pubertal development by age 8, while the mean age of onset of menses occurred at 12.2 years in African American girls and 12.9 years of age in Caucasian girls.

Herman-Giddens was very surprised to see how many girls were developing earlier. But earlier than what? Epidemiological research proves that the average age of puberty in women has dropped by four to six years in the past 100 years. A century ago the average pubescent female was 17. Now, girls are becoming women between the ages of 11 to 13. This has caused an increase in teen sexuality, not to mention the risk of early pregnancy. Why is this happening?

Developing Bad Habits

Obesity researcher Dr. Douglas L. Foster reported in a 1995 Experimental Biology meeting that the levels of glucose (sugar) in our blood is the real culprit when it comes to the onset of puberty. The average person in North America consumes almost 70 kg of sugar a year. In his research, Dr. Foster was able to delay puberty in sheep by reducing the levels of blood glucose, and he was able to induce early puberty by increasing the levels. This precipitous reduction in the age of puberty closely approximates the major increase in the dietary consumption of high-carbohydrate diets in the last century. Many parents complain that their children, especially girls, are growing up too quickly. With the link made between a high-carbohydrate diet and early puberty, we now have another piece to the sugar puzzle.

By the time our teenagers are in their twenties, many continue their teenage habits. Their diet now consists of take-out meals or home delivery food. Many young parents are so tired when they come home from work that they sit in front of the TV until bedtime. Mindless snacking becomes a nightly habit. At night working parents are so exhausted that heating up TV dinners in a microwave seems to be a quick-fix solution. These lifestyle habits become firmly entrenched and premature aging continues to accelerate when these folks reach their thirties, forties and fifties, the time when biological aging really makes its impact on our future. This is also when most people notice that they are breaking down a lot faster than they used to, and they can't seem to repair the damage as easily either. This is when catabolism really emerges as our biggest enemy in fighting the effects of cellular aging.

THE ATHLETE, THE SENIOR AND THE CHILD

In stark contrast to this all-too-familiar way of living, athletes are a special group of individuals that are great to study when it comes to biological aging. An athlete can either resemble the physiology of a child or an aged person. A true athlete is constantly pushing to excel, always training to run a little faster, to jump a little higher, get a little stronger or put on a little more muscle. If the athlete is successful at increasing his or her perform-ance, then the athlete is in an anabolic state, or one that resembles a child. A child's anabolic metabolism is always superseding its catabolic one.

Unfortunately, many athletes push themselves to a point where their bod-ies begin to break down faster than they can rejuvenate. This is often referred to as overtraining or the critical point. When an athlete experiences this overtraining spiral, their physiology can begin to resemble that of an aged person. The energy level drops precipitously, lean body mass becomes compromised and is quickly replaced by fat, blood glucose levels rise and stress hormones such as cortisol begin to dominate the hormonal system with a subsequent decline in the sex hormones.

Inspiring Examples: The Masters Athletes

Some shining examples of athletes who are young at heart are the active, robust and healthy masters athletes, who come from all backgrounds and are usually over 40 years old. They are fathers, mothers, grandparents and even great-grandparents. Sometimes they are doctors, business people or lawyers. Many are former Olympians and some former cardiac surgery patients. They have learned to train with discernment and wisdom. The main lesson they have learned along the way is not to overdo it.

Some are world-class North American fitness experts such as Jack La Lanne and his wife Elaine, who are now in their late eighties and still in per-fect shape and health. Then there is Arnold Schwarzenegger, who is over 50 and perhaps the greatest bodybuilding champion of all time. Even heart surgery couldn't slow him down. Schwarzenegger just completed a live-action part in a film doing most of his own stunts. Dennis Tinnerino, now in his sixties, is still in excellent health. He has won almost every bodybuilding title in the world, some twice!

In an October 1999 article in *Sport Medicine*, L.G. Maharam wrote about the increased interest in the performance of masters athletes. Masters ath-letes give us new hope as they challenge many beliefs about normal aging. Studies on masters athletes have proven that you don't have to experience the common symptoms of old age like loss of lean body mass, increase of fat, degenerative joint diseases, osteoporosis, heart problems and difficulty in breathing. This confirms that what we as a society consider "normal" aging is in fact "sedentary" aging, which is directly related to an inactive lifestyle. We've all heard the saying, "If you don't use it, you'll lose it."

According to Stephen Seiler, author of *Masters Athlete Profiles*, 75-year-old Paul Randall, one of the first subjects in the Masters Aging and Rowing Study, was consistently ranked in the top three rowers in the world in the 70–79 age group. Paul has improved his best performance in the grueling 2500-m race consistently over the last four years. Mr. Randall trains for rowing by lifting weights, stretching, running and doing 100 sit-ups each day. When Mr. Randall is not in training, he visits his six children, six grandchildren and five great-grandchildren.

The masters athletes, individually and as a group, prove beyond any doubt that if you use it, you are not going to lose it. These athletes continue to demonstrate that muscle strength and flexibility can be greatly improved in as little as eight weeks of resistance training, even in 90-year-old individuals. Stronger muscles further enhance function by stabilizing osteoarthritic joints. The Masters Athlete Studies show that seniors, not just athletes, can reduce their biological age by as much as 20–30 years less than their chronological age, especially where measures of blood profiles, hormonal levels, heart rate and lung capacity or V02 max (one's maximum capacity to take in and use oxygen) are concerned.

We are not trying to convince any of you to become masters athletes here. Instead, we want to emphasize that "normal" aging is in fact sedentary aging and the key to healthy longevity is to understand this distinction and then act on it! You can increase your life expectancy and the quality of your life with something as simple as weight lifting exercises and a simple walking program, which will be discussed in Parts II and III of this book.

Age as an Adventure

Betty Friedan, recognizing the power of choice in her book *The Fountain of Age,* suggests that we tend to "deny the reality and ignore the triumphs of growing older." In her book, Friedan conceptualizes a much different picture of aging and calls it "Age as Adventure." She describes an active, robust, healthy group of men and women in their sixties, seventies and eighties who are discovering extraordinary new possibilities, the benefits and joys of growing older.

But what age should we realistically be able to achieve? In his best-selling book, *The Power of Superfoods,* fellow anti-aging researcher Sam Graci states that "After a quarter of a century of nutritional research I have concluded that progressive deterioration can be slowed down, and that the human body can operate efficiently in a youthful state well into its 90s or maybe even to 120."

A study recently published in the respected medical journal the *Lancet,* which evaluated the health histories of 37 centenarians, found that most experienced a low rate of hospitalization and freedom from cancer and Alzheimer's disease, and that nearly 90% were able to live independently into their tenth decade. Dr. Thomas Perls, one of the study's authors and coauthor of the book *Living to Be 100*, commented that of the 10% of the subjects who became infirm, most only began to require more health care and assistance when they reached their nineties; they spent 90–95% of their lives in good health. These centenarians had made relatively wise health choices throughout their lives, which ultimately contributed to their healthy longevity. This study confirms the observation that growing older does not necessarily mean experiencing more illness, and emphasizes the importance of maintaining healthy habits to avoid illness.

HEALTHY LONGEVITY IS ON THE RISE

The number of centenarians is rising every year. According to a July 1999 census report, there are about 72,000 people older than 100 in the U.S. alone, a number that is expected to reach 834,000 within the next 50 years. Even more important, says Richard M. Suzman, associate director for Behavioral and Social Research at the National Institute on Aging, which funded the study, "the rate of disability in all populations, including the oldest of the old, has been dropping since 1982."

Duke University published a paper at the beginning of 1998 stating that the limit of the human life span is now around 135 years, but we seem to break down long before we have to. Since the average life span in North America is approximately 80 years, according to this study we are only experiencing on average around 60% of our potential life span. Making healthy choices along our journey would give us a much greater chance of reaching our full potential.

2

Assessing
the Damage

A friend of many years, Shara, called the other day. It was her birthday and she had just blown out the candles on her cake. Forgetting that it's rude to ask somebody their age, Brad blurted out, "So, how old are you today?" She replied, "I'm 39." Then he remembered she has been 39 for as long as he'd known her. As a matter of fact, Brad soon found out her chronological age is 62! No wonder she felt and looked like she was still 39; she lived a healthy lifestyle.

In this chapter we take a closer look at the aging process, and we'll have you ask yourself how you look, how you feel and how you perform. You will go through a self-test containing important questions about the changes taking place in your body. To successfully reverse your biological age, you have to listen to the early warning signs, many of which we will outline in this chapter.

The Baltimore Longitudinal Study of Aging, one of the first (and one of the most influential) comprehensive investigations of healthy people from middle to later life, has revealed much about the visible and invisible biomarkers (biological signs) of aging. Yes, aging can be slowed down and, in many cases, some of the catabolic processes associated with aging can even be reversed, but first, you need to know what you're looking for. Later on, in Part III, you will find detailed information on concrete steps you can take to achieve a younger, more vital Bio-Age.

RECOGNIZING AND REVERSING THE BIOMARKERS OF AGING

Don't we all wish we could slow down or reverse the destructive effects of aging in our body? Wouldn't we appreciate knowing how we can age without becoming a burden to our family and to society, all the while enjoying the last part of our lives in good health and free of disease? Living—isn't that what life is all about? Then why do so many of us die before our genetic makeup dictates that we have to? The answer seems to be surprisingly simple.

Increasing Our Bodies' Repair Budget

We are each given a repair budget at birth, which allocates repair funds to our fragile bodies. This repair budget encompasses anabolism. As mentioned in the last chapter, it is the process that allows us to build complex things from simpler things—to rebuild and repair rather than to wear or tear down. We have learned much about this process from observing animals of much shorter life spans. The fact is, the current life expectancy (or repair approximation) for both men and women is around 80 years. Unfortunately, our bodies often begin breaking down long before our lives end. Why do we experience such a decline in our health as we age, and are the effects of this decline inevitable? To answer these questions, let's explore a useful analogy.

Wouldn't it be amazing if you were just given a brand-new, expensive sports car designed by the world's most brilliant engineer? Of course it would. But there is one catch. This incredible machine has a specific manual for you to follow with regard to high-grade fuel, fluids, checkups and maintenance. Without the proper care, the vehicle will most certainly begin to malfunction or break down. The engineer designed the vehicle and knows what the engine requires for performance. Would you follow these guidelines? Now think of your own incredible vehicle, the one called the human body. It was just given to you. The engineer who designed your vehicle is brilliant, but the question remains: do you follow the care and maintenance instructions that came with it? If you are like many modern-day humans who break down through the aging cycle, the answer is probably no. The amazing thing is that we were all given a magnificent body to take us through life in style, giving us peak performance every step of the journey. Though our genetics and environment have a strong influence on how we age, we still have the opportunity to enhance the original gifts with which we're endowed. *Bio-Age* offers three basic biological markers of aging, which represent the way we look, the way we feel and the way we perform. We have developed the following self-test to help you discover what shape your vehicle is in by assessing these three markers of aging.

How Have I Aged?

As you go through this self-test, please consider an important aspect of mid- or late-life. Heart disease and cancer are two of the most prevalent causes of death today. We recognize that the best anti-aging program on the planet won't deliver even if you do all the right things, yet succumb to cancer, heart disease or another serious illness. Some of the signs below may be warning signs of disease, so make sure you pay attention to all of them.

Also, if you're 35 and check more than one box in each section of the test, there is greater reason for concern than if you are 55. This is because many of the signs below should not be present in younger people, as they are often indications of illness or a clear signal that your biological aging is advancing at a much faster rate than it needs to be.

Please remember that the test below is an informal look at the signs of aging. There are much more exhaustive surveys, but this one will be useful as a "pulse" to keep in mind as you journey through the pages of *Bio-Age* and consider what it might mean to pursue healthy longevity.

Self-Test Checklist

You can learn to recognize signs of aging by taking a close look at yourself in the mirror. The skin is the largest organ of the body and will clearly show signs of premature aging.

HOW DO I LOOK?

☐ Am I overweight, resembling a pear or apple shape?
☐ Do I have a spare tire around my waist?
☐ Is my face showing signs of wrinkling?
☐ Do I have dark age spots on my face, hands, arms, etc.?
☐ Is my skin excessively dry, looking paper-thin?
☐ Has my skin lost its elasticity?
☐ Is my hair thinning or falling out in patches?
☐ Am I losing hair, especially on the top of my head?

HOW DO I FEEL?

☐ Do I suffer from dry mouth or periodontal disease?
☐ Do my teeth ache, especially when drinking hot or cold beverages?
☐ Do my joints ache before or after exercise or both?
☐ Do I cry easily and suffer mood swings?
☐ Do I live in constant fear, worry or anxiety?
☐ Do I anger easily? Do I lose my temper often?
☐ Do I feel tired most or all of the time?

How do I perform?

☐ Do I no longer walk briskly or do I walk with a shuffle?
☐ Do I have a difficult time climbing stairs?
☐ Can I no longer run, even if I have to?
☐ Is my sex drive on the decline?
☐ Do I lose sentences in the middle of a conversation?
☐ Have I begun to consistently forget names, phone numbers, addresses or lose my keys, glasses, etc.?
☐ Do I have difficulties concentrating?

HOW DO I EVALUATE WHETHER I'VE BEEN AGING NORMALLY OR PREMATURELY?

To recognize whether we have aged before our time, we need to understand what it means to age normally. The most important and common biomarkers of aging are the loss of muscle, strength and vital energy. As you grow older, there is obvious wear and tear on your body. We begin to breathe more heavily and get short of breath. Many of us have trouble sleeping. We take longer to heal, which means that our repair and rebuild function (our anabolic function) declines and begins to malfunction, and the catabolic process of breakdown begins to destroy cells at an accelerated rate. Our youthful energy production slows down and many of us need a nap every afternoon. If you have these signs well before age 60, you know you are aging before your time. At age 60, these signs become more common, but there is convincing evidence that a smart rebuilding program can minimize many of the aging biomarkers. This has been shown with masters athletes who compete in rigorous competition well into their seventies and eighties.

The Bio-Age Markers of Aging

According to recent evidence gathered from the Baltimore Longitudinal Study of Aging, our bodies age in similar yet unique ways. Factors such as genetic disposition, lifestyle and stress influence the way we age. The Baltimore study has isolated biomarkers of aging, as listed below, together with some of their research findings. Maybe you checked off several boxes in the Self-Test Checklist; before you move to Part III where we discuss what you can do to reverse these signs of aging, here's a look at what happens to your physiology when you let a sedentary lifestyle set in.

Muscles

Muscle mass declines anywhere between one third and one half of its original mass, followed by a decrease in metabolism, ultimately leading to unwanted fat gain. Hand-grip strength may fall by 45% by age 75.

Oxygen Capacity

Our body's ability to take in and utilize oxygen (referred to as our V02 max or our vital capacity) declines by about 1% a year after the age of 16. By the time of retirement age we may only have one third to one half of our natural ability to take in and deliver oxygen to all of our tissues. Oxygen consumption during exercise on average after the age of 25 decreases 5–10% per decade. Our breathing capacity diminishes by 30–50% between the ages of 20 and 80.

Bones

Bone mineral loss begins to outstrip replacement around age 35. Loss speeds up in women during and after menopause. Men are also increasingly affected during andropause (that is, the loss of testosterone; see Chapter 3).

Blood Vessels

Arterial walls thicken and narrow. Systolic (first reading) blood pressure rises 20–25% between the ages of 20 and 75.

Pancreas

Glucose metabolism declines progressively with an ever-increasing level of insulin. Cells become more resistant to the binding of insulin. Digestive enzymes decline.

Kidneys

The kidneys begin to shrink in size and function around age 40. The bladder loses its elasticity and capacity to eliminate urine.

Brain

Memory and reaction time may begin to decline any time between ages 40 and 70. Forgetfulness increases, and it becomes difficult to process more than one train of thought at a time. Short-term memory usually fails first.

Heart

As we age, our heart rate while exercising falls by 25% between the ages of 20 and 75. Heart rates in young healthy people have variability, which is healthy. As we age, we begin to lose this variability.

Eyes

Difficulty focusing on close objects begins in the forties; farsightedness begins in the fifties; susceptibility to glare increases; the ability to see in dim light and to detect moving targets decreases. Degenerative changes in the retina become more common past age 60; the ability to see fine detail decreases in the seventies.

Ears
The ability to hear high-frequency tones may decrease in the twenties and low frequencies in the sixties. Between the ages of 30 and 80, men lose hearing more than twice as quickly as women.

Other Signs of Aging
The following are additional biomarkers of aging related to the self-test and are not covered in the Baltimore study.

Weight
Weight gain is a consequence of sedentary aging and it's a particularly insidious symptom because being overweight triggers the aging process to really kick in. Maintaining a healthy weight is one of your most powerful anti-aging tools, but, according to recent statistics, about 58 million North Americans are clinically obese (at least 20% heavier than their ideal weight). About 50% of all women and 25% of all men are overweight. Each year over 300,000 people die from obesity-related complications, a figure exceeded only by smoking as the leading cause of preventable death in North America. As other chapters will detail, obesity contributes to aging in many ways: it makes joints deteriorate more quickly; it promotes free radicals (more on this in Chapters 5 and 9); it encourages insulin-related disorders, culminating in Type 2 diabetes; it breaks down the cardiovascular system, clogs and inflames blood vessels, raises blood pressure; wears down the immune system; and depresses important hormone levels.

Excessive weight is not only the most visible but also one of the most serious factors in premature aging. It used to be that the muscle–fat ratio began to decline after age 30 with fat deposits showing around age 45, but now the muscle–fat ratio begins to show in the late teens and early twenties. Many senior citizens lose muscle mass and add fat deposits, which in men is seen mostly in their abdominal area, and in women around their hips, thighs and upper arms.

Sarcopenia
Related to weight gain is sarcopenia, which is probably the most serious sign of premature aging. By age 30, most of us begin to lose muscle strength. As we continue aging, from age 40 and perhaps up to 90 and beyond, this process known as sarcopenia (muscle wasting, or "vanishing" flesh) sneaks up on even

the healthiest individuals. Many of us don't recognize the warning signs until it has progressed; the gradual loss of different types of muscles accounts for part of the slowing of our movements with age. According to Ian Smith, M.D., emeritus professor in the Department of Internal Medicine at the University of Iowa, skeletal muscle makes up over half of our lean body weight. We lose about 1 kg of muscle each decade starting at age 30. So, as we reach 75, we only function with about 75% of our original muscle mass. Therefore, muscle loss can have a crippling effect. In Dr. Smith's research, he discovered a "disuse syndrome" that leads to musculoskeletal fragility, obesity, depression, cardiovascular vulnerability and early aging even in the younger age groups. Sarcopenia can be reversed with the Biocize program (see Part III).

Take the example of Bob. Bob is a stockbroker with whom Brad used to exchange pleasantries at lunchtime. The conversation was always the same. "Hi Brad, how are you? How are things going? Are you still working out at the gym?" My reply was, "Yes, still working out five times a week." Bob would brag, "I'm still the same weight I used to be in college. Haven't gained an ounce. Lucky me, because I'm far too busy to exercise!" I didn't say much, but I wondered whether Bob ever had time to look in the mirror. I repeated, "Same weight, huh?" Bob assured me, "Yeah, same weight! Although the funny thing is my old clothes no longer fit me. I guess I've gained a little extra muscle through my old age." Little did Bob realize he was in for a shock. His daughter was getting married in a few months and he needed to be fitted for a tuxedo.

The next time I saw Bob he asked me what gym I was working out at. Taken aback, I replied, "Just curious, why the sudden interest?" Bob explained that he was shocked when he went to be fitted for his tux and saw himself in a full-length mirror. "For the first time I noticed that my chest had dropped to my drawers. I noticed my arms were very thin, and my muscles looked like they were gone. How could that be? I weigh the same as I did since high school, and I'm only 49 years old. What looked back at me from the mirror was an image of an old man with my face. I was shocked and decided I'd better start exercising before I lose any more muscle."

Bob is not alone. This is the norm for many men around age 50 whose weight hasn't changed, but their body measurement and shape have. Bob committed himself to reshaping his body, and within six months he added 5 cm of muscle to his chest and another couple of centimeters to his arms. His energy level increased and he felt like and performed as well as a much younger man. Inspired, his wife Jan also began to work out to keep up with Bob. They both noticed that their skin began to tighten and regained a healthy look.

Skin

One cannot hide the most visible signs of aging in the canvas that covers our bodies, our skin. Most men and women's skin loses elasticity as soon as they reach their twenties. Because collagen decreases by age 50, the skin begins to thin and sag, especially due to excessive sun exposure, smoking, lack of exercise and the sugar–protein interactions described in Chapter 16, "AGEing with Sugar."

Hair

Almost 50% of men have some signs of balding. By age 40, 25% of women have hair-thinning problems and some are losing hair. (Balding in the crown area can be a sign of arteriolosclerosis, a hardening of the walls of the arteries.) Premature graying of hair can be a sign of a vitamin and mineral deficiency. Stress and smoking are other contributing factors to hair loss.

PAYING ATTENTION TO THE WARNING SIGNS OF PREMATURE AGING

Many people are too busy to notice the signs of premature aging and many more pay with their health. One of the main reasons the warning signs tend to be ignored is that they may be invisible. You don't notice bone loss, high blood pressure, high cholesterol readings or elevated blood sugar until it is severe enough to cause medical problems.

Sometimes, even the family doctor tells older adults that their blood pressure or blood sugar is a little on the high side, so they are told, "It's natural for your age. There is nothing to worry about." This implies that the criterion for health is age-related and that normal aging carries no risks other than early death. When we pay attention to the early warning signs, we can prevent possible disease. A preventive health measure is one of the most important actions we can take to ensure vibrant health. It is also the driving force behind the Bio-Age program that we propose in Part III of this book. Research shows that it is almost never too late to begin a series of healthy habits that are both simple and powerful. Health promotion and disease prevention in the older adult has become very popular in the exercise business. Therefore, fitness professionals are focusing on ways to help older adults maintain vitality and wellness. There is no reason to age before your time for a lack of knowledge.

There is a remarkable capacity for the older adult to recover lost functions, such as walking, stair climbing, muscle size and strength. The goal of healthy longevity is to avoid disability, which is typically experienced near the end of life and characterized by invalidism, dependency on family or society, frailty and pain.

WE *CAN* IMPROVE THE QUALITY OF OUR LIVES

The baby boomers, now in their fifties, are looking for ways to create vitality for this phase of their lives. They are not alone; people of all ages are exploring ways to slow down aging and improve their health. Regular check-ups and helpful tests play an important part in recognizing the invisible warning signs of aging.

We can choose to listen to the leading warning signs, such as modest increases in systolic blood pressure, abdominal fat, elevated blood glucose levels and decreases in lung, kidney and immune function and do something about them. In addition, we can remedy loss of bone density and loss of muscle mass associated with "normal" aging.

3

The Three Pauses

WHY DO WE AGE?

As we outlined at the beginning of Part I, when the late Russian aging researcher Vladimir Dilman developed his neuroendocrine theory of aging, he hypothesized that as we age, our endocrine (hormonal) balance begins to falter. The body's hormones are controlled by the hypothalamic-pituitary axis in our brains. This axis, located in the center of the brain, regulates the secretion of growth hormone, the activity of the adrenal glands, which are responsible for controlling the body's stress, and the activity of the sex and thyroid glands. This axis forms a kind of neuroendocrine "clock" of aging. Since hormones are the regulators of our biochemical functions, and our ability to manufacture a steady supply of hormones declines with age, then this neuroendocrine clock regulates the rate of aging in the body's organ systems. And we are only as strong as our weakest organ!

A Balancing Act

No one knows the exact cause of aging. Aging may actually be a combination of many things that cause the body to move away from the one thing it strives most for: homeostasis (balance). Dr. Dilman believed that if you could recreate the homeostasis of youth, then you would hold the key that controlled aging. Since hormones are the main controllers of overall biochemical balance, perhaps hormones are the missing keys.

In the next three sections of this chapter we will keep Dr. Dilman's philosophy in mind and look at three of the most important areas of concern when it comes to premature aging and the neuroendocrine axis. We will explore this hormonal decline toward premature aging in a man's body beginning with male menopause or, as it is now referred to, andropause. We will look at the many changes that take place along the way in a woman's body that eventually lead to menopause or the cessation of the menses. And we will explore a fascinating aspect of aging known as somatopause or the decline of one of our most powerful anti-aging hormonal allies, human growth hormone (HGH).

In Part III, we will give suggestions on how to "naturally" overcome the many obstacles in our hormonal pathways as we are faced with these three pauses.

PAUSE #1: ANDROPAUSE, THE MALE TRANSITION

If the word "andropause" sounds familiar, it's probably because it resembles that transitory time in a woman's life called menopause. Andropause is actually called male menopause in many circles, which, when you think about it, does describe the situation a little better since we are talking about a pause in a man's life, thus *men-o-pause*. But the word "andropause" first appeared in the literature in 1952 and is commonly defined as the *natural cessation of the sexual function in older men due to a marked reduction in male hormone levels.*

Andropause also happens to be one of the primary reasons some men age prematurely by losing a great deal of muscle while gaining excess fat. Unlike menopause during which women lose most of their female hormones almost overnight, andropause works ever so slowly, creeping up over many years until you wake up one morning as a completely different person. The man you once were has been replaced by a softer, mushier and sometimes grumpier one.

Taking Andropause to the Polls

In a recent Angus Reid survey, 78% of family physicians polled said they believe men can experience something similar to menopause as they age. And 71% of doctors polled agreed that male menopause, or andropause, could affect a man's quality of life the way menopause affects a woman's. Seventy percent of the general public polled by Angus Reid said they believe men experience the condition, and 67% think it affects the quality of a man's life the way menopause affects women.

"We have spent the last 20 years talking about accepting and treating female menopause," said John Wright, senior vice president of Angus Reid.

"And now both physicians and the public are recognizing that physiologically, men go through a similar phase." The president of the Canadian Andropause Society said there should be no question about the validity of the condition.

Testosterone: It's More Than Just a Sex Hormone

Just as menopause reflects a decline in a woman's hormonal cascade, andropause reflects a decline of male hormones called androgens. Testosterone is the principal "male" hormone with which most people are familiar. Ninety-five percent of a man's testosterone is made in the testes, with a meager 5% produced in the adrenal glands. Testosterone is a fat-soluble steroid hormone that is synthesized from cholesterol.

Testosterone is vital to men since it is required to maintain muscle mass and stave off the deposition of fat throughout the body. Since over two thirds of middle-aged men possess excess body fat, the issue of adequate testosterone is crucial. Moreover, testosterone has a powerful regulatory effect on protein synthesis and is vital to the development and integrity of the male genitals. An adult man's testicles normally produce 7–10 mg of testosterone per day, but as a man takes on more body fat, his ability to sustain this level of production falls. As testosterone levels fall, his capacity to burn fat falls as well. A vicious cycle is set in motion where body fat lowers testosterone and falling testosterone limits the ability to burn fat. This is, in part, due to the manner in which fat affects an enzyme called aromatase. As you will learn a little later, aromatase is responsible for converting androgens into estrogens and is primarily located within fat cells. Fortunately, our knowledge of natural ways to alter levels of this enzyme raises hopes of thwarting this downward spiral.

After about age 35, a man usually begins to experience a slow decline in his testosterone levels of about 1% a year. This slight dip in normal levels at first goes unnoticed and causes only modest changes in body composition, which may cause only a minor increase from year to year in those love handles. The decline in testosterone is not felt just in the tummy area. There is also a weakening of muscle strength and bone tissue. Declining testosterone secretion also causes the body organs to begin to shut down, resulting in memory loss and increased irritability. A man will also notice more and more fatigue-related deficiencies. But it is the noticeable increase in body fat that will sound the first alarm that things are not as they should be.

The Importance of Testosterone

Testosterone is much more than just a sex hormone. There are receptors for testosterone in all parts of the body. This hormone is crucial for protein synthesis and is one of the key factors that sustains muscle mass from adolescence to old age. Without adequate testosterone, one cannot maintain adequate bone density. Also, testosterone is known to influence memory and cognition in very important ways. Testosterone improves oxygen uptake throughout the body, revitalizing all tissues. Oxygen is a fundamental ingredient in the burning of body fat through a biochemical process called betaoxidation.

Testosterone helps control blood sugar, and as you will see in both the "Insulin" and the "Aging with Sugar" chapters, excess blood sugar not only causes us to store more fat than we would ever care to, it also sets us up for a whole host of problems that greatly accelerate the aging process.

Testosterone may be the most important health factor in the male body. When naturally abundant, testosterone is at the core of energy, stamina, sexuality and a lean body. But when it is deficient, it is at the core of fatigue, aging, disease and obesity. Without adequate testosterone you can experience:
- decreased energy
- lowered metabolism
- decreased muscle mass
- increased body fat, especially a potbelly
- diminished sex drive or sexual ability
- depressed mood or lack of motivation

Restoring optimal levels of testosterone has been proven to:
- lower body fat
- increase muscle mass and size
- boost brain function, including memory, visual acuity and concentration
- protect the heart; it reduces virtually every cardiovascular risk factor, including cholesterol, blood sugar, abnormal clotting and stress response
- strengthen the bones
- lower insulin levels

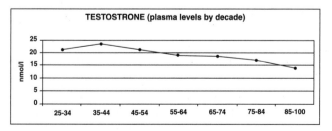

The above figure shows the mean blood level of testosterone for different age groups. Notice that between the ages of 25 and 45 testosterone levels are at their highest. Levels then decline significantly with each decade. With this decline comes many of the negative events associated with declining health and vitality.

Testosterone and Obesity

As mentioned in the book *Fat Wars* by coauthor Brad King, one of the most detrimental effects of reduced testosterone production is the decline of muscle mass, which ultimately results in a decrease in our anabolic metabolism. Since we are in a never-ending battle to control the breakdown—or catabolic sequence—of our metabolism, keeping adequate levels of testosterone is paramount in slowing down the deterioration of our fat-burning engines. Muscle tissue cannot be built without testosterone, and since muscle is the key metabolic engine of the human body, we must understand its importance in our war against our 30 billion fat cells.

In a startling study published in *Obesity Research* in 2000, of the 284 middle-aged men tested, low testosterone levels were discovered to be indirectly or directly related to the amount of fat the men were carrying around their midsections. Abdominal obesity, or visceral adiposity as it is described in the medical literature, is clearly associated with major health problems like diabetes and heart disease. In another study published in the journal *Atherosclerosis* in 1979 involving 76 men, the higher their testosterone levels, the better their levels of good cholesterol (HDL) and the lower their levels of bad cholesterol (LDL). This same study showed that men with higher testosterone levels also had lower levels of triglycerides, which are fats that travel around our bloodstreams and are too easily stored as body fat.

Another study, this one appearing in the journal *Metabolism* in 1998, discovered that in a population of 51-year-old men abdominal obesity, anxiety and depression were found to be closely related. There have been several other studies that have favored this correlation.

All Tied Up with Nowhere to Go

You certainly can't ignore the research when it comes to the anti-aging, fat-fighting potential of testosterone, but not all testosterone is created equal because not all testosterone in the body is biologically active. It is only the free, unbound testosterone that exerts its wondrous effects on men's bodies. It is also the free, physiologically active testosterone that declines the most with age. In one study involving 372 males aged 20 to 85, age was found to be directly related to body mass index and fat mass. Specifically, the younger the subjects, the lower the fat levels and the higher the amounts of muscle tissue. This study also revealed that the younger subjects had much higher free testosterone levels than the older ones, indicating that free testosterone positively influenced body composition.

The decline in free testosterone is due to the increased binding effect with age of a transport protein called sex hormone binding globulin (SHBG).

Testosterone is unable to elicit its physiological responses once it is bound to SHBG. It is not uncommon for free testosterone to decline by about 1% per year after the age of 35, and it is interesting to note that SHBG is regulated in part by insulin levels (we'll be discussing this in Chapter 5). This implies that dietary carbohydrate levels, blood sugar and blood insulin actually affects testosterone levels over the long haul. This is another reason to be careful about carbohydrates, as we'll see later.

In one study appearing in the *Journal of Clinical Epidemiology* in 1998 involving 52 men over 65 it was discovered that the increase in SHBG was directly related to the increase in the age of the men. On average, there was a 13% increase in SHBG per five years, making it harder and harder for elderly men to lose weight.

Testosterone and Prostate Disease

Since we've highlighted the benefits of increasing men's natural free testosterone when it comes to slowing down biological aging and increasing fat loss, some of you may be thinking, "Hey, doesn't testosterone cause prostate disease in men?" But prostate disease increases exponentially in men past 40, even though their testosterone levels are declining precipitously. Contrary to popular belief, it is not testosterone in and of itself that leads to prostate disease; rather some maintain that prostate disease is caused by the conversion of testosterone to an active metabolite called *dihydrotestosterone* (DHT). An active metabolite is a substance produced when one chemical is converted to another. The metabolite of testosterone called DHT is known to stimulate cell growth within the prostate gland. The culprit responsible for this biochemical conversion is an enzyme known as 5-alpha-reductase. Commonly used medications for prostate disease are the natural herb saw palmetto and the drug Proscar™, both of which have been shown to inhibit 5-alphareductase activity.

But DHT is not the only culprit in prostate enlargement. Even more compelling is new research that shows us that estrogen may play an even greater role in prostate disease by latching onto SHBG, the same binding protein that testosterone is bound to. Once estrogen is bound to SHBG, it can interact with androgens to cause cell proliferation (cell growth). Bound estrogen can stimulate certain growth factors such as IGF-1 and IGF-2, which can speed the growth of prostate cells, leading to prostate disease and even cancer. However, SHBG must first adhere itself to the supporting tissue of the prostate known as the stroma, before it can exert any negative effects. If this process is stopped, then in theory prostate enlargement may also come to an end.

Men and Estrogen

Losing testosterone or having it bound up are far from the only problems men face as they get older. As men experience a drop in their testosterone levels, or a rise in their SHBG levels, they usually experience a rise in their estrogen levels too. And you women who are reading this chapter thought you had problems! In men as well as in postmenopausal women, most estrogens are produced directly from androgens. Androgens and estrogens have similar metabolic effects in the liver, where testosterone is enzymatically converted into estradiol or E2. There are actually three subtypes of estrogen in the body: estrone (E1), estradiol (E2, the active "female hormone") and estriol (E3). Estriol is the protective estrogen of the body and its deficiency directly causes the hot flashes and nervousness associated with menopause in women.

It is the estrogen known as estradiol that is responsible for a great deal of the mayhem. The conversion of androgens to estrogens is called aromatization and is carried out by the enzyme aromatase. The aromatase enzyme creates trouble as men age because it lives in their fat cells. These fat cells literally become aromatase factories because the larger the fat cells become, the more aromatase they churn out. More aromatase means *less* testosterone. In essence, men with extra body fat make more of an enzyme that converts their testosterone to the "female" hormone estrogen. This is also how women produce most of their estrogen after menopause. As stated earlier, as we age we lose muscle and gain fat. The more fat, the higher the conversion of testosterone to estrogen. The less testosterone you have, the less muscle you make.

Aromatization

Aromatase is also one of the main culprits behind the ineffectiveness of testosterone-replacement therapy for many men over 35. Exogenously administered testosterone can convert (aromatize) into even more estrogen, which can potentially cause a worsening of the hormone imbalance already being experienced in the aging male. There are certain studies showing that testosterone-replacement therapy does not increase estrogen beyond normal reference ranges; however, the standard laboratory reference ranges do not always address the issue of estrogen overload.

Another complication of excess estrogen is that it increases the body's binding of free testosterone by increasing the production of sex hormone–binding globulin. In order to effectively increase the amount of natural testosterone in the body, men must also look at inhibiting this aromatization, the conversion of valuable testosterone into estrogen. As you can see, women are not the only ones who experience transitory problems as they age. As a matter of fact, it is not uncommon for a man of retirement age to have higher estrogen levels in his body than a woman of the same age, provided the woman isn't on estrogen-replacement therapy, so it stands to reason that the myriad natural compounds available today may soon be a staple of any man's anti-aging regimen.

Natural Remedies

In Part III, we will look at stinging nettle, one of nature's most powerful tools in preventing this unfortunate conversion from taking place. In addition, natural relief for testosterone depletion is recognized in studies of specially developed elk velvet antler extracts—these studies have shown that the extract may be able to boost natural testosterone levels in the body. On a different front, there is a new paradigm of anabolic supplements on the market that use natural herbs found primarily in the Brazilian rainforest, which allow the body to increase the availability of its own naturally produced testosterone. These supplements do not increase testosterone *per se*, but increase its availability to a man's body (for more information see Appendix II).

What Are the Real Risks of Testosterone Replacement?

Testosterone replacement therapy has been available in Europe for years. In North America, however, choices have been more limited. Recently, new classes of testosterone applications have become available in the form of testosterone patches and creams; we will outline these in Part III. Men who are deficient in testosterone can apply natural testosterone safely in larger doses. These higher doses of natural testosterone seem to present no apparent health risks but instead offer many increased health benefits. In Part III, we offer some natural remedies to counter declining testosterone levels. The following are some possible risks of testosterone-replacement therapy.

Prostate cancer

Autopsies have revealed that most men by age 50 have nests of atypical cells in their prostate, which look like prostate cancer cells. There is a great deal of concern among urologists that increasing testosterone levels might activate prostate cancer. On the other hand, there is a good screening test called prostate-specific antigen (PSA), which all men over 50 should have performed annually and which is relatively effective in detecting early prostate cancer (see tests in Appendix I). *There is no evidence in the medical literature that testosterone replacement therapy increases the risk of prostate cancer.*

Heart Disease

There is a major concern that increasing male testosterone levels could also increase serum cholesterol and serum LDL cholesterol levels. This increases the risk for coronary artery disease. Men using testosterone supplementation should have their serum lipids carefully evaluated and rechecked periodically. A serum lipid panel should include total cholesterol, LDL, HDL, triglyceride and lipoprotein (a). Lipoprotein (a) is a protein-bound form of LDL cholesterol with potentially damaging effects on the cardiovascular system.

Liver Disease

Some of the orally available forms of testosterone for men in the USA and Canada contains methyltestosterone. Unfortunately, if used for sustained periods of time, it can damage the liver. The *Physicians' Desk Reference* cites several different forms of liver damage from high-dose methyltestosterone, including liver cancer, cholestatic hepatitis and other liver diseases.

Suppression of Testicular Function

As a general principle, whenever any hormone is administered, the gland that normally produces it can cease to function and recovery may be variable. Patients with borderline low testosterone levels may commit themselves to lifelong therapy if they start with medical testosterone replacement.

The Latest in Pharmaceutical Testosterone Replacement

In today's media- and corporate-driven world, physicians learn most about new trends, techniques and medications through pharmaceutical-sponsored education and popular media exposure. With the release of the new testosterone replacement therapy, now available commercially in the U.S. as AndroGel® (testosterone gel) 1% CIII, men may have a viable pharmaceutical approach to raising their testosterone levels. Data compiled from a study conducted by 16 research centers in the United States and presented at the annual meeting of the Endocrine Society showed encouraging results in the areas of increased sexual function, mood, lean body mass, bone density and muscle strength.

Pharmaceutical marketing and positive public relations for testosterone therapy have increased in the last few years and are getting more aggressive all the time. It may take a few years, but testosterone will eventually get its due respect. Some experts have even speculated that the use of testosterone-replacement therapy for men may one day rival estrogen-replacement therapy for women.

PAUSE #2: MENOPAUSE

Menopause is the transition in a woman's life when the ovaries stop producing eggs; the production of estrogen and progesterone (the hormones responsible for sexual and reproductive function) declines; and menstruation ceases for 12 months in a row.

The Roles of Estrogen and Progesterone

The ovaries produce estrogen, which stimulates the uterine lining and prepares it for receiving a fertilized egg. Estrogen also renews bone tissue, keeps skin supple and protects premenopausal women from heart disease.

Progesterone, also produced by the ovaries, is crucial for ensuring that the uterus can successfully maintain a pregnancy. Like estrogen, it too is involved in maintaining bone health.

On the first day of a woman's cycle, the brain secretes a follicle-stimulating hormone, which prompts the ovaries to produce estrogen. The rising level of estrogen stops the pituitary gland from producing the follicle-stimulating hormone and instead begin producing luteinizing hormone, which starts ovulation and stimulates the ovaries to produce progesterone. If a woman is not pregnant, the estrogen level decreases, the uterus's lining deteriorates and a period occurs.

The Start of Menopause

This change usually takes place by the age of 51, although some women experience it in their forties and others in their sixties. Premature menopause (before the age of 40) can be hereditary or the result of surgical removal of the ovaries. About 5% of women experience late menopause (after the age of 52).

Some Effects of Menopause

Hot Flashes

Hot flashes—profuse sweating and sudden heat on the chest, neck and face—can last on average for about four minutes. They can occur several times a day and at any time of the day or night.

Mood Changes

The unexpected mood swings, anxiety, tearfulness and irritability are similar to premenstrual syndrome and may be related to a decline in estrogen levels. Some women may suffer depression, viewing menopause as the end of their youth and the onset of old age.

Sexual Problems

The onset of menopause may bring about a decreased sex drive and vaginal dryness caused by reduced estrogen. Some postmenopausal women, however, feel free from the fear of pregnancy and therefore enjoy a greater sex drive.

Osteoporosis

Bones are constantly renewed, but after menopause they begin to break down. Lower levels of estrogen and progesterone can reduce bone density, making them thinner and more vulnerable to fracture. About 25% of post-menopausal women will suffer from osteoporosis. Those who are predis-posed to osteoporosis include small-boned Caucasian or Asian women and those who smoke, drink excessive alcohol, have a poor diet with insufficient calcium, avoid exercise or take certain medications.

Alleviating the Symptoms of Menopause

Hormone Replacement Therapy

Hormone-replacement therapy (HRT) is not for everyone. Estrogen-replace-ment therapy reduces osteoporosis, but must be taken for many years for maximum benefit; if a woman under 65 stops taking estrogen, her bones will deteriorate quickly. Estrogen also protects from cardiovascular disease, but, as is the case for osteoporosis, must be taken over the long term for the most beneficial effects. Other advantages of estrogen therapy include the elimina-tion of hot flashes, vaginal dryness and mood swings. However, there are also risks involved with HRT. Long-term estrogen therapy with moderately high doses increases the risk of breast cancer, especially for women who have a family history of the disease. Progesterone therapy for the prevention of endometrial cancer may, when combined with estrogen, further increase the risk of breast cancer. All women should consult with their doctor when weigh-ing the advantages and disadvantages of HRT.

Alternative Therapies

The discomforts of menopause can be alleviated with natural treatments using a variety of herbs such as black cohosh, red clover, dong quai (for vagi-nal dryness); kava, valerian root and St. John's wort (for mood swings, anx-iety and irritability); Korean ginseng (for fatigue); and kava, valerian root and hops (for insomnia). Women should consult a health professional con-versant in integrated medicine to determine which approach would be best for them (For an alternative to HRT, refer to Appendix II for a supplement designed for menopausal transition.)

Lifestyle Changes

1. Quit Smoking: Smokers go through menopause two or three years earlier than non-smokers and are at greater risk of osteoporosis.
2. Exercise Regularly: Exercise to maintain ideal body weight, reduce stress and anxiety and improve mental outlook. Weight-bearing exercise will help prevent osteoporosis.
3. Healthy Diet: Monitoring dietary fat, calcium and vitamins will strengthen bones and maintain physical fitness.

Soy Protein Isolates

Soy foods and flaxseeds contain phytoestrogens, natural plant estrogens. Women in Asia who ate a diet high in soy foods had fewer menopausal symptoms and a lower incidence of breast cancer. A study at Bowman Gray Medical School showed that 20 g of soy daily decreased the incidence of hot flashes and lowered blood pressure.

Soy protein isolates, available as a supplement, increase bone density in postmenopausal women by increasing the level of estrogen and decreasing osteoclasts, which destroy bone tissue. Use only water-extracted, non-GMO soy protein isolates because they will retain their natural isoflavonoids, genistein and daidzein, which reduce the risk of osteoporosis and cardiovascular disease. (For supplement recommendations refer to Appendix II.)

Sensible, healthy lifestyle changes, a good diet and hormone replacement therapy, if necessary, can go a long way toward reducing the discomforts of menopause and making this life experience a positive one. In Chapter 12, Dr. Michael Zeligs discusses menopause and possibilities for natural treatment.

PAUSE #3: SOMATOPAUSE

HGH: One of the Most Abundant Hormones

Aging in a very real sense starts in our heads. Our brains control the way our bodies function. The brain is one of the key control centers where aging is concerned, and it usually all begins with messages sent out by our hypothalamic-pituitary axis. The pituitary, the body's master gland in the center of the brain, consists of an anterior lobe that secretes 10 hormones that regulate such activities as growth, reproduction and metabolism. Human growth hormone (HGH), also known as somatotrophin, is the most abundant of the 10 and has been the focus of many studies on why and how we age.

Why Is HGH So Important When It Comes to Our Bio-Age?

Don't let the name fool you. Though one of growth hormone's key roles in your body is to regulate growth, especially at puberty, its role goes far beyond that. It is also responsible for increasing lean body mass (muscle) and decreasing stored body fat by freeing it up as an energy source. Don't forget that as we age we lose our vital muscle tissue and gain fat (like we had to remind you once again).

HGH is secreted in rhythmic pulses from the pituitary gland throughout the day and night, but primarily while we sleep. In fact, up to 75% of HGH is produced while we are in our deepest phase of sleep (stages III and IV). It is also produced in response to intense exercise (see Chapter 17). The pulsing effect of HGH is regulated by two opposing hormones produced in a gland that sits just above the pituitary in an area called the hypothalamus. The first hormone is called growth hormone-releasing hormone (GHRH) and is responsible for increasing the amount of HGH into the bloodstream. The second hormone is called somatostatin and is responsible for decreasing or halting the production of HGH.

As HGH is pumped into our bloodstream, it only hangs around for a few minutes, but don't let its fleeting appearance deceive you. It is very powerful. In these few minutes growth hormone has a mission—it must make its way to two locations. One is the fat cells, where it latches onto specific growth hormone receptors, activating the release of stored fat for energy.

The other location is the liver, where it stimulates the release of a special set of hormones called insulin-like growth factors (IGF) or somatomedins. There are actually three of these growth factors, referred to as IGF-1, IGF-2 and IGF-3. Researchers are still not 100% sure as to the functions of IGF-2 and IGF-3, so most of the focus at this time is on IGF-1. These growth factors bear a close resemblance in structure to the hormone insulin, thus their names. Insulin-like growth factor 1 (IGF-1), also referred to as somatomedin C, is required for the growth of the cells, bones, muscles, organs and the immune system. Even though HGH stimulates the release of these growth factors, they are also created independently of this hormone.

The Ultimate Aging Therapy

According to Dr. Ronald Klatz, the president of The Academy of Anti-Aging Medicine and coauthor of the book *Grow Young with HGH*, hundreds of doctors have started using HGH for anti-aging purposes. In fact, doctors are the largest single class of users—proof of the dictum "Physician heal thyself."

HGH is the first substance that has been clinically shown to reverse the effects of aging. The substance is amazing; too little makes us dwarfs, and too much turns us into giants. But the right amount at the right time may help us reverse the aging process.

HGH has been called the ultimate anti-aging therapy. It affects almost every cell in the body, rejuvenating the skin and bones; regenerating the heart, liver, lungs and kidneys; and bringing organ and tissue function back to youthful levels. HGH revitalizes the immune system, lowers the risk factors for heart attack and stroke, improves oxygen uptake and helps to prevent osteoporosis.

It may be the most powerful aphrodisiac ever discovered, reviving sexuality and potency in menopausal women and andropausal men. The list of benefits includes:

- 8.8% increase in muscle mass on average after six months without exercise
- 14.4% loss of fat on average after six months without dieting
- higher energy level
- enhanced sexual performance
- regeneration of heart, liver, spleen, kidneys and other organs that shrink with age
- greater cardiac output
- superior immune function
- increased exercise performance
- better kidney function
- lowered blood pressure
- improved cholesterol profile, with higher HDL and lower LDL
- stronger bones
- faster wound healing
- younger, tighter, thicker skin
- hair regrowth
- wrinkle reducer
- reduction of cellulite
- sharper vision
- mood elevation
- increased memory retention
- improved sleep

On the Decline

After our early twenties, HGH declines approximately 14% per decade until by the age of about 60 we have an 80% decline in the hormone. IGF-1 levels follow closely behind, with a decline of nearly 50% soon after middle age (40). It is widely believed that this prodigious decline of HGH and IGF-1 is directly responsible for not only robbing us of our youth, but for the body transformation that we have all come to fear with increased age.

This transformation can be likened to a hard, young McIntosh apple turning into a soft, old, mushy one. This loss of lean body mass is a biological trait shared by the majority of the population as we age. What if this transformation could be stopped or even reversed? In a sense we would have an answer to one of the biggest problems of aging.

You Can't Fool the Body

Many studies have demonstrated both physical and mental improvements, particularly in the elderly, following the use of HGH injections. It is important to mention that there can also be side effects such as diabetes, hypoglycemia, disturbance of homeostasis and disfigurement following improper use of the hormone. Many users do not achieve the desired effects. One of the reasons is that your body has an uncanny ability to slow or even stop its natural release of the hormone by increasing its levels of the anti-growth hormone, somatostatin. Most disturbing, however, is the finding that hormone injections can suppress the normal GH response. Study suggests that you and your doctor should take a very cautious approach to growth hormone therapy, especially if you have elevated blood glucose levels. In our opinion, anyone with a fasting blood glucose above 125 is not a good candidate for growth hormone therapy.

Carrier Proteins

The publicity regarding HGH has a tendency to misinform and overlook the biochemical fact that it is actually the liver's production of insulin-like growth factors that produces the most benefits from HGH. The real secret to optimal health benefits is achieving a balance between HGH and IGF-1. This can only occur via special IGF serum-binding proteins. These carrier proteins are essential to maintain equal distribution, create a long-term circulating reservoir and delivery of the IGF growth factors to the correct target tissues and, in the right amounts, to provide a control mechanism for anabolic (anti-aging, muscle-building, fat-burning) functions.

It is important to maintain sufficient amounts of these carrier proteins in order to prevent a range of side effects from using HGH and to achieve optimal benefits. In summary, the IGF-1 carrier proteins regulate the correct bioavailability of IGF-1. But the stability of all this depends upon the concentration of another serum protein called albumin. When this essential serum protein is low, the entire HGH–IGF-1 balance fails and your Bio-Age goes way up. (See Chapter 15 for more on albumin.)

Nature's Way to Higher HGH Levels

Nearly 50% of the pituitary gland where HGH is produced comprises growth hormone–producing cells called somatotrophe cells. The amazing thing is that these cells can be stimulated to produce youthful amounts of this hormone at any age. Dr. William Sonntag and colleagues at the Bowman Gray School of Medicine in North Carolina recently completed a study showing that the decline in HGH secretion with age is actually reversible. But as described earlier, the best approach for increasing growth hormone and its growth factor family is to supply the body with ways in which it can increase its supply naturally. That way the body won't build up a defense mechanism that can eventually cut off the supply of this essential hormone. Well, nature as well as the specially devised exercise program discussed in Chapter 17 may just hold some of the answers we're looking for.

As was mentioned earlier, the age-regulating hormones of our body, HGH and IGF-1, decline about 80% by the average time of retirement age. Bioavailable IGF-1, and its growth factor friends taken orally, are naturally occurring and in exceptionally high concentrations in life's first food, colostrum (see Chapter 13 on colostrum). Anti-aging clinics around the world have isolated growth hormone and its growth factor family, charging exorbitant fees for something found naturally and in perfect balance in colostrum. The added benefit of colostrum is that these muscle-building, fat-burning growth factors are not degraded by our systems; instead they enter our bloodstreams intact. Given that two thirds of our population will lose one third of their muscle by the time they are 60, we can use all the natural help we can get!

HGH and Male Sexuality Before, During and After Andropause

According to the Kinsey Report, a famous study of sexuality:

1. Growth hormone is at its peak at adolescence.
2. Somewhere in a man's late twenties or early thirties the time between erections begins to increase. Men usually can have sex once a day, sometimes twice or more times a day.
3. By age 40 men have sex only two or three times per week.
4. By age 60 men are down to once or twice a week or less (usually this is when impotence starts to increase).

The Kinsey Report also claimed that 2% of men under the age of 40 are impotent. By age 80 7.5% are incapable of having or sustaining erections. From a study of 1290 men, the Massachusetts Male Aging Study (MMAS) reported that complete erectile dysfunction increased from 5% at age 40 to 15% at age 79, with difficulty having erections experienced by 52% in the older age group. Was the decline in growth hormone and sexual performance a coincidence, or is there a cause-and-effect relationship between the two? The first clinical analysis of the effects of HGH replacement in 202 people, including 172 men, by Dr. L. Cass Terry and Dr. Edmund Chein, showed that fully three quarters of the participants said that they had an increase in sexual potency or frequency. Sixty-two percent of the men reported that they were able to maintain an erection for a longer period of time. The vast majority on growth hormone therapy reports an increase in sexual appetite and performance.

HGH AND FEMALE SEXUALITY

Women do not usually have a comparable decline in sexual menopause function to that of men in andropause. Usually a healthy woman can experience orgasms into old age, but sometimes certain health conditions associated with menopause and aging can interfere with her sexual pleasure. As early as age 35 and definitely by age 45, there is a loss of estrogen, so many women begin to experience vaginal dryness and sometimes atrophy of vaginal tissues. This condition can cause discomfort that can lead women to avoid intercourse, or have it less frequently.

Many menopausal women also report a lack of libido. If they have a partner, they may wish to have sex less frequently. Some single women say they have lost interest in men and sex. These feelings are often related to hormonal deficiency of estrogen, testosterone, dihydroepiandrosterone and HGH. By replacing these hormones and adding HGH therapy, women reported increased libido, heightened pleasure and multiple orgasms.

Dr. Klatz adds in his educational book, *Grow Young with HGH*, that an associate, Vincent Giampapa, M.D., admits that the sexual effect of growth hormone is so strong that if both husband and wife are not on it, it can create a great discrepancy in libido between the two partners.

The Real Sex Organ

Have you ever noticed that when we are relaxed, when we feel good, we become aware and open to the sensual world all around us? The sights, the smells, the sounds, the touch, the tastes and the sensual feelings that delight the mind, all light up our sensual erotic center, and desire and arousal flow naturally. The most important sexual organ is our mind. How we think and feel influences sexual functioning in both men and women. Human growth hormone has a direct effect on the biochemistry of the brain, which in turn controls cognition and our emotions. HGH also raises the cellular metabolism and energy level. People taking HGH sometimes have difficulty deciding whether their increased sexual performance is due to psychological or physiological reasons. The truth is the answer is both, since there is little real separation between mind and body. The three pauses discussed in this chapter are a fact of life, but how we act and react during this Act Three part of life is up to us. In Part III of this book, you will find a complete plan to help you enjoy your life, ensuring a minimum of discomfort and more pleasure along the way. But next, you'll discover the crucial importance of peace and tranquility because few things will age you more quickly than stress.

4

Stress: The Invisible Saboteur

Contending with chronic stress at work or at home is an all-too-familiar scenario for many of us. Combine this fact with a diet of stress-producing food and a lack of exercise and we can unfortunately find ourselves on a sure path to premature aging. Of course, stress is an unavoidable feature of daily life but, as we'll discuss, not all stress is necessarily bad. However, the physiological effects of unremitting negative stress can be devastating to the goal of healthy longevity.

STRESS CAN BE DEADLY

Continuous negative stress has been linked to North America's five leading causes of death: heart disease, cancer, lung disease, accidents and cirrhosis of the liver. Author and stress researcher Kenneth Pelletier has contended that, in America, between 80–90% of all illness is linked to stress and that 75–90% of all visits to the doctor are for stress- and anxiety-related concerns. Many other researchers in this field have emphasized the pervasive problems stress can create. As Lori A. Leyden-Ruenstein, author of *The Stress Management Handbook*, has pointed out, chronic stress can have a powerful impact on our emotional, physical and material well-being by negatively affecting our health, job, finances and relationships. Stress costs North American industry more than $300 billion each year in absenteeism, reduced productivity, stress-related accidents and workers' compensation benefits.

THE EVOLUTIONARY DEVELOPMENT OF STRESS

One reason that levels of stress and stress-related disease are so high is that our evolutionary development produced a stress response that functioned as a method of survival. The stress response or, as it is commonly referred to, the fight-or-flight response, served early humans well in primitive times. For example, let's imagine that primitive man just finished a lunch of fresh berries and leaves. Since this kind of meal will not sustain him for very long, he must find his next meal. As he prowls his territorial domain, oblivious to any impending danger, he suddenly comes face to face with a predator. For a split second he freezes in his tracks, but then almost as quickly, something miraculous happens in his body. There is a sudden surge of newfound energy and all of his energy reserves become instantly mobilized.

Glucose, amino acids from protein structures and fats come pouring out of his fat cells, liver and muscles, all to feed the muscle groups that will be used in his fight for life. Since the body has already mobilized an abundance of glucose, it needs to deliver the fuel to the critical muscles as quickly as possible. His heart rate, blood pressure and breathing rate instantly increase to ensure a rapid delivery of fuel and oxygen that will form energy. The digestion of his earlier meal is abruptly halted. His body has more important things to do at this moment, and digesting food isn't one of them. His body is interested in only one thing—focusing his energies on the problem at hand, and that problem right now is survival. Time to bolt!

Now let's move the scenario into modern day. This time *you* are facing a difficult situation, only it's a danger of a different kind. You just happen to be stuck in one of the worst traffic jams ever. It's the hottest day of the year, and you don't have air conditioning. The driver next to you is in a convertible with the loudest stereo you've ever heard, and it's playing the kind of music you detest. Needless to say, you're upset. We can all relate to a scenario like this. Whether you are in prehistoric times running from a predator, or in the here and now stuck in a traffic jam, your body reacts physiologically to the situation in the same way. Stress causes a massive release of stress hormones, which cause an immediate drainage of your energy reserves. The only problem is that most of this energy is coming from stored glucose (sugar) taken from tissues and the liver.

During a stressful situation, broken-down fatty acids from stored fat are used to a much lesser extent than is the case in non-stressful periods. In times of stress, the body has a very hard time letting go of its fat reserves since stored fat has been and always will be eminently important for survival. That is why fat is stored—so we can survive in times of famine. The stress response was never meant to do anything more than help us survive life-or-death situations, but this built-in survival mechanism is also responsible for a great deal of the diseases many of us currently suffer from. Whether the stressor is psychological or physical, the outcome will invariably be the same—degradation to our bodies' systems. To further understand the problems we face when we are under chronic stress, we will have to explore the stress response further.

ADRENALINE: YOUR FRIEND AND FOE

The main hormone produced during the stress response is epinephrine, also known as adrenaline. Adrenaline is responsible for that jolt of energy the body requires during emergencies. Remember the damaging process of oxidation discussed in the introduction to Part I? When produced in excess, adrenaline is one of the most oxidizing hormones. Too much adrenaline can overtax our antioxidant defenses, causing us to age prematurely. We have evolved from a time when there were great physical challenges to face; it was a definite survival advantage for us then to have a system that quickly "up-regulated." Adrenaline and other hormones became the messengers necessary to activate that famous fight-or-flight response. But in this day and age, we are hardly faced with the same threats we routinely encountered long ago. For the long-term stresses we confront now, we still rely on stress hormones to get us through. No matter what situation we are facing, we still use the same hormones as our ancestors did when a predator was chasing them. The only difference is that our ancestors used the hormones to get out of danger, and therefore used large quantities of them more quickly. We still produce tremendous amounts of these hormones, but use them over a much longer time. As you will see, the longer the stress response is activated, the more problems we are faced with.

CORTISOL: THE STRESS DEMON

The other hormone produced during the stress response is cortisol. Both adrenaline and cortisol are produced by the adrenal glands that sit on top of our kidneys. Many diseases and cases of obesity have been blamed on excess cortisol production in response to stress. Cortisol can be likened to that one person who was never invited to the party, but showed up anyway, the same one who didn't understand when the party was over and it was time to leave! Yes, the party is over and everyone else has gone home, but cortisol is still there sitting on the edge of your bed, talking to you as you try to sleep! Cortisol is produced easily enough, but it is very hard to get rid of once it's in your system. Cortisol causes most of its damage at the molecular level by altering the production of specialized hormone-like substances called eicosanoids, which are produced by every cell of the body.

Eicosanoids are specialized messenger molecules that help cells talk to one another. They are made from essential fatty acids—essential because our body cannot produce these fatty acids from within, so they must be taken in through diet. Linoleic acid and arachidonic acid are two such fatty acids. Cortisol dramatically affects eicosanoid synthesis and may disrupt this vital messenger system in ways that contribute to inflammation and disease. In effect, it fosters the breakdown of many body systems.

Cortisol: The Muscle Destroyer

We all know people in the gym who work out religiously each week, who seem to eat well and follow all the rules but never seem to get more muscular. For many, the problem is cortisol. Cortisol will steal muscle faster than you can build it. Here's how.

Cortisol is produced along the same biochemical pathway as other hormones, including sex hormones, and will always win out over the others to keep itself in abundance during times of stress. For instance, cortisol will compete with testosterone—ever wonder why you don't have a sex drive when you're stressed out, or why you lose muscle mass and strength? Testosterone is needed for muscle tissue synthesis and without muscle, fat cannot be burned. Have you ever wondered why you gain weight when you're under stress for long periods? Cortisol will compete with progesterone, one of the reasons why women have irregular menstrual periods when they are stressed out. Cortisol will also compete with dihydroepiandrosterone (DHEA), your anti-aging hormone, which is why people seem to age so drastically when they are under stress for long periods. DHEA is also needed to burn fat.

The second problem in this sequence is that adrenal hormones are immediately life sustaining and therefore are given precedence over testosterone. Cortisol especially gets the lion's share of progesterone. Testosterone production gets only the leftovers, so increasing your cortisol output is a double-whammy for muscle loss. First, the cortisol and other adrenal hormones use up most of your supply of progesterone, leaving only a dribble to make testosterone. Besides competing with the muscle builders, cortisol attacks muscle directly by stealing its valuable nitrogen and converting the leftovers into sugar for energy.

To demonstrate how cortisol can munch on muscle, let's look at some medical problems that cause severe muscle loss or cachexia. Diseases with both elevated cortisol and loss of muscle include diabetes, Cushing's Syndrome, multiple sclerosis, myasthenia gravis, most forms of cancer and chronic painful diseases such as arthritis.

Many of these diseases give us a good clue to the mechanism that elevates cortisol in normal folk—chronic stress. The original definition of aggressive, driven Type A personalities specified their high levels of cortisol.

Many studies show that athletes who are angry or too driven also show elevated cortisol. A 1994 study at St. Bartholomew's Hospital in London found that high cortisol levels significantly reduce growth hormone output. The researchers concluded that reduction of stressors in life could be essential for optimal training.

Now, how does all this information on stress pertain to premature aging? Let's go back in time again to the prehistoric man who narrowly evaded his predator and is now safe for the time being. After utilizing all of his glucose reserves, his body will be sending out ravenous feed-me signals in order to replenish the fuel. Time to hunt again! But let's assume that our friend here was out of luck and food was nowhere to be found this time. Energy waits for no one; it must be created for life to go on; this is built into our genetic codes. In times of famine, the body looks to alternative fuels, even if they must come from within. Our caveman friend will start to create sugar for energy by breaking down bodily protein, and muscle tissue is first in line. (Remember sarcopenia in Chapter 2?) Our physiology operates in the same way today, only our stress reactions are not necessarily triggered by life-and-death situations. Constant high-level stress creates a significant obstacle to achieving our optimum Bio-Age.

THE PHYSICAL REACTION TO STRESS

In their book *Stress Management*, Edward A. Charlesworth and Ronald G. Nathan explain what happens when a person is faced with a fight-or-flight (i.e., stress) response.

- Your digestive system slows so blood may be directed to the muscles and the brain. It is far more important to be alert and strong in the face of danger than to digest your food. Have you ever felt this as butterflies in your stomach? You can imagine what it feels like when you are faced with daily continual stress, such as traffic jams, misunderstandings and arguments at home, even before you leave for work. Your digestive juices are used to putting out the daily constant stress fires instead of digesting your usual fast-food lunch. Before you know it, you may find you're suffering from indigestion, malnutrition or ulcers.
- Stress, the invisible saboteur, also affects your breathing, which gets faster to supply more oxygen to every part of your body, especially your brain and muscles. Can you remember trying to catch your breath after being frightened? Shallow breathing creates a lack of oxygen going to the

brain, creating the domino effect of poor concentration that usually affects your memory.

- The heart speeds up, and your blood pressure soars, forcing blood to parts of the body that need it. When was the last time your heart was pounding?
- Perspiration increases to cool the body.
- Muscles tense in preparation for important action. Have you ever had a stiff back or neck after a stressful encounter with another person, or just a stressful day?

Of course, stress plays a positive and crucial role in protecting us in real emergencies. For instance, chemicals are released to make the blood clot more rapidly. If one is injured, this clotting can reduce blood loss. Have you noticed how quickly some wounds stop bleeding? Sugars and fats also pour into the blood to provide fuel for quick energy. Have you ever been surprised by your strength and endurance during an emergency?

STRESS AND SEROTONIN

Over-eating and weight gain, other important consequences of stress, are due to a neurotransmitter in our brains called serotonin. Constant stress can easily deplete the levels of this important neuropeptide. Research shows us that when serotonin levels are low or when they are unable to remain in their special pockets called synaptic junctions, chronic cravings for sweet and starchy foods can ensue. These cravings exist, in part, because of the insulin-enhancing effects created by the sugars these foods release. As insulin escorts all the other amino acids from the bloodstream into the cells, an essential amino acid called tryptophan (the precursor of serotonin) is able to make its way into the brain to manufacture serotonin.

While the body does not manufacture tryptophan, it is available in a number of foods (pineapple, chicken, turkey, yogurt) and when ingested with carbohydrates it becomes an effective serotonin producer. And serotonin plays a crucial role in achieving a youthful Bio-Age.

Through extensive research over the past 40 years it has been established that the activity of serotonin has a material impact on levels of insomnia, pain sensitivity, stress, anxiety and depression; all of these being important factors in biological aging. Serotonin has also been demonstrated to have appetite-suppressant qualities.

Because of its high ratio of tryptophan, alpha-lactalbumin from whey protein has shown great promise in improving our ability to deal with excessive daily stress and elevate our moods.

In a 2000 study published in the *American Journal of Clinical Nutrition* 29 highly stress-vulnerable subjects participated in a double-blind, placebo-controlled study that subjected them to excessive stress. The participants were first given a diet enriched with either alpha-lactalbumin or sodium caseinate (another milk protein). Measurements of mood, pulse rate and cortisol were assessed both before and after the stressor. The researchers reported a 48% higher increase in plasma tryptophan levels after the alpha-lactalbumin diet as opposed to the casein diet. In the stress-vulnerable subjects, this increase in plasma tryptophan was accompanied by a decrease in cortisol and a reduced depressive state. The researchers concluded that consuming alpha-lactalbumin–rich whey protein increased plasma tryptophan ratios and, in stress-vulnerable subjects, improved their ability to deal with excessive stress by altering their serotonin levels. As you'll see in Part III, incorporating these and other substances into your diet is an excellent step on the path to healthy longevity.

CHRONIC STRESS AND PREMATURE AGING

As we have emphasized, the results of chronic stress form a huge barrier to healthy longevity. To sum up, if you have frequent and repeated exposure to high-stress levels, the body is not able to expend the energy it creates by taking physical action. The stress hormones therefore remain circulating in the system and the body continues to sound its alarm, eventually causing a breakdown of the body's system.

Additionally, after repeated or ongoing activation of the stress response, energy stores of glucose and amino acids (protein) become depleted. Without adequate protein supplies, the immune system's ability to produce white blood cells and virus-fighting antibodies is impaired, leaving the body susceptible to disease. If, because of negative stress, fatty acids continue to be released into the blood system as part of the stress response, they promote the formation of plaque in the arteries, which leads to arteriosclerosis (a hardening of the walls of the arteries). The possible increase in blood pressure jeopardizes the cardiovascular system. Each time the stress response system is triggered, the body begins to break down and show signs of aging.

The Stages of the Stress Response

Dr. Hans Selye, the author of *Stress Without Distress*, is often referred to as the "father of stress research." He has classified reactions to stress as the General Adaptation Syndrome. This syndrome typically has three stages: alarm reaction, resistance and exhaustion.

The Alarm Reaction

During the alarm reaction, the stress activates the body to prepare for fight or flight. Heart rate, breathing and perspiration increase. The eyes' pupils dilate, and adrenaline and cortisol are released. Stored energy floods the bloodstream. According to Selye, if stress is intense enough, death may result during the alarm reaction.

Stage of Resistance
After the resistance stage of adaptation to stress, the signs of the alarm reaction become diminished or non-existent. Resistance to toxic stimuli and illness such as infectious diseases increases above its normal level (for the short term).

Stage of Exhaustion
The stage of resistance is followed by a stage of exhaustion. The signs of the initial alarm reaction reappear, but they do not abate. Resistance is decreased, and illness or death may follow. Other stress effects are not so dramatic.

THE POSITIVE SIDE TO PHYSICAL AND EMOTIONAL STRESS
In order to deal with stress effectively, we need to understand the difference between physical and emotional stress.

Physical stress is different from emotional stress. An example of good physical stress is the stress felt by your bones during exercise. This kind of resistance stress is actually necessary to stimulate your bone-building cells, the osteoblasts, to make new bones. It's a fact; the bones in the racquet arm of professional tennis players are 15–20% more dense than the bones in the other arm. Now on the other side of the coin when it comes to resistance stress, if you overdo it in the gym lifting heavy weights day in and day out, you will most certainly suffer from a degradation of cartilage sooner rather than later in your life.

Emotional stress occurs when we look at any situation as one of impending doom. For example, if you had a deadline to finish an important project for work and you knew there was no way you were even going to come close to your deadline, you would most certainly suffer from symptoms of excess stress. Because in our day-to-day life such scenarios are all too common, managing your stress by modifying your attitude, your behavior and your habits becomes all-important. We also need to appreciate that not all stress is harmful or negative; in certain doses stress can sometimes serve as a source of motivation; "healthy" stress can spur us on to creative work and enrich the activities that give us pleasure. There is, of course, an important difference between life's stimulating thrills and overwhelming anxieties. In Part III we discuss methods that you can use to alleviate the burden of unhealthy stress.

CAFFEINE AND STRESS

Though the body's hormonal response to stress is complex, the ways in which we trigger it are sometimes tied to some of our simplest habits. In a ground-breaking 1999 study performed at Duke University in England, people who drank four or five cups of coffee throughout the morning were shown to have slightly elevated blood pressure and higher levels of stress hormones all day and into the evening. This high caffeine intake fooled the body into acting like it was continually under stress.

In another study, which followed 72 habitual coffee drinkers, the researchers found that the subjects produced more stress by-products (adrenaline and noradrenalin—the adrenaline in the brain) and had higher blood pressure on the days they consumed the coffee compared with days they abstained. The researchers concluded that moderate caffeine consumption can make a person overreact to day-to-day events, responding with an unwarranted level of stress. The problem can become exacerbated for those who consume excess coffee.

This study, as well as others, points to caffeine's ability to boost blood pressure, heart rate and stress hormones in subjects who drink four or five cups of caffeinated coffee per day. But this latest study also showed that the subjects' blood pressure and stress hormones stayed elevated right until bedtime, even though their last cup of coffee was between noon and 1 p.m.

THE PREMATURE AGING STRESS TEST

Before we look at ways to manage stress in Part III, the following test may give you an idea if your stress level is contributing to premature aging. It will also heighten your awareness of your most common stress triggers:

Mental Stress

1. Do you know the difference between good and bad stress?
2. Do you watch violent TV shows late into the night, causing you to have sleep disturbances?
3. Does it take you an hour or more to fall asleep because your mind is racing?
4. Do you spend time daily indulging in negative thinking? Do you hold on to negative thoughts that you've imagined?
5. Is your life cluttered with too much stuff, so you can never find lost keys, lost wallet, etc., when you are in a rush?

Emotional States

6. Are you aware that neurotransmitters called endorphins affect your emotions, that is, they give pain relief, relief from fatigue and a feeling of energy-producing well-being?
7. Are you overly sensitive? Do you overreact to other people's criticism at work, at home, in your relationships?
8. Do you lose your temper over little things? (The newsboy throws your paper too far from your door, for example.)
9. Are you aware that your mind and body are connected so that what you feel has a direct impact on your physical well-being?
10. Have you considered that both negative thinking and emotional states bring on stress, which can suppress the immune system enough to increase your risk of getting sick?
11. Do you realize that being involved in relationships with negative people or situations, over a prolonged period of time, can cause stress and affect your immune system and start to prematurely age your physical body?
12. Are you still living in the past? Do you hold on to grievances against parents, bosses, close relationships?

Physical Health

13. Do you understand that the right kind of exercise can help you manage stress and prevent premature aging?
14. Do you work out strenuously in the evening?
15. Are you aware that compulsive overexercise can cause major stress in the body, including aging in bones and joints, and wear and damage to internal organs?
16. Do you know that a carefully planned exercise program, practiced faithfully, may prevent the need for hip or knee replacements?
17. Have you considered the fact that by exercising consistently, you oxygenate your brain, heart, etc., which will help with stress management?
18. Have you considered how important it is to drink at least eight to 12 glasses of water daily? That proper water intake is essential for cleansing, balancing and giving necessary energy to prevent stress? Are you aware that water transports oxygen to every part of your body?
19. Do you read and put into practice the latest information in current health articles and books about eating right?

HOW TO AVOID AND CONQUER STRESS, THE INVISIBLE SABOTEUR

Now that you recognize the many faces of stress, the invisible saboteur becomes visible. The good news is you have the power to change your habits, to make necessary lifestyle changes to halt and reverse premature aging caused by stress. In Part III there are suggestions that will help you to manage your stress in a healthy way for life.

5

Insulin: A Hormone of Aging?

When we set out to write *Bio-Age*, we knew we had to put together an inclusive look at the aging process. An inescapable component of this approach is diet. We quickly realized that how one's diet is structured is paramount to the overall success of our *Bio-Age* plan, or for that matter, any successful anti-aging plan. This is not to say that we have the perfect diet for everyone on this planet. If we did, this book would probably be titled *The Bio-Age Miracle Diet*, but it's not.

However, we do have a sincere obligation to provide the latest science on the foods that alter our biochemistry in favor of slowing down our Bio-Age. As Barry Sears, the best-selling author of *The Zone* and its follow-up series of books, puts it, "Eating is indeed a hormonal event." In order to best describe the concept of how foods alter our biochemistry, we need to focus our attention on a food group we hear so much about—carbohydrates.

Over the past two decades, many of us have bought into the idea that carbohydrates give us energy, fat makes us fat and protein in excess causes kidney damage. We are here to tell you in no uncertain terms that the matter is not so simple. There is no doubt that carbohydrates have the potential to add important calories and nutrients to our diet, but people were not made to eat processed carbohydrates, for it's these carbohydrates that wreak havoc with our hormonal systems and contribute greatly to the aging process. (This is discussed in detail in the "AGEing with Sugar" chapter.) One only has to go back in time to learn why this is so.

FATLESS CAVEMEN!

In spite of a lack of today's comforts, early humans were quite healthy. Fossil remains of our prehistoric ancestors show us that they were very strong and robust indeed. Our ancestors had lean physiques with strong, dense skeletal frames to hold them up. No excess lard here!

According to Dr. Boyd Eaton, a recognized expert in evolution and the diet of early humans, 99% of our genetic structure was formed before our biological ancestors evolved into *Homo sapiens* about 40,000 years ago, and 99.99% of our genes were formed before the advent of agriculture about 10,000 years ago.

Our individual genetics have evolved through millions of years of evolution that have shaped our need for specific nutrients. In fact, your genes, which control every function of your body, are essentially the same as those of your early ancestors. If you feed these genes well, they in turn will do their job well, which ultimately means keeping you healthy for a long, long time. But if you consistently expose these genes to substances with which they are unfamiliar or to nutrients in the wrong ratios, they may eventually behave in ways that are not at all compatible with healthy longevity.

So just what did early humans eat? They consumed a diet far different from what we are eating today. Because of the pervasiveness of convenience and fast foods, we are overly dependent on the modern diet, which is rich in refined carbohydrates and overprocessed fats. Genetically we are better suited to a diet of wild game and unprocessed fruits and vegetables.

THE CARBOHYDRATE CONNECTION

Things have changed in the last 100 centuries. In this time, we seem to have reversed the fundamental law that shaped our physiology and have gone against the principles that got us this far to begin with. Now, instead of eating like our ancestors, we have become carbohydrate addicts, consuming carbohydrates as our main source of food with protein as the supplement food. So what does this have to do with healthy longevity, you ask? A lot!

According to geneticists, it takes almost 100,000 years for any substantial genetic alteration to become part of our new cells. Since we've been consuming carbohydrates as our main food source for only 10,000 years, it may take another 90,000 years for our genes to catch up with a high-carbohydrate diet. Dr. Eaton believes that the less you eat like your ancestors, the more susceptible you'll be to many of the diseases of modern civilization—diseases like diabetes, heart disease, arthritis and cancer—the same diseases we have come to expect after middle age.

In order to attain your optimum Bio-Age, you must eat what your body is genetically receptive to. Since our hunter-gatherer brothers and sisters from centuries ago functioned best on a diet rich in proteins from meat (from wild game), supplemented with whole fruits and vegetables, we would be wise to do the same. If you are a vegetarian, there are many ways you too can incorporate high-quality proteins into your diet without eating meat. We will discuss this in greater detail in the next chapter. The forces of natural selection allowed us to evolve to function optimally on these foods. And since food was then not always in abundance, and we didn't have the convenience or guarantee of at least three balanced meals per day, we developed an incredible storage capacity within our 30 billion fat cells. Each and every one of those 30 billion fat cells can expand 1000 times in volume, and if that isn't enough, they can also increase in number when they're stuffed.

But wait! How can simply eating different foods be so effective in slowing and reversing biological age? Well, read on to discover one of the greatest weapons ever developed when it comes to combating premature aging.

A DOUBLE AGENT: INSULIN

We'd like to introduce you to a very powerful hormone that has a strong influence on all of metabolism, insulin. Insulin is a protein-based hormone that is secreted from the pancreas immediately following a meal and during periods of elevated blood sugar. Insulin is the Dr. Jekyll and Mr. Hyde of metabolism. On the positive side, insulin performs functions necessary for life, including the deposit of sugar (glycogen) in muscle so that you have an ample source of energy. In addition, insulin promotes the synthesis of proteins for building enzymes, hormones and muscle. But there is also a negative side of insulin. When it's produced in excess, insulin plays a major role in the prevalence of obesity, as well as cardiovascular disease and Type 2 diabetes. Premature aging is linked to the negative side of insulin.

When most of us think of insulin, we tend to think of diabetes. There are several types of diabetes, but there are two with which we are most familiar. Type 1 is often referred to as juvenile onset diabetes and accounts for only 10% of those who have the disorder known as diabetes. Type 1 diabetes is due to a dysfunction of the pancreas, which secretes insulin. In Type 1 diabetes, for some reason the pancreas is either unable to secrete enough insulin or may not produce it at all.

Type 2 diabetes is a whole different problem, accounting for almost 90% of overall diabetes. Type 2 diabetes, or adult onset diabetes, usually strikes after the age of 40 and is caused when the insulin receptor sites on the cells become resistant to insulin, rendering it non-effective. Insulin's job is to direct the excess blood sugar into the cells via receptors that reside on the cells' surface. The problem, however, is that these receptor proteins are not fixed entities on the cells but are produced as the cells need them. When there is a constant excess of sugar in the bloodstream, the receptors down-regulate (meaning that these regulators are not made as abundantly as when there is less sugar in the bloodstream) due to the overproduction of the sugar. This is when the problem of insulin resistance occurs. What this means is that your cells, which store the blood sugar as glycogen, don't work with insulin so well. Because blood sugar cannot enter the cells, blood sugar as well as blood insulin levels remain elevated, which over time can lead to a whole array of body changes collectively called Syndrome X.

How Insulin Can Make You Fat

Because insulin is especially sensitive to carbohydrates from the diet, the more carbohydrates you eat at one time, especially the refined kinds (processed foods), the greater the amount of insulin is needed to clear it from the bloodstream. Besides becoming insulin resistant, the transport proteins inside the cells that help bring in the sugar begin working at a slow pace, and more insulin is needed to jam the sugar into the cells. But here's the kicker—insulin is the major fat-storage hormone as well.

In addition to enhancing the uptake of blood sugar into cells, insulin also shoves fatty acids into muscle and fat cells. The body must get the fat out of the bloodstream so that blood sugar doesn't become too low. Excess insulin makes you fat and keeps you fat! In order to free up the fat so it can be burned in the muscle cells, you've got to lower your insulin levels—it's really that simple. How do we know this? Because people with Type 1 diabetes, whose pancreases produce little or no insulin at all, cannot gain weight. It is insulin that stimulates the cells' insulin receptors and puts carbohydrate energy into fat cells.

There are about 18 million people with Type 2 diabetes in North America, about half of them undiagnosed. By dropping excessive body fat via the *Bio-Age* plan, we suspect that 15 million of those afflicted with diabetes would likely take less medication, have more energy, greatly improve their health and live longer. Of the roughly 90% of people with Type 2 diabetes, perhaps 85% are over-fat, many obese. In North America alone, over 12 million over-fat people are destined for a whole slew of nasties, including a two- to three-fold increase in the risk of blindness, amputations, kidney failure and heart disease. The fact that diabetes and over-fatness go hand in hand should tell us that if we can control fat, we can prevent or control diabetes. Research is now confirming this.

Where's the Fat At?

Many researchers believe that it's not just *how* fat you are that affects your risk of getting a disease like diabetes as much as *where* most of that fat is located. Recent research has shown that visceral fat (abdominal or belly fat), as opposed to fat on the thighs and butt, is one of the top markers of premature aging and future disease. According to research at the U.S. National Institute of Health, this gut-centered fat is related to an overproduction of hormones (insulin, cortisol, adrenaline, etc.), which surge into the bloodstream during the stress response and cause the body to store more abdominal fat, further exacerbating the problem. The more belly fat you have, the higher your mortality risk. In addition, tummy fat cells seem to be especially good at dumping lipids (fats) into the bloodstream.

These lipids find their way to your muscle tissue, where they inhibit the uptake of blood sugar, causing a spike in the output of the hormone insulin from your pancreas. Since insulin is a storage hormone, one of its main jobs is to drive blood sugar into cells for storage or for use as energy at a later time. Since excessive blood lipids from belly fat reduce the effectiveness of insulin (also known as insulin resistance), more insulin must be produced to drive the blood sugar into the cells. It is this excessive insulin, also known as hyperinsulinemia, which is directly related to the damage caused by over-fatness and obesity.

In addition to higher insulin levels, people with excessive tummy fat are especially good at releasing another hormone called cortisol under stress conditions (we discussed this extensively in Chapter 4). Men and women with potbellies tend to produce more cortisol throughout the day, which is directly related to an increased risk of disease and accelerated aging. So if you're trying to live longer, belly fat is no longer in style.

INSULIN AND CORTISOL: A DAMAGING ALLIANCE

Insulin is also of vital importance to our Bio-Age because of the way in which it operates in conjunction with cortisol. Most of our one hundred trillion plus cells can burn either fat or glucose as fuel, but the brain (under non-fasting conditions) relies heavily on available glucose for continual energy. Our brain uses approximately 100 g a day of glucose (almost one half our total circulating blood sugar). Unlike the other organs of the body that require insulin to pump glucose into their interiors, our brain is able to absorb glucose independent of insulin, which gives it first priority over the other cells of the body. That is unless insulin levels are kept high by consuming insulin-spiking foods throughout the day.

Many researchers believe that insulin resistance often develops as we age because of a built-in safeguard that diverts insulin from the body's tissues in order to feed the brain. In other words, to compensate for years of chronically high insulin levels, the tissues of the body are made insulin resistant for the sake of the brain. This is because high levels of circulating insulin have been shown to inhibit the release of an important brain-feeding hormone called glucagon. So the body must have a back-up plan to raise blood sugar levels for the brain. This is where cortisol enters the picture.

As we pointed out in the last chapter, excess cortisol can wreak havoc on the best-laid anti-aging plans. Often in producing cortisol, the body is just trying to help compensate for low blood sugar levels by stimulating cortisol release. Here's why: cortisol is able to manufacture more glucose by cannibalizing existing body structures (mostly muscle, skin and organ tissue) in a process called gluconeogenesis. But cortisol helps the brain in another way, by blocking the amount of glucose used by other cells, thus causing insulin resistance.

The problem is that even though cortisol may be trying to help the brain in one way by raising blood sugar and cutting off the supply to the other structures, it often backfires. Cortisol has been shown to negatively affect the hippocampus, the key memory center in the brain.

Insulin and Hormonal Communication

You will recall that hormones are the generals of our systems. But they are, in a very real sense, only the messengers. Most hormones relay their "message" by latching onto specific docking sites (receptors) on the outside of cells. Most hormones, including glucagon, use a second messenger called cyclic AMP (cAMP). Insulin uses two other messengers. When insulin levels are too high, its messengers dominate the cell's communication system. In response, the messengers needed by other hormones become too low.

While this may seem a bit complicated, there is a basic strategy. We can strive to increase the messenger cyclic AMP. This can be done by natural means that include:

- Decreasing insulin levels throughout the day and especially at night
- Increasing levels of omega-3 fatty acids (which we cover in Chapter 7 and in Part III)
- Exercising through Biocize and other properly devised programs (see Chapter 17 and Part III)
- Losing excess body fat
- Supplementing with Coleus Forskohlii extract (see Appendix II)

Free Radicals: Creating More Problems Than We Can Handle

Another big problem associated with complications due to excessive insulin production and glucose overload is the production of excess free radicals. Free radicals are those harmful fragments of oxygen that are important known causes of tissue damage and have been associated with many aspects of aging, including inflammatory diseases, cataracts, diabetes and cardiovascular diseases. Increased free radical formation and lipid peroxidation are common in Type 2 diabetes and are among the key reasons for premature aging associated with this disease. Ingestion of sugars, fats (saturated and trans) and sodium have been linked to decreased insulin sensitivity, while caloric restriction, carbohydrate restriction, exercise, ingestion of the trace minerals chromium and vanadium, soluble fibers, magnesium, essential fatty acids and certain antioxidants are often associated with greater insulin sensitivity. Many top researchers believe that through diet manipulation, the glucose/insulin system may increase life span and reduce the incidence of chronic disorders associated with aging.

So just how do you lower insulin levels? How do you get rid of the evil Mr. Hyde? You can lower insulin by changing your diet, by exercising using the principles explained in the Biocize chapter and by taking certain nutrients outlined in the nutrient section of Part III. For now, let's focus on the foods you eat on a daily basis so that you can understand just how the foods you never suspected could increase your Bio-Age actually do!

Restricting Carbohydrates

One of the greatest ways to affect insulin levels is to take away, or at least restrict, the food source that causes its greatest rise, carbohydrates. There are many diet and life plan books available espousing the benefits of carbohydrate restriction in reducing many of the complications associated with advanced age. Many of the followers of these low-carbohydrate diets will gladly tell you that when nothing else seemed to work for their fat loss, high cholesterol, high blood pressure, high triglyceride levels (the major form of fat that is found in the bloodstream) and other problems, the low-carbohydrate approach seemed to do the trick. This would make sense since carbohydrates are the main stimulators of insulin in the first place.

To better understand the health benefits of reducing carbohydrates, we can look to the studies confirming the benefits of caloric restriction. The effects of caloric restriction (CR) on life span, disease and aging in physiological systems have been documented in almost every animal species ever studied except humans. Studies of CR and aging using our closest biological relatives, rhesus monkeys, have been ongoing for several years at the

National Institute on Aging and the University of Wisconsin-Madison. Most of the data published from these studies show the myriad benefits of restricting calories to approximately 30% less than what would be deemed normal. These monkeys have less body fat, almost as much muscle, lower body temperature, lower fasting blood glucose, lower insulin and lower serum lipids than other monkeys that are allowed to eat as much food as they want. In addition, insulin seems to function more effectively in monkeys on CR.

One of the reasons behind the amazing benefits of CR is that it lowers the overall amount of carbohydrates in the diet. Once again, carbohydrates are the main stimulators of insulin and if the overall amount is being reduced due to a balance of the other two macronutrients, protein and fat (don't worry, you'll be learning about these in the next two chapters!), then it would stand to reason that insulin production would be kept in check. But an easier way to control the overproduction of insulin is to watch the overall amount of carbohydrates you consume (we give you guidelines in Part III), especially the ones that break down and release their sugars too quickly.

Low Fat = Low Weight: A Bad Misconception!

Over the last 20 years, we've all seen the explosion of low-fat diets hit the market. We are led to believe that if you replace saturated fat–laden foods with low-fat carbohydrates, all our weight problems would be solved. Over the last decade we have become even fatter, with nearly a 30% jump in obesity. If we are truly becoming more conscious of our fat intake, lowering it all the time and still getting fatter, you're probably wondering why it isn't working.

Here's a little statistic to put things into a better perspective: Most North Americans consume approximately 1 cup of sugar daily; that's almost 70 kg of sugar each year. Also, many carbohydrates you consume (bagels, potatoes, carrots and breads) are quickly metabolized into glucose (sugar) in your system. The higher your glucose load, the higher your insulin levels. Understanding how insulin levels relate to increased Bio-Age will give you the knowledge you need to experience healthy, disease-free longevity, not to mention the power to evict the fat living in the nearly 30 billion fat cells that call your body home.

FAST AND SLOW CARBS: THE GLYCEMIC INDEX

Every time you eat a meal, your blood sugar rises. When you eat a meal high in carbohydrates, your blood sugar rises faster than if you had eaten mostly proteins and fats. Certain carbohydrates pass into your bloodstream faster than others. The concept of the "glycemic index" (GI) has been developed to describe just how fast a certain food turns to blood sugar. The higher the glycemic index rating, the faster the food turns to blood sugar. A glycemic index of 100 is for the sugar glucose, and this sugar is used as the standard from which all other foods are measured. Every other food falls somewhere between 0 and 100. Foods with a rating of 50 or less are considered low glycemic. Foods higher than 70 are considered high glycemic and should be reduced in your diet or avoided entirely.

Carbohydrate foods come mainly from plant foods, such as cereal grains, vegetables, beans and fruits. In addition, milk also contains a carbohydrate sugar called lactose. Since carbohydrates, when compared with proteins and fats, raise the blood sugar level the fastest, the plant-based foods will tend to have the higher glycemic index. In general, foods with the highest glycemic index are those with a low fiber level, a high starch level, and those that are highly processed. Foods with the lowest glycemic index are proteins, fats and unprocessed fruits and vegetables that have their fiber intact. Sounds like the diet of early humans doesn't it? Fruits and vegetables are for the most part low glycemic (with some exceptions). But if they are part of a processed food such as vegetable pies or rice cakes, they would most probably become high glycemic. In those cases, their original food values have been changed.

High GI: Watch Out for These

What may surprise you is that many of the so-called "diet foods" you have been told are good for you are actually the worst foods you can eat when it comes to the glycemic index and the resulting rise in insulin levels. These include rice cakes (GI 82), most breads such as white or wheat (GI 70), baked potatoes (GI 93), many sports drinks (GI 70–90) and white rice (GI 72). Ouch! Eat too many of these foods and you might blow up like a blimp.

How many of us eat rice cakes as a snack and a baked potato for dinner? And those fat-free snack foods that are so popular today are also high in refined flour, which makes them a prime stimulant of insulin. No wonder most of us end up experiencing less-than-optimum health in our later years.

You can use the glycemic index as a guide in your Bio-Age plan against premature aging and unwanted fat gain. By consuming more foods with a lower glycemic index, you'll lower your insulin levels and free up more fat so it can be used as fuel instead of just having it sit there on your hips, butt and legs. You'll also be reducing your risk of heart disease and diabetes, which are two more Bio-Age markers. In the case of heart disease, high insulin levels greatly increase the risk. In the case of Type 2 diabetes, for years you could be setting the stage for diabetes without even knowing it. You could actually be in a phase called normoglycemic because your insulin level is elevated and is pushing blood sugar into cells, keeping it normal in the blood. Then one day, your pancreas, after pumping out gobs of extra insulin every day for several years, decides that enough is enough and whammy! Suddenly there is a big rise in blood sugar with nowhere for it to go. The result is diabetes. Many overweight individuals are either prediabetic or have Type 2 diabetes.

Moderation Is Key

On pages 71–72 we've listed a number of foods and ratings on their respective glycemic index. Now you can arm yourself with the necessary weapons against some of the top Bio-Age markers. All you have to do is glance at the foods listed in the index now and then and you will have a good perspective on which foods you should consume and which foods you should reduce or avoid. Does a high glycemic index mean you should avoid a particular food altogether? No. We all want to live a happy and healthy life, and part of living is enjoying a favorite meal (or two, or three) now and then, but not every single day. Moderation is the key.

We have truly conditioned ourselves to crave sugars, and this habit must be refocused toward foods with a low glycemic index. In addition, many of the high-glycemic foods we eat are among the tastiest and cheapest foods we can buy, so we are drawn to highly processed foods as well as to a number of low-priced starches, cereals, grains and breads, all with a high glycemic rating. If you do decide to indulge in a little high-glycemic food during a meal, try combining it with other foods that have a low glycemic index so you'll lower the overall insulin effect.

Abstaining from every single high-glycemic food may be too stressful and not realistic, so don't worry if you deviate from the low-glycemic path every now and then. Just do it in moderation and avoid excess. If you crave something sweet, a piece of low-glycemic fruit can do the trick. Try sticking with the berry family of fruits, an apple, orange, peach or grapefruit. Notice we didn't recommend fruit juice. Most fruit juices are low or void of fiber, which makes them high glycemic. Avoid purified fruit juices and stick with water, milk or juice with a high pulp content. In addition, other researchers suggest adding acidic foods to a meal. The acidity seems to lower the glycemic index. Acidic foods include fresh lemon juice, grapefruit juice and red wine vinegar. This doesn't mean that you can eat a large pile of french fries as long as you drown them in vinegar. But this may be something to consider when eating a salad or a stir-fry vegetable dish, for example.

You can use the glycemic index to roughly predict the yield from a mixed meal. Higher glycemic index foods can be balanced with low-glycemic index foods. A rule to remember is to never consume high-glycemic index foods all by themselves. They'll raise your blood sugar fast, resulting in a fast rise and long run of the pro-aging, fat-storing hormone, insulin.

Just in case it hasn't sunk in yet, fat is not always the criminal you've been led to believe, so let's summarize the point. Fat doesn't make you fat (unless you're eating gobs of it) and, as you will see in Chapter 7 on "Fatty Acids," some fats are actually necessary for fat loss and decreasing your Bio-Age! It is usually the excess levels of insulin from high-glycemic carbohydrates and excessive calories that age you before your time, make you fat and keep you fat for life.

AN ESSENTIAL TRACE MINERAL AND INSULIN

Although there are many nutrients we discuss in the nutrient chapter of Part III, chromium deserves an initial mention in this chapter. More than 90% of North Americans are deficient in the trace mineral chromium. When you combine low chromium consumption with high blood sugar levels due to a high consumption of sweets, grains and refined foods, the result is a staggering increase in Type 2 diabetes, over-fatness, obesity and premature aging. Most soils contain low or no chromium. As a result, the plants we eat contain very little chromium as well. Except for supplemental chromium, there is no good way to boost the level of chromium in your cells.

If you are over-fat, there is a good chance you are insulin resistant. Your cells just don't let the sugar enter their interiors as well as they used to. This results in the pro-fat insulin spike that keeps the fat pounds on, even during the toughest of exercise and diet routines. Chromium is an essential key in correcting the cells' resistance to insulin. It helps your cells function better, allowing blood sugar and amino acids in easier and keeping blood insulin levels lower.

Two of the most popular forms of chromium, chromium polynicoti-nate (niacin-bound chromium) and chromium picolinate, should both perform well and have been researched extensively. A recent study comparing the two forms of chromium in conjunction with exercise gave the nod to niacin-bound chromium as the preferred form. The recommended dosage is 200–400 mcg of elemental chromium per day. In some studies with people with diabetes as much as 1000 mcg daily was needed, but these levels should be used only under doctor's supervision.

LOW-GLYCEMIC FOODS: Rated 20–49 (Allies)

- All-bran cereals
- Apples
- Apple juice
- Barley
- Berries
- Black-eyed peas
- Bulgur
- Butter beans
- Cherries
- Grapefruit
- Milk
- Muesli cereal
- Navy beans
- Oranges
- Peaches
- Peanuts
- Pears
- Peas
- Plums
- Soybeans
- Strawberries
- Wild rice
- Yogurt (no added sugar)

MODERATE-GLYCEMIC FOODS: Rated 50–69 (Limit consumption)

- Basmati rice
- Beets
- Buckwheat
- Carrots
- Cereal (low sugar)
- Corn on the cob
- Grapes
- Ice cream
- Lima beans
- Oatmeal
- Pasta (soft cooked)
- Peas
- Potato chips
- Potatoes (red, white)
- Pumpernickel bread
- Raisins
- Sourdough bread
- Sucrose (table sugar)
- Sweet potato
- Whole wheat bread (100% stone-ground)

HIGH-GLYCEMIC FOODS: Rated 70–100 (Eat at your own risk or with low GI foods)

- Apricots
- Bagels
- Bananas (ripe)
- Breakfast cereals (refined with added sugar)
- Corn chips
- Cornflakes
- Corn syrup solids
- Crackers and crispbread
- Doughnuts
- Glucose and glucose polymers (maltodextrin-based drinks)
- Hamburger and hotdog buns
- Honey
- Jelly beans
- Maltose
- Mango
- Muffins (due to the processed flour)
- Pancakes

- Papaya
- Parsnips
- Puffed rice or wheat
- Potato (baked)
- Rice cakes
- Shredded wheat
- Soft drinks and sport drinks (added sugars)
- Toaster waffles
- Watermelon
- White bread
- White rice
- Whole wheat bread

While we offer the glycemic index as a useful guide, we would also like to point out that it has some limitations as well. These are described below:

- The GI of raw versus cooked food of the same kind can be different. (Cooking helps to loosen up or release the molecules of sugar from the food in some cases, like cooked carrots.)
- How a food is cut can affect the GI.
- The GI of a food may vary between people.
- Length of cooking time can alter the GI, with longer times usually raising GI.
- Ripeness of a fruit can alter its GI; the riper the fruit, the higher its GI.
- Combining foods can lower or raise the collective GI.
- Some foods with low GI are very damaging to the body.

THE EFFECTS OF GLYCATION

This latter point deserves special consideration because the sugar fructose has a GI of only 32. Fructose, sometimes known as fruit sugar, has become one of the most common sweeteners, with each North American consuming roughly 22 kg per year. Under the GI concept, fructose would appear to be acceptable, even desirable. In fact, the very popular book *The Glucose Revolution* raises little concern over fructose because of its low glycemic index and makes no mention whatever of the dark side of fructose, namely, glycation. Glycation is a damaging sugar–protein reaction that is a hallmark of the aging process. (We'll explore this in Chapter 13.) Yes, fructose (and its metabolic cousins) is a very powerful glycating agent, which can trigger the formation of AGE proteins throughout the body. Fructose may contribute to the browning, wrinkling and stiffening of ligaments, tendons, cartilage, skin, bone, eyes, brain, heart muscle, blood vessels and virtually any tissue within the human body. Even your DNA, the genetic blueprint that guides your structure and function, can be damaged by these fructose-derived changes. We strongly urge that whenever you see fructose or high-fructose corn syrup on the food label—stay away! In Part III's step 5, we offer some suggestions about safe and effective alternative sweeteners.

So, is the glycemic index a useful tool? We believe it can be a helpful guide to keep a check on the amount of insulin-spiking foods you consume. Limiting your total carbohydrate intake and making general use of the glycemic index are key steps to take on the path to healthy longevity.

6

Aging with Protein

Chances are you've heard of the latest high-protein diet books that have flooded the bookstore shelves. While many knowledgeable people have taken on the complex subject of protein, diet and well-being, we believe the *Bio-Age* concept offers new insights that will inspire readers to a better understanding of ways to improve health. Protein no doubt plays a key role in health and fitness, but we want to make it clear that a balance between high-quality proteins, fats and, yes, even certain carbohydrates is the answer when it comes to the overall success of reducing your Bio-Age.

Many people come face to face with an inevitable dilemma as they pass that middle-age mark: Should they diet to lose added fat? Most never reach their fat-loss goals because of an all-or-nothing approach to these diets. Overwhelming research has confirmed that if you consume a proper balance of foods while lowering your overall high-glycemic, insulin-spiking carbs, you will lose fat, even through increased age.

Most of the high-protein diets you see on the market are really low-carbohydrate diets in disguise. Many of these diets fall short of the ideal meal plan. Although many carbohydrates do cause us to gain unwanted fat, removing them altogether from the diet is certainly not going to solve the problem; a few bad apples don't spoil the whole bunch.

A number of recent research studies support additional dietary proteins to replace high carbohydrates and saturated fats. Studies have shown that the low-fat and high-carbohydrate diets recommended in the past have been a big failure, and based on our genetic heritage, such diets are likely to fail us in the future. To a large extent this is due to our inability to utilize artificial carbohydrates in the amounts we have become accustomed to. Remember, we didn't hunt and forage Twinkies™ and rice cakes 100,000 years ago, so we cannot expect to have the biochemical tools necessary to process these foods effectively today.

As mentioned in the insulin chapter, high-carbohydrate diets, especially those that do not mention the glycemic index, keep your triglyceride and insulin levels high throughout the day and create sluggish cells that are poor fat burners. All of these factors may contribute to an increase in your Bio-Age. To reverse this process, many researchers now recommend scaling back on the carbs and increasing the quality proteins (more on this a little later). But why is protein so important to Bio-Age success in the first place?

ESSENTIAL CARBOHYDRATES?

Every day your body builds and rebuilds close to 300 billion cells with the raw materials found in protein. Carbohydrates can supply energy for building these body proteins, but they don't supply the actual raw building materials. Only protein and certain fats can do that.

Protein is absolutely essential for life and reducing your Bio-Age. And we know that certain fatty acids are also essential to life (we'll be discussing the importance of fatty acids in Chapter 7), but what about carbohydrates? Some carbohydrates, as we have pointed out, are *desirable*, but have never been proven to be *essential*. There has never been an RDA (recommended daily allowance) or an RDI (recommended daily intake) established for carbohydrates.

PROTEIN: ANOTHER CHAIN IN THE LINK

Protein is second only to water as the most plentiful substance in the body. In fact, well over 50% of our body's dry weight is protein (though the brain's dry matter is nearly 60% fat). The proteins you consume from the foods you eat are made up of subunits called amino acids. Amino acids form three-dimensional peptide chains called dipeptides, tripeptides or polypeptides that provide our bodies with a constant supply of nitrogen and sulfur, and a constant supply of nitrogen and sulfur is what we require if we want to remain highly anabolic. Amino acids contain approximately 16% nitrogen. It is the chemical component of nitrogen that separates amino acids from the two other basic nutrients, carbohydrates and fatty acids.

There are about 20 amino acids that are considered biologically important. Eight of these amino acids are considered essential because the body cannot produce them on its own and they must be obtained from our diets. The other 12 amino acids can be synthesized in the liver from these original eight.

The Biological Factory

A molecule of protein is actually a chain of anywhere from a few amino acids (oligopeptides) to several hundred amino acids linked together as a polypeptide. These proteins are formed by the chemical reaction of one amino acid combining with the acid end of another, forming a peptide bond. These polypeptides serve as the building blocks for your organs, muscle cells, transport proteins and enzymes. Your body has the incredible ability to manufacture protein structures comprising hundreds of amino acids in different sequences in only a few seconds. This is a continual process known as protein synthesis.

In nature, there are approximately 300 amino acids, but only about 20 are interwoven throughout most life forms. An average body uses anywhere from 300–500 g of protein a day, but the average diet in North America, according to the RDA, should contain only 0.8 g of protein per kilogram of body weight. Even with this figure, most North Americans take in approximately 100 g per day, so where does this leave the other 200–400 g the body uses?

THE ANABOLIC/CATABOLIC CYCLES

The body is a biological factory that is able to recycle approximately 300–400 g of its own protein stores per day. Even though the body is very adaptable at tearing down proteins and reusing their amino acids to rebuild new proteins, only about 75% of the amino acids obtained through this process are recycled. This leaves the other 25% or so dependent on outside supplies (foods). This process of breaking down proteins is called catabolism, which, as we've outlined, is defined as any process in which complex substances are converted into more simple compounds with the release of energy. Its counterpart, anabolism, is defined as any process in which living cells convert simple substances into more complex compounds, especially into living matter. This elegant dance between catabolism and anabolism is one of the key factors to sustaining life.

Protein synthesis, or the creation of new proteins from simple amino acids, is one of our most vital anabolic processes. As we've discussed, when we are young and vital protein synthesis runs very efficiently, so we are predominantly anabolic. But as we age, our catabolic metabolism begins to exceed our anabolic metabolism, and the body's ability to construct protein starts to slow down. In fact, a well-accepted theory is that aging can be deemed a malfunction of the body's ability to repair itself; in other words, catabolism exceeding anabolism.

Forever Young

Aging causes a decline in the anabolic function of protein synthesis, which inevitably leads to disability and death. Huge amounts of research dollars have been spent investigating the role that protein synthesis plays in the development of disease and aging. In the May 1998 issue of the *Journal of Clinical Investigation*, scientists found that administering certain mixtures of amino acids to older people increased their net muscle protein synthesis. For these elderly people, the increased amino acid delivery into the cells was able to stimulate muscle protein synthesis. According to the study, amino acid ingestion results in a net protein deposition and the restoration of youthful anabolic metabolism at the cellular level.

The scientists concluded that there is a dietary basis to explain the loss of muscle mass that occurs with aging. They also determined that a lack of amino acids is more likely the problem, rather than the inability of cells to utilize amino acids once ingested. An anabolic response achieved with amino acid therapy indicates that muscle mass could be preserved or restored in the elderly if adequate protein or amino acids were ingested on a regular basis (see Appendix II for recommended protein formulas). In other words, those who have lost muscle mass can regain it by consuming a diet high in bioavailable protein or free amino acids, especially if weight-bearing exercise is added to the mix.

Prehistoric Protein

Almost everyone has heard the saying, "You are what you eat." This statement is only partly true. We are not only what we eat, but more importantly, we are also what our ancestors ate. And guess what? Our ancestors ate protein and lots of it. As we discussed in the previous chapter, we have evolved to run best on the same foods as our prehistoric ancestors—and their diet consisted of at least 30% protein.

Of course, the protein our ancestors ate was a little different from much of the protein we consume today. Early man consumed protein from "lean game meats," which also contained the essential fatty acids and many other nutrients we are lacking in our contemporary diets. Other research indicates that we were predominantly hunters and then gatherers. It is interesting that the research also indicates that our early ancestors were much healthier than the people of the agricultural revolution, who consumed a diet high in carbohydrates.

Protein Helps to Burn Fat

Protein consumed with every meal increases your level of alertness. While high-carbohydrate meals have the opposite effect, leaving you feeling dull and sleepy, protein helps to elevate your resting metabolic rate throughout the day and night even while you sleep. Compared with a high-carbohydrate meal, the thermic response (that is, the energy produced) from a high-protein meal can be 40% greater, and that's a lot of heat (increased heat equals increased calories burned). Research also shows that protein meals increase the oxygen consumption by two to three times that of a high-carbohydrate meal, indicating a much greater increase in the metabolic rate. If you don't get enough protein from the foods you eat, you'll slow your metabolism down to a snail's pace.

Protein is especially important to help with recovery and growth after proper exercise, especially weight resistance and Biocize (outlined in Chapter 17). As we've outlined, research shows that a diet rich in proteins contributes to greater gains in muscle during resistance training than does a high-carbohydrate diet. Higher protein meals are also more satisfying, filling you up more effectively than a high-carbohydrate meal and consequently decreasing hunger. Proteins that are very effective at curbing your appetite are the ones containing high levels of the whey protein isolate alpha-lactalbumin, as well as special proteins found in specific whey isolates called glycomacropeptides (GMPs). One of the most important things you can do on the *Bio-Age* plan is to consume high-quality protein with every single meal. Later in this chapter we will be discussing whey protein more extensively.

Muscle, Protein and Aging

The link between protein, muscle and aging has a very important element we should never forget as we embark on a path to healthy longevity. That is, muscle is the engine of metabolism. Muscle is the tissue that is rich with tiny little energy-burning factories called mitochondria. In well-conditioned muscle, each muscle cell may contain 1000 or 2000 mitochondria. Mitochondria take dietary fuel such as sugars, fats and amino acids and turn them into energy.

The more muscle you have, the more mitochondria you have available to burn dietary fuel of any kind. Well-conditioned (aerobic) muscle contains even more mitochondria, so the more you use the muscles you have, the more efficient you become at burning all fuel. As stated earlier, good-quality protein is an absolute requirement for building this added muscle.

Thus, your formula for healthy longevity looks something like this: Consume high-quality protein to support muscle building. Exercise that muscle to increase its energy-producing capability. Consume high-quality nutrients in a healthy balance to support the efficient system you've worked so hard to create.

Stress and Protein

As we mentioned in an earlier chapter, cortisol, your predominant stress hormone, becomes elevated in the face of physical or psychological stress. It robs us of our youth, our vitality and is one of the biggest contributors to depleting our muscle mass and making us gain weight. In other words, stress keeps us fat. Cortisol functions by stealing nitrogen from the protein in our muscle structures. It then turns the amino acids into sugar for increased energy. If there is not a sufficient supply of new protein (amino acids) in the system, cortisol will have no other choice but to take it from our body tissues, and muscle tissue is the first to go. Remember, loss of lean body mass (muscle) is one of the top Bio-Age markers. If you haven't gotten the point by now, we'll say it one more time: You can't afford to lose a gram of muscle if you want to decrease your Bio-Age.

Getting the Most from Protein

Medical journals are full of research-based reports detailing the all-important condition of maintaining a positive nitrogen balance for muscle growth and superior health. Nitrogen balance refers to the difference between the amount of dietary nitrogen that is deposited in the muscle tissue and the amount that is lost or excreted. If nitrogen balance is positive, this indicates that there may be a net growth in body tissues. If nitrogen balance is negative, however, this will indicate that our protein intake is inadequate and that the body may be cannibalizing its own muscle tissue. This nitrogen-depositing aspect of protein gives us the opportunity to measure the nitrogen balance of different proteins in order to determine which sources are the most beneficial for optimum health.

The actual value of the various protein foods is measured in the net protein utilization index (NPU), which reflects the biological value and percentage of digestibility of a specific protein. The biological value of protein is the efficiency with which the protein deposits the right amino acids required for the building process of anabolism. And as you know by now, increasing your anabolism is a crucial step in attaining a younger Bio-Age. For peak anabolic function, it is not the total amount of protein consumed that's crucial, but the amount of protein that is finally available to the body following consumption.

Ecdysterones and Protein

Research has confirmed that specific extracts called ecdysterones from certain plants can have a very positive effect on anabolism. In fact, a Russian study conducted in the 1970s over a three-week period found that subjects taking ecdysterones along with pure protein were able to lower their body fat percentage and increase their muscle size. Refer to Appendix II for recommendations about anabolic-enhancing supplements containing ecdysterones.

THE BEST SOURCES OF PROTEIN

Our bodies all have their own specific amino acid profile, and there is not one food that fits that profile exactly. Mother's milk is rated the best, perhaps a "perfect" protein. Other than mother's milk, all other proteins are compared to egg, the next best thing with regard to NPU. The only food to have a higher NPU than whole eggs is whey protein. However, whey protein is considered an isolate, not a whole food, so NPU is still measured against the egg.

The NPU of various foods (from highest to lowest)

Protein	Biological Value (i.e., % digestible)
AlphaPure® whey protein isolate	159
Whey protein concentrate (lactalbumin)	104
Whole egg	100
Supro® non-GMO soy protein isolate	100
Cow's milk	91
Egg whites (egg albumin)	88
Fish	83
Beef	80
Chicken	79
Caseinate and milk protein isolates	77
Soy	74
Rice	59
Wheat	54
Seeds, nuts, legumes (beans), sea vegetables (spirulina and chlorella)	49

As you can see, plant-based proteins are very low on the list. This means that if you are a strict vegan (only consuming 100% plant-based foods) and an active person (exercise, athlete, etc.), you will have a more difficult time building and repairing muscle tissue, especially with advanced age. Many studies have shown that if you replace an athlete's essential protein supply with an exact amount of plant-based protein, that athlete will begin to lose quality muscle and strength almost immediately.

Many vegetable proteins are not very high-quality sources of amino acids to begin with, and many of these foods like beans, peas and corn are loaded with carbohydrates. Nuts and seed proteins are also low on the list. Sizable portions of proteins from vegetables are never absorbed because the fiber in these foods binds to the protein.

Supplementing one's diet with high-quality protein isolates that contain whey protein, soy protein or a mix of these two is a fast and convenient way to supply your body with growth- and repair-enhancing nitrogen. In addition, some of these isolates are rich with valuable sulfur groups, which we'll describe shortly (see Appendix II for supplemental protein recommendations). You will read about specific recommendations for fine-tuning your eating strategies in Part III.

AGING THE RIGHT WHEY

Whey protein is a by-product of the cheese industry. Years ago, most of the whey was simply disregarded as waste. That is until scientists researched the profiles of its protein structure. Whey protein isolates are the highest-quality protein known to modern science. This is because of their superior amino acid profile, which gives them the edge over other proteins when it comes to their digestibility potential and incorporation into muscle tissue. Whey proteins are extremely anabolic, and are able to increase protein synthesis faster and better than other proteins. And, as we've noted, consuming proteins that support anabolic function contributes greatly to your repair budget and helps to maintain an optimum Bio-Age.

The most exciting potential of whey protein isolates comes from their ability to modulate our internal army, the immune system. Our immune systems are extremely busy, and the older we get, the harder it is for them to spring into action and defend us (one of the reasons we don't see 60- and 70-year-old soldiers fighting in our armies). Cancer researchers have known for years that numerous cells mutate into cancerous cells each and every day. If our immune systems are strong, they are able to kill those mutated cells each day, but that's just the tip of the iceberg for our immunity. Millions of organisms—like viruses, parasites, bacteria and fungi— are also trying to gain a foothold and take over. Anything that can increase the function of the immune system is highly recommended in the *Bio-Age* plan.

The Whey to Strong Immunity

Here are a few incredible things that whey isolates have been shown to do:

- In 1996, anti-cancer research showed that the growth of breast cancer cells are strongly inhibited by low concentrations of whey protein.
- Another 1996 anti-cancer research report showed that glutathione in cancer cells is much higher than in surrounding normal cells. This makes it harder to kill cancer cells with chemotherapy. When whey protein is introduced, cancer cells respond by losing their glutathione, while normal cells actually increase in glutathione, adding more protection against chemotherapy.
- In a 1988 paper published in the *Journal of Nutrition*, animals that were fed whey protein before being exposed to a strong cancer-causing agent (dimethylhydrazine) mounted an incredible immune response. Tumors were smaller and far fewer in number.

Other Benefits of Whey Protein Isolates

- They are lactose-reduced, allowing those with lactose intolerance to also benefit from whey's superior amino acid profile.
- They help to stimulate the release of the hormone glucagon, which in turn stimulates the body to burn fat for energy, thus increasing one's metabolism.
- They stimulate the liver to release special polypeptides called somatomedins or insulin-like growth factors that control the steady rate of muscle growth and are produced under the influence of the anti-aging hormone HGH.
- In clinical settings whey has been shown to increase immune response by up to 500% due to its high levels of the amino acid cysteine, which is a precursor to the tripeptide glutathione, one of the strongest antioxidants in the body.
- They are been shown to decrease appetite due to their ability to stimulate the release of cholecystokinin (CCK), an appetite-suppressing hormone.

ADVANCES IN PROTEIN SCIENCE

Recent technological advances have allowed scientists to split whey proteins in order to isolate the alpha-lactalbumin portion. This results in a protein that has three to four times the alpha-lactalbumin content present in a typical whey protein isolate product.

Whey proteins have been researched for years and particular emphasis has been placed on the alpha portion due to its high levels of concentration in human milk. If there's anything we have learned about nutrition and the human body, it is that the closer something resembles our own innate human structure, the more it will be accepted into those structures. The alpha portion of whey constitutes up to 25% of the total proteins in human milk, making it the major single component of mother's milk.

As we look at the many attributes of the new whey protein isolates available today, we can't help but be amazed. But what exactly do we mean by the new whey isolates? Whey hasn't always been as powerful a protein supplement as it is today. It took a few decades to reach the potential of the newest whey isolates available. Early whey proteins contained as little as 30–40% protein. They were filled instead with huge amounts of fat, lactose (milk sugar) and undenatured proteins (damaged proteins). These earlier whey products were referred to as whey concentrates.

A good majority of the products available today come from the newer advancements of ion-exchange and cross-flow membrane extraction, but the newest generation of whey isolates are very expensive to produce. If properly isolated, they can contain upwards of 90% pure protein with almost no fat and minimal levels of lactose.

Due to the increased cost (double the price of high-quality concentrates) of the newer isolates, many manufacturers tend to mix the isolates with less expensive concentrates and still call them isolates. There are only a very small percentage of companies using 100% isolates.

These high alpha levels are key to anabolism (protein synthesis) as they are a perfect source of protein—instantly bioavailable. This means that the protein goes immediately into use by the body in the repair process, slowing catabolism and cellular aging. When taking some of the new whey protein isolates, your increased anabolic rate means you will look, feel and perform better longer even as your chronological age increases. We'll describe some of the specific sources of these isolates in Part III and in Appendix II.

TRYPTOPHAN

Through extensive research over the past 40 years, it has been established that the activity level of a brain chemical (neurotransmitter) known as serotonin has a material impact on levels of insomnia, pain sensitivity, anxiety and depression. Serotonin has also been demonstrated to have appetite-suppressant qualities.

As we discussed in Chapter 4, tryptophan, an essential amino acid, is necessary for the brain to manufacture serotonin. Since the U.S. Food and Drug Administration banned the sale of L-tryptophan as an amino acid supplement in 1989, the market has been forced to replace it with expensive prescription drugs. Whey protein powders are excellent natural sources of tryptophan. The higher the alpha-lactalbumin portion of the whey, the higher the tryptophan levels. Adequate tryptophan equals balanced neurotransmitter levels, enhanced moods, cortisol reduction and better sleep. These benefits of tryptophan go a long way to lowering your Bio-Age.

In a new research report, alpha-lactalbumin has shown great promise in improving our ability to deal with excessive daily stress and elevate our moods. It is through several biochemical mechanisms that stress not only contributes to a depressive state, but also causes us to age drastically on a biological level. As noted in Chapter 4, consuming alpha-lactalbumin resulted in a 48% increase in blood tryptophan levels, which was accompanied by an improvement in depressive symptoms. Also noticed was a reduction in cortisol, one of the body's chief catabolic stress hormones. Thus, alpha-lactalbumin is a valuable mood-stabilizing substance that helps support the anabolic state so important to a vital Bio-Age.

PROTEIN AND GLUTATHIONE

One hallmark of aging is a sharp decline in a protein-based substance called glutathione. Glutathione is one of our key sentinels because it has critical antioxidant properties and is one of our chief detoxifying molecules. For every toxic molecule removed by glutathione, we lose one molecule of glutathione. Thus, this vital protector is regularly removed from the body as it is used. Glutathione is also one of the main nutrients that protects us against damaging sugar-protein reactions called glycation (discussed in Chapter 16). In essence, glutathione is one of the most important substances in the body. A brief list of the benefits of glutathione is below:

- improves liver function
- prevents cancer
- promotes longevity
- ameliorates bronchitis
- provides immune support
- ameliorates psoriasis
- ameliorates chronic fatigue syndrome
- promotes general disease prevention

CYSTEINE: AN ALLY IN HEALTHY LONGEVITY

Of the three amino acids the body uses to manufacture glutathione—cysteine, glycine and glutamic acid—cysteine is the most important since it contains the crucial sulfur molecule. Cysteine is a dietary amino acid that is found in almost all proteins. When there is adequate cysteine in our diet, our bodies can make the much-needed glutathione and the powerful antioxidant enzyme discussed in Chapter 1, glutathione peroxidase. With inadequate dietary cysteine, glutathione cannot be manufactured and we become more susceptible to free radical damage and the effects of toxic exposure. Moreover, our repair budget suffers enormously. In a sense, as our glutathione levels fall we are more prone to fall into a catabolic cycle of breaking down.

Certain whey protein isolates contain high levels of cysteine and other factors crucial to building our glutathione reserves. Alzheimer's disease, Parkinson's disease, liver disease and many other conditions are associated with low glutathione levels. Also, people with low glutathione have poorer exercise tolerance and often feel terrible when they exert themselves. If glutathione levels are low, it makes building your muscle reserves that much harder. Some whey isolates are much higher in their capacity to create an anabolic environment for enhanced repair, which will be discussed in Part III.

HOW MUCH PROTEIN?

Now that we have extolled the many virtues of supplying your body with high-quality protein throughout the day, let's find out how much we should have. As mentioned earlier, according to the RDA for protein, we shouldn't be taking in any more than 0.8 g per kilogram of body weight. While this amount may be all right for sedentary people, many researchers, including us, believe that it is much too low for someone who wishes to gain muscle and slow biological aging.

The amazing thing about the RDA is that it recommends that all adults, regardless of their weight or activity levels, consume the same quantity of protein. We don't have to tell you how crazy this sounds. We recommend a much higher intake of protein than the spartan measures listed in the RDA, especially if you want to gain fat-burning muscle and reverse your Bio-Age. But just how much is enough?

We are all biochemically different and therefore our protein requirements are different as well. Simply put, the more active you are, the more protein you will need to repair your body. Exercise physiologist Dr. Lee Coyne points out in his book, *Fat Won't Make You Fat*, that according to some of the most respected researchers in the field of nutrition, the RDAs in many instances can be low by at least a factor of three. This assumption is further backed up by research by Dr. Emanuel Cheraskin. After assessing the Cornell Medical Index Health Questionnaire filled out by 1040 dentists and their spouses, Dr. Cheraskin found that those who consumed two or three times the RDA of protein had the least medical health problems and therefore were the healthiest.

Individual protein intake and absorption are also affected by the way the proteins are prepared (raw, cooked) as well as by the accessory nutrients that are available for the assimilation of the protein. For instance, protein requires a full array of the B vitamins in order to be properly utilized and incorporated into body tissues.

As we have tried to stress throughout this book, one of the most effective ways to decrease your Bio-Age is to increase your anabolic metabolism (anabolism). Protein is a driving force behind anabolism due to its ability to supply the nitrogen necessary for repair.

Bio-Age Anabolic Daily Protein Requirements

When figuring out your protein requirements, keep in mind that not all body weight is the same. For instance, fat is inert and doesn't require protein, whereas muscle is part of your metabolically active lean body weight and requires plenty of protein. In order to find out proper protein requirements for your lean body mass and anabolic metabolism, you will first have to get your lean body mass measured. There are many ways you can have this done, such as at a doctor's office, a university or your local fitness club. There are also many different methods for measurement, some better than others. For your convenience, we have completed a section on a recommended body-fat testing method in Appendix I, along with recommendations for what the results mean for your protein consumption.

7

Fatty Acids

Some years ago, Dr. Sidney Baker, a former professor at Yale University School of Medicine, undertook a curious experiment with one of his colleagues. They set out to determine the total area that would be covered if you took the covering off every one of the body's cells and laid them out side by side. They learned that the total surface area covered by our cells is the equivalent size of 10 football fields.

What makes this more interesting is the fact that our cell membranes, the covering that surrounds each cell, are made primarily of fat. It is astounding to think that the nutrient most of us have grown to hate is the champion of our cell structure and comprises such a vast surface area. Even more extraordinary, as mentioned in Chapter 6, is that the dry weight of brain is nearly 60% fat. Maintaining proper heart rhythm requires the right balance of fat. Building our bone density and strength is dependent upon the right kinds of fat.

Our inflammatory system allows us to respond to physical or biological insults and to initiate repair. When the inflammatory system is out of balance, inflammation runs unchecked, contributing to a broad spectrum of aging-related changes. Orchestrating the inflammatory system's complex web of activity is also the domain of fatty acids.

Imagine a nutrient that regulates bone formation, heart rhythm, mood, behavior, energy, immune function, energy production and the virtual foundation of the entire inflammatory system within the body. This is the elegance of the fatty acid family.

FATTY ACIDS AND THE YOUTHFUL BRAIN

Over 50 different conditions of the brain may be associated with fatty acid imbalance or insufficiency. Dr. Schmidt has described the extraordinary ways in which fatty acids can be used to heal a variety of brain-related conditions in his book *Brain-Building Nutrition: The Healing Power of Fats and Oils*. Consider this abbreviated list of brain-related conditions that may be influenced by fatty acids:

- age-associated memory impairment
- aggression
- Alzheimer's disease
- anorexia nervosa
- anxiety
- attention deficit
- autism
- bipolar disorder
- brain tumor (glioma)
- cerebral palsy
- chronic fatigue
- depression
- developmental delay
- diabetic retinopathy, neuropathy
- hostility
- hyperactivity
- learning disability
- lower IQ
- memory problems
- multiple sclerosis
- phobias
- postpartum depression
- retinal disease
- schizophrenia
- slower information processing and reaction time
- predisposition toward suicide
- tremors

These conditions of the brain are only a fraction of the maladies in the human body that may be influenced by fatty acids.

Balancing Act

One remarkable aspect of the human body is the way balance is required to maintain our inflammatory system in working order. This is achieved by the right balance of essential fatty acids from the omega-6 and omega-3 families. These families are the foundation of a sophisticated messenger system throughout the body.

These messengers tell the immune cells whether to wake up or settle down. They tell the blood vessels whether to narrow or widen. The messengers tell the blood platelets whether to stick together or separate, thus affecting the clotting of blood. The messengers regulate inflammation. For every messenger that performs one function, there is another that performs the opposite function. In a sense, the messengers are like a town crier, signaling a call to action or signaling that all is well.

These messengers come under a variety of technical names, but each of them has something in common: they are made from essential fatty acids that come from your diet. Some messengers are formed from omega-6 fatty acids, while others are formed from omega-3 fatty acids. In many cases, the messengers that are formed from omega-6 fatty acids perform the opposite function of those formed from omega-3 fatty acids.

BUILDING THE MESSENGERS: FROM DIETARY FAT TO PROSTAGLANDINS

The membranes of your nerves, blood cells and blood vessels are made of untold trillions of fatty acid molecules. The balance of these fatty acids within the membranes is determined largely by your diet. When your diet is balanced in omega-6 and omega-3 fatty acids, your cells are balanced in these fatty acids as well. When your diet has too few omega-3 fatty acids, your cell membranes have too few omega-3 fatty acids.

Fatty acids that form the structure of your cell membranes become messengers when a call to action is sent out. This call can be prompted by a trauma, a virus, a bacteria, a free radical, a toxic chemical, a heavy metal or some other trigger. Once the call to action has been sent, your cell's fatty acids are released from the membrane and are chemically transformed into highly active hormone-like substances. Once the hormone-like messengers are released, they exert powerful and profound effects on a vast array of functions within the brain.

Prostaglandins from Fatty Acids

These messengers are given the name "prostaglandins" because they were originally discovered in the prostate gland. Now we know that prostaglandins are produced throughout the body. Prostaglandins (PG) are formed directly through a series of steps from dietary fatty acids. Those we're concerned with are called PGE1, PGE2 and PGE3.

PGE1 is formed from dietary linoleic acid. This is the fatty acid predominant in corn oil, sunflower oil, sesame oil and safflower oil. PGE2 is formed from the fatty acid called arachidonic acid. This fatty acid is found only rarely in plants and is most common in animal meat. PGE3 is formed from the fatty acid eicosapentaenoic acid (EPA), found in krill, salmon, mackerel, herring, sardines and other fish. Another form of PG3 is formed from the fatty acid docosahexaenoic acid (DHA), found in the same fish as EPA.

PGE1 is important in the nervous system as it affects the release of compounds from nerve cells that transmit nerve impulses. It tends to have anti-inflammatory properties and is immune enhancing. It can reduce fluid accumulation and has a significant effect on the nervous system. Some doctors have manipulated the PGE1 pathway to improve depression, multiple sclerosis, PMS-related mood changes, schizophrenia and other conditions.

PGE2 is a highly inflammatory substance. It can cause swelling, increased pain sensitivity and increased blood viscosity. Some of the other compounds associated with PGE2 can cause blood platelet clumping, spasm of blood vessels, accumulation of inflammatory cells in an area and over the long term can change the way in which nerve cells communicate. These compounds can also cause an overactive immune system within the nervous system, encouraging your own immune cells to attack you.

Substances called leukotrienes are related to PGE2 in that they are made from the fatty acid arachidonic acid, the same fatty acid from which PGE2 is made. However, leukotrienes are an even more potent inflammatory substance. They have been estimated to be 1000 to 10,000 times more inflammatory than histamine, the substance associated with the runny nose and watery eyes of allergy and hay fever. Leukotrienes signal white blood cells to travel to an area. This is good when you need them, but white cells can do a lot of damage when present in excess amounts.

The PGE2 family is sometime viewed as a "bad guy" because of the powerful inflammatory potential they possess. In reality, we need this family for many vital functions. The problem arises when the system is out of balance, when there is too much activity in this family. This balance is tied to fatty acid balance.

PGE3 tends to be mildly anti-inflammatory and immune enhancing. It is thought to counter the effects of the powerfully inflammatory PGE2 substances. It prevents blood platelets from clumping and helps prevent blood vessel spasm. Fatty acids important in PGE3 formation, like EPA and DHA, can also reduce arachidonic acid in the cells. This reduces the chance of producing messengers from arachidonic acid and is one way that these fatty acids can alter the production of highly inflammatory messengers.

FOOD SOURCES OF EFA AND THEIR MESSENGERS

PG Series	Fatty Acid	Fatty Acid Family	Food Sources
1	linoleic	omega-6	sunflower, safflower, sesame and corn
1	gamma-linolenic	omega-6	primrose, borage and black currant seed oil
2	arachidonic	omega-6	animal meat, milk, eggs, squid and warm-water fish

3	alpha-linolenic	omega-3	flax, canola, pumpkin, chia, walnut and brazil nut
3	EPA	omega-3	cold-water fish, krill and algae (some)
3	DHA	omega-3	cold-water fish, krill and algae (some)

Primed for Inflammation

This messenger system is necessary to control a remarkable array of functions within the body and the brain and it is generally able to do so as long as the fatty acid *balance* is appropriate. Should one family of fatty acids be present in greater amounts than another, the scales are tipped toward the fatty acid type that predominates. The most common scenario of imbalance is that relating to arachidonic acid and the PGE2 pathway.

For example, if you consume a diet high in arachidonic acid, this fatty acid becomes predominant in your cell membranes. When an event happens in the body that might trigger inflammation, the inflammatory portion, of which arachidonic acid is a part, works very effectively. However, once its work is done and the process needs to be subdued, there may not be an adequate balance of other fatty acid messengers to do the job. In one sense, the cells are "primed for inflammation" with inadequate messengers to shut off the system properly. This is why consuming foods or supplements with the omega-6 to omega-3 balance in mind is crucial to good health.

TOO MUCH OF A GOOD THING

Your immune system responds to invaders by releasing a vast network of chemical messengers. One of these, called interleukin-1 (IL-1), is a key first messenger that triggers a robust immune response. Because of this interleukin-1 is a vital health partner at all stages in life. However, sometimes IL-1 production persists at high levels over long periods. When this occurs, IL-1 can be damaging to health. In the *Journal of Neuroscience*, researchers state that an increase in IL-1 may be the trigger underlying a number of aging processes, especially in the brain. IL-1 is now considered by some to be the "predominant proinflammatory and catabolic" messenger in the progression of arthritis. IL-1 levels are also increased in many disorders of the brain and heart that are common to the aging process.

It turns out that fatty acids may be among the most critical factors that limit the excess production of IL-1, so that it does not elevate to damaging levels. Numerous studies have shown that flax seed oil and fish oil decrease IL-1 levels in a variety of inflammatory conditions. Flax seed oil reduced IL-1 levels by 30%, while fish oil reduced IL-1 by 74%. In people with inflammatory arthritis, fish oil reduced IL-1 levels by 90%. On the other hand, too much of the harmful omega-6 fatty acid arachidonic acid leads to *increased* IL-1. It appears from this and other research that fatty acid balance is crucial to maintaining the proper balance of immune messengers so that these signals do not cause catabolic damage to the body as we age.

Conditions of Fatty Acid Imbalance

The omega-6 to omega-3 ratio is a comparison of the amount of omega-6 fatty acids in the diet (or in the body) to omega-3 fatty acids. Though experts disagree on the precise ideal ratio, most agree that it lies somewhere between 1:1 and 4:1, for example, four parts omega-6 fatty acids to one part omega-3 fatty acids.

The problem today is that the ratio has shifted much too far in the omega-6 direction. Modern estimates place our adult dietary ratio somewhere in the vicinity of 20:1 or higher. In essence, modern diets consist of far too much omega-6. Linoleic acid is one of the valuable fatty acids of which we get too much. Linoleic is concentrated in warm-weather vegetable oils such as sunflower, corn and safflower.

Here is just a sample of studies showing what can happen when there is too much linoleic acid in the diet or when the omega-6 to omega-3 ratio gets too high:

- Tissue from brain tumors contained more than four times as much linoleic acid (and only half as much DHA) than normal brain tissue.
- Dutch men whose diets were highest in omega-6 fatty acids were more likely to suffer from dementia than those with high omega-3 levels in the diet.
- People with depression had higher omega-6 to omega-3 ratios.
- The higher the level of omega-6 oils in the diet, the greater the risk of melanoma (skin cancer).
- Women with higher levels of omega-6 fatty acids were at greater risk of dying from breast cancer.
- People with diets high in linoleic acid were more than three times as likely to die from cancer as those with diets high in olive oil (oleic acid).

Don't let this evidence scare you away from linoleic acid. Remember, you need it in order to survive. The key is to balance the intake of this fatty acid with that of the omega-3 fatty acids. Using supplements or oils that contain linoleic acid along with some of the other omega-6s and omega-3 is fine as long as the ratio stays below 4:1. Switching to oils high in oleic acid and rich in omega-3 fatty acids is the best way to lower linoleic acid and calm the storm that can arise with too much linoleic acid.

FATTY ACIDS AND TOTAL HEALTH

Thus far, we've emphasized the important role of fatty acids in the brain and have described how fatty acids may affect things like cancer, but there is a growing list of other conditions related to fatty acid imbalance. In short, fatty acid imbalance can be at the core of a vast array of health complaints that seem entirely unrelated at first glance:

- asthma
- cystic fibrosis
- diabetes
- eczema
- gum disease (gingivitis)
- heart arrhythmia
- hypertension
- IgA nephropathy (kidney disease)
- immune suppression
- infection
- inflammatory bowel disease (Crohn's)
- lupus
- obesity
- osteoporosis
- PMS
- polycystic kidney disease
- psoriasis
- pulmonary disease
- rheumatoid arthritis
- Syndrome X

It is beyond the scope of this chapter to describe in depth the way fatty acids affect all these conditions and more. However, the science is very clear: Fatty acids can affect *all* body systems. None are spared from the effects of fatty acid deficiency.

DOES FAT MAKE YOU FAT?

Most people are worried that if you increase your fat intake you automatically risk becoming fatter, but this depends largely on the types of fats you consume, the amount of total carbohydrates and the total amount of calories. In general, consuming the right balance of omega-6 and omega-3 fatty acids actually supports weight loss because it makes your metabolic machinery run more efficiently. In addition, eliminating trans fatty acids from the diet improves your insulin response, which is key to losing or maintaining optimum weight. (We discuss the dangers of trans fatty acids on pages 94–95.)

A study conducted at University Hospital in Geneva, Switzerland, examined the fat intake question with relation to weight gain. One group of overweight patients was placed on a diet of only 26% fat. The other embarked on a generous 45% fat diet. Each diet contained a very low 1200 calories per day. (We do not advocate a 1200-calorie diet.) Both groups were carefully monitored in the hospital. In the end, the high-fat group had lost slightly more body fat (8%) than the low-fat group (7.2%). Remember, decreasing body fat is one of the key targets for healthy longevity.

When you restrict fat, not only do you limit the beneficial fatty acids vital to health, but you must make up the caloric difference with something else. This something else is usually carbohydrates. But what is the consequence of this shift to more carbohydrates? This very question was raised during a study at Rockefeller University.

Normal-weight people were placed on either a 40% fat diet or a 10% fat diet and monitored every 10 days to see how much fat they were making. Yes, the body is very good at making *fat* from carbohydrates (as covered in Chapter 5, "Insulin"). Those on the high-fat diet were making little or no fat, as measured by triglyceride levels and triglyceride content. Those on the low-fat diet, however, had quite a different story to tell. Doctors discovered that between 30–57% of the fatty acids in the triglycerides was saturated fat *manufactured* by the body. In short, those eating low-fat, high-carbohydrate diets *made more of their own saturated fat*!

How is this possible? The body's requirement for fat is crucial. When the subjects were deprived of fat in their diets (the 10% fat group), their bodies said, "It looks like starvation is underway. I'd better make up some more fat to store for the long haul." The subjects then used their elaborate biochemical pathways to take carbohydrate and turn it into fat. This is one of the body's elegant tools to ensure we continue to survive and reproduce despite shortages of vital fat molecules that may occur from time to time.

Studies like these point out that eating fat does not necessarily make you fat. Be careful how you restrict fat because you may just deplete the needed essential fatty acids that will sustain your health during a long life. At the same time, you might be telling the fat cells to "load up," which is one of the crucial enemies of healthy longevity.

Trans Fatty Acids: Stiffening with the Harmful Fats

Given that fat is so vital to the body's structure and function, it is remarkable that instead of concentrating on the "good" fats, we consume so much of a dreadful fat called the *trans fatty acids*. Trans fatty acids are formed from our normal dietary unsaturated fatty acids through the process of hydrogenation or other methods of adulteration. French fries, potato chips, chicken nuggets, deep-fried fish burgers and doughnuts contain anywhere from 8–13 g of trans fatty acids per serving. That's a whopping 2–4 tsps of trans fatty acids. Doughnuts have been found to contain up to 13 g of trans fatty acids. Foods that say "partially hydrogenated oil" on the label also contain trans fatty acids. Margarines can be very high in trans fatty acids, though some members of the food industry have taken steps to reduce trans fatty acids in their foods.

Some calculations have shown that an adult male consuming 145–250 g of fat per day, which is not unheard of, might consume nearly 50 g of this fat as trans fatty acids.

One of the problems with trans fatty acids is that they are *solid* at body temperature once they are incorporated into cell membranes or fat cells. They pack more densely in cells, making your cells more rigid and inflexible. Several animal studies have shown that trans fatty acids may cross the blood-brain barrier and end up nestled snugly in the nerve cell membrane. Trans fatty acids have been associated with heart disease and stroke. Trans fatty acids have also been found to lower testosterone in male animals and increase the number of abnormal sperm. In our opinion, trans fatty acids should be minimized or eliminated from the diet.

CHOLESTEROL: FROM VILLAIN TO HERO

If cholesterol were a human being, you would see its picture plastered all over the post office wall as public enemy number one. We have vilified this essential substance to near mythic proportions. Is it possible for cholesterol to be so dangerous? The scientific evidence points to the contrary. For instance, the myelin sheath that surrounds your nerve cells is roughly 75% fat, with 25% of this fat made up of cholesterol, but what is cholesterol? How does it differ from fatty acids? And what happens to the brain when cholesterol levels get too low?

Cholesterol, while typically called a "fat," is really a steroid. Chemically it is a complex set of ring structures that form the backbone for all steroid hormones in the body like cortisol, estrogen, testosterone and progesterone. Without adequate cholesterol we do not make adequate steroid hormones. Cholesterol is also a vital *structural* molecule in all cell membranes, including, as noted earlier, the brain. Your body is capable of making tremendous amounts of cholesterol daily.

Fatty acids are very simple chain-like molecules with tiny gaps called double bonds. This is partly what distinguishes one fatty acid from another. They are also distinguished by their length. Saturated fats have no gaps in their structure. Monounsaturates have one gap, or double bond. Polyunsaturates have two or more gaps, or double bonds. This feature is what gives all the oils their different properties of taste and texture. It also dictates the myriad vital functions in the human body. Thus, fatty acids and cholesterol are vastly different both structurally and functionally. We must have both to thrive.

We know from numerous experiments in all domains that the nerve cell membrane fluidity changes when cholesterol levels get too low. What is the effect? Biochemically, the effects are numerous, but one observed effect on people is disturbing. Dr. Beatrice Golomb set out to answer the question of problems associated with low cholesterol. Fifty percent of men whose cholesterol levels were below 150 mg/dl had more violent deaths than men with higher readings. In all, Dr. Golomb reviewed 163 studies that connected *low* cholesterol levels to violence and suicide. Cholesterol-lowering medications were also associated with increased risk of death by violence. While a cholesterol level below 200 mg/dl appears to be ideal, we believe that cholesterol levels below 150 mg/dl can be dangerous, especially if coupled with insufficient or imbalanced essential fatty acids.

So we cannot simply view fat as a harmful substance. The very fabric upon which the human being is built is wholly dependent upon fat.

WHICH FATS AND HOW MUCH?

Devising a diet that incorporates the best balance of fats is tricky, given with all the conflicting opinions. It is important to note, however, that almost none of the low-fat advocates have studied or addressed the brain's fatty acid requirement in their work. The low-fat advocates have focused principally on heart disease and have not addressed the very diverse needs of certain fatty acids in brain function.

Dr. Artemis Simopoulos, director of the Center for Genetics, Nutrition and Health in Washington D.C., advocates the following approximate breakdown of fats in the daily diet:

- 75% of fat from monounsaturates (olive oil being one of the best sources)
- 8% of fat from saturated fat
- 17% of fat from polyunsaturates

It may seem confusing that we have so strongly emphasized the importance of polyunsaturated fatty acids for the brain, yet they comprise such a small part of the total fat picture. But we emphasize this part because of the vital role that specific unsaturated fatty acids play in regulating brain function, immune function and many messenger systems within the body.

Additional considerations for your fat intake include:

- the omega-6 and omega-3 fatty acids in a balanced ratio that falls somewhere between 1:1 and 4:1; some supplements contain a ratio of 1:2, which is just fine since it errs on the side of caution, i.e., extra omega-3 fatty acids
- oleic acid to support the absorption of this fatty acid
- the brain's two main long-chain unsaturated fatty acids (especially DHA)

In Part III, you will find details on the specific foods you need to include in your diet to get maximum benefit from your intake of fatty acids and keep your Bio-Age young!

Part II

The Bio-Age Research: Views from Our Experts

These next 11 chapters feature the contributions of top researchers in key areas of anti-aging science. Each contributor is an expert in his field, and each outlines some of the most up-to-date and advanced information on anti-aging strategies.

In addition to authors Brad King and Dr. Michael Schmidt, the *Bio-Age* contributing experts are:

Fereydoon Batmanghelidj, M.D.

Dr. Fereydoon Batmanghelidj received his medical education and training at St. Mary's Hospital Medical School of London University. He has spent most of his scientific life researching the link between pain and disease and chronic dehydration. Dr. Batmanghelidj discovered the healing powers of water 21 years ago when he was serving time as a political prisoner in an Iranian jail. He successfully treated 3000 fellow prisoners suffering from stress-induced peptic ulcer disease with the only medication he possessed—water. This is when he made his discovery that the body indicates its water shortage by producing pain. Since his prison experience, he has focused his full-time attention on dehydration-produced health problems in the body, which has helped hundreds of thousands of people suffering from a variety of pains and degenerative diseases regain their health.

Dr. Batmanghelidj has presented his findings at several international conferences, and they have been published in a number of scientific journals. His findings are now available to the public in an easy-to-understand form in his four books, and his videotapes and audiotapes of his lectures. You can find out more information at www.watercure.com.

Stephen Cherniske, M.Sc.

Stephen Cherniske is a nutritional biochemist with over 30 years of academic, research and clinical experience. He has taught clinical nutrition at two southern California universities and directed the nation's first FDA-licensed clinical laboratory specializing in nutrition testing. Stephen Cherniske is a member of the American Medical Writers Association and Who's Who in American Professionals, and has published numerous scientific papers and a nationally syndicated newspaper column. He was an advisor to the U.S. Olympic team and served on the faculty of the American College of Sports Medicine. His book *The DHEA Breakthrough* (Ballantine 1996) was an international bestseller. *Caffeine Blues* (Warner Books) was published in 1998 and *The Metabolic Plan* (Random House) is scheduled for release in 2001. Presently, Stephen serves as president of Oasis Wellness Network in Broomfield, Colorado.

Edward J. Conley, M.D.

Dr. Edward J. Conley is the director of The Fatigue & Fibromyalgia Clinic of Michigan. He is a board-certified family practice physician. He has served as a consultant to Olympic athletes on how to improve their performance and is an Assistant Clinical Professor of Medicine at Michigan State University. Dr. Conley has treated thousands of patients with Chronic Fatigue, Fibromyalgia, Candida, allergies and other related disorders at his clinic. He has seen most of them return to a higher quality of life based on the treatment program at the clinic and described in detail in his book *America Exhausted*.

Daniel Crisafi, Ph.D.

Born and raised in Montreal, Dr. Daniel Crisafi earned a Bachelor's degree, a Masters of Science and a Ph.D. He also attended the Institut Naturopathic du Québec and has obtained his Master Herbalist degree. Dr. Crisafi has served on numerous health-related advisory boards. He is a former vice-president of the École d'Enseignement Supérieur de Naturopathie du Québec. Dr. Crisafi has also received an honorary degree from the École d'Enseignement Supérieur de Naturopathie du Québec for his contribution to the advancement of naturopathy in that province as well as an award from the Canadian Natural Health Society for his humanitarian work in promoting health.

In addition to his regular lecture appearances, Dr. Crisafi is the editor-in-chief of *Vitalité Québec* and *Health and Vitality* magazines. He is the author of the first Canadian book on candidiasis (*Candida Albicans-EdiForma*). He is also a coauthor with Sam Graci of *Les Superaliments* (Chenelière McGraw-Hill). Dr. Crisafi has been featured in numerous publications, including *Natural Health Products Report*, *La Presse*, *The Ottawa Citizen*, and *Chatelaine*. He has also appeared on a variety of radio and television stations across Canada and the U.S. As a consultant for the health food and natural supplement industry for over 15 years, Dr. Crisafi's objective is to raise awareness about the value and need for natural products and services offered by health food and natural health circles.

Sam Graci, M.A.

Sam Graci is the founder and president of Graci Research Ltd., a company committed to nutritional research and development. He is the creator of greens+, an award-winning concentrated green food that contains a variety of organic greens and herbs. His research into medicinal plants, produce, grains and organic growing techniques has taken him around the world.

Sam Graci is a graduate of the University of Western Ontario, where he studied adolescent psychology and chemistry. He holds additional degrees in education and counseling. He is the author of the best-selling *The Power of Superfoods* and has written numerous articles on health and nutrition for magazines and newspapers. Mr. Graci has appeared frequently on television and radio talk shows. He lives on Saltspring Island in British Columbia. His forthcoming book, *The Food Connection*, will be available in fall 2001.

Donald Henderson, M.D.

Dr. Henderson is the Chief of Staff at the Daniel Freeman Memorial Hospital in Los Angeles, specializing in gastroenterology. He has coauthored numerous articles about diseases and the treatment of the gastrointestinal tract, including gastric cancer. Dr. Henderson has conducted many clinical studies on the treatment of a variety of GI problems, and is currently working on studies involving the use of colostrum for such treatments. He is a coauthor of *Colostrum, Nature's Healing Miracle*. Dr. Henderson serves as a consultant to the American Cancer Society and many other healthcare-related companies.

Kenneth Seaton, Ph.D., D.Sc.

Australian-born research scientist Kenneth Seaton, Ph.D., D.Sc., has spent the last quarter century researching the origins and nature of common diseases, and is the developer of the concepts of Advanced Hygiene.

After graduating from Sydney University, Dr. Seaton went on to spend 12 years as a research fellow with the Popular Science Syndicate School of Sciences, graduating with degrees in microbiology, nuclear physics, biology and physiology. In 1989 he received a Doctor of Science degree for the discovery of the relationship between serum albumin levels, mortality/morbidity and personal hygiene.

Dr. Seaton is the author of three books: *Life, Health and Longevity*; *Breaking the Devil's Circle* and *Is It Possible to Prevent the Common Cold, AIDS, Cancer & Slow the Aging Process?* He has written over 100 articles that have been published in the *Journal of the National Medical Association*, the *Australian Medical Journal* and other professional and popular publications. Dr. Seaton is in demand as a public speaker and has appeared on such television programs as *Tony Brown's Journal, Good Morning Australia, Good Morning Sydney, Dr. Whitaker's Health Show* and others.

Michael A. Zeligs, M.D.

Dr. Zeligs is a physician working in the fields of preventive nutrition and aging intervention. Dr. Zeligs has broad expertise in clinical medicine and scientific training in physiology and molecular biology. This background has allowed him to become a leader in the new field of Phytonutrition. He has pioneered new uses for phytonutrients from cruciferous vegetables, creating nutritional approaches to hormonal health, cancer prevention and healthy aging.

Dr. Zeligs earned a Masters degree in stress-physiology from the University of California, Santa Barbara, and an M.D. degree from the University of California, Irvine, College of Medicine. He has completed specialty medical training in Anesthesiology, Pediatrics and Molecular Immunology. As a physician-investigator, he sponsored Investigative New Drug Filings with the FDA, studying early uses of dehydroepiandrosterone (DHEA) to improve metabolism and immunity. His nutritional research has resulted in numerous patents covering vitamin-hormone combinations, hormonal eye drops, and new formulations for phytonutrients that are otherwise insoluble and poorly absorbed.

Dr. Zeligs is the founder and CEO of BioResponse Nutrients, a research and development group creating innovative nutritional products and natural medicines.

8

The Metabolic Model
of Aging

Stephen Cherniske, M.Sc.

BACKGROUND ON AGING

As more than 76 million American baby boomers (and 1 billion worldwide) reach their fifth decade of life, you've no doubt noticed the soaring interest in anti-aging. After all, boomers have enjoyed the longest period of peace and prosperity in modern history, and they don't want to give it up. "We walked on the moon for Pete's sake. Why do we have to grow old?" And in fact, we may not have to, at least not on the schedule that our grandparents and parents followed.

I was born in 1948 when life expectancy was 65 years. Today, it's pushing 77, but that mark hasn't budged in the last decade and a half. What this means is that we've achieved as much benefit as we could squeeze out of advances in sanitation, decreased infant mortality, vaccinations and antibiotics. In order to get beyond the 77 mark, we're going to need dramatic new developments.

This may bring to mind genetic engineering (GE), since that area of research is continually highlighted in the news. The sobering truth, however, is that practical GE therapies are decades, perhaps many decades, away. More than 2500 people have received GE treatments for diseases in which specific gene targets have been identified, (e.g., cystic fibrosis, Down's syndrome, sickle-cell anemia), but as of this writing, no one has been cured.

The real question for boomers is: *What can I do today?* And the answer is: *Pay attention to your metabolism.*

A METABOLIC OVERVIEW

Draw a horizontal line, on paper or in your mind. At the left end write *birth*. At the right end, put *death*. Right now, you're somewhere between those two points, but the question is where? This line represents your life span, but not just in terms of years. More important, it represents a *metabolic shift* that takes place from the most anabolic state (childhood) to the most catabolic state (old age).

Anabolic metabolism is the rebuild, repair and restore activity of your body. Catabolic activity refers to breakdown and degeneration. At every stage of life, your health is determined by the balance of these two forces. We now know how to alter the balance in favor of rejuvenation and youthfulness. In other words, no matter where you are on this line, you can move to the left.

It's done by resetting the time signals that determine how your brain and body interact. These signals, originating from a variety of tissues and organs, are sent to the brain, which acts as a data analysis and command center. The brain, in effect, constantly polls the body for information as to how the entire organism is performing. There are two distinct reasons for this.

First, this information helps the brain run things at maximum efficiency. If muscle mass and physical activity are low, for example, the brain assumes that very little energy is required to maintain that system. Consequently, when the brain hears that the stomach has received 800 calories (the average dinner), instructions to the gastrointestinal tract and liver are, "Convert those calories to fat." If, on the other hand, muscle mass is maintained and those muscles are worked through regular exercise, the brain's instructions are, "Convert those calories to energy."

The significance of such a dialogue is obvious in terms of health, fitness and longevity, and this is not a metaphor or a simplistic view of physiology. These "messages" actually take place biochemically. The above muscle–stomach–brain dialogue, for example, can be quantified by measuring hormone signals from insulin, cholecystokinin, fatty acid oxidase, carnitine palmitoytransferase, acyl-CoA dehydrogenase and lipoprotein lipase. Because you probably don't want that level of detail, I'll use more familiar terms to illustrate how the human body functions and, more importantly, how to help it work better and last longer.

HOW OLD ARE YOU REALLY?

The second facet of the body–mind dialogue relates to *mortality*. Beyond determining the metabolic fate of dinner, the brain needs to know *how old we are* so that it can most effectively control the vast array of hormones and biochemicals relating to growth, repair, sex, immunity and energy. It is quite accurate to say that this dialogue is *the primary factor that determines how we age and when we die*. The body–mind communications that foster optimal health and maximum life span are known as *longevity signals*. Quite simply, when the brain receives longevity signals from the body, it in turn sends anabolic (rebuild, repair, restore) instructions to the cells, tissues, and organs. On the other hand, if the brain receives over-the-hill signals from the body, it responds with catabolic (wear down, tear down, breakdown) instructions.

You may be asking why. That's normal; everyone asks that. You see, life is a game, and it's Mother Nature's game, not ours. The team we're on is the *Homo sapiens*, an extraordinarily successful team, possibly the best in the league. But this game is much different from the ones we're used to. In the games we've invented (sports, education, careers) you first learn the rules, then the fundamentals and finally strategies for winning. We're so used to doing this that we think *everything* works this way. Then one day you look in the mirror and notice that your hair is thinning, there are deep lines in your face, you don't have the energy or drive you once had, and then it hits you: there is another game being played here. All the while you were working so hard to win the career game, you were losing nature's game . . . and we all know how it ends.

What makes nature's game so difficult is that we were all placed on this team without our consent or knowledge. *No one told us the rules*, and so we went our merry way and grew up to behave much the same as our parents behaved. And unless we depart in some fundamental way from this age-old behavior, we will suffer much as our parents suffered and die at about the same age.

This fundamental shift has to do with understanding the game. In nature, the name of the game and the single objective is *survival*. Not your survival, but survival of the species—all species. The flowers that bloom today will die tomorrow to contribute nitrogen and carbon to the soil, which supports thousands of soil-dwelling species. They in turn support the growth of plants, which create oxygen that supports millions of species. All thinking persons at one time or another have marveled at the astoundingly beautiful and unbelievably complex game that Mother Nature plays.

The problem is that most of these people fail to understand that they are *part of the game*. We think we're different because we own computers, drive cars, fly in space shuttles and talk on cell phones. But Mother Nature couldn't care less about technology. She's into survival; the really basic motivation that hasn't changed in millions of years. The brain shifts your body into a catabolic tailspin after age 40 because it is simply doing what it was programmed to do millions of years ago. Your DNA does not know about hospitals, miracle drugs and refrigerators packed with food. All it knows is that in the past, when muscle mass and activity decreased and immunity started to fail, it was not a good sign. So the primordial conclusion—the instructions hard-wired into your genes—initiates the shutdown sequence. Nothing personal. It was fun while it lasted.

Think about that the next time you're sitting on the couch, munching on some high-fat, artery-clogging snack, watching television. You think it's entertainment, but a part of you (the ancient part that hasn't changed in 30,000 years) is getting a biochemical read-out on your heart rate, hormone levels, muscle mass and respiration and concluding that something is *terribly wrong*. Thus begins the shutdown sequence that will put you in your grave in your mid-seventies, terribly premature compared with what you *could* experience if only you had known.

THE METABOLIC PLAN

If we are in fact players in nature's game, the only way to enjoy this game—and win—is to learn the rules. I define winning as achieving maximal life span *and* high-level wellness, the combination of health extension and longevity. This can only be done by resetting the signals that control metabolism. While no one can stop aging, this strategy will enable you to slow dramatically the rate at which you age.

Changing the signals is accomplished in one of two ways. You can maintain an extraordinarily high muscle mass through daily strenuous exercise. This signals the brain that you are young, thus maintaining anabolic metabolism. Jack Lalane is a perfect example of this strategy. Now 86 years old, he regularly performs 900 push-ups in a day, something that few college athletes could do. The result? When Jack's brain asks his body how old he is, and the muscles report that they just did 900 push-ups, the brain concludes that he must be in his thirties.

DHEA: A CAUSE OR AN EFFECT OF AGING?

If you're not willing to devote hours a day to strenuous exercise, you might like to hear about an alternative strategy, wherein one alters the hormone signal going from the body to the brain. The most comprehensive anabolic influence in human metabolism is dehydroepiandrosterone (DHEA), a hormone produced primarily by the adrenal glands and influencing more than 150 different biochemicals throughout the body and brain. It's important to understand that DHEA levels typically start falling after age 30, and the decline accelerates dramatically with advancing age. DHEA levels of the average 70-year-old will be only 10–15% of what they were at age 28.

For decades, scientists looked at this and said, "Oh well, that's just the way it is. That's aging." In other words, they assumed that plummeting DHEA production was an unavoidable *effect* of aging. Then a few of us started asking the question, "What if declining production of DHEA is actually a *cause* of aging?" Early experiments with animals showed that restoring levels of DHEA had dramatic effects on immunity, body composition, brain function and metabolism. Twenty years later, with more than 6000 studies in print, here is what we know:

1. Restoring youthful levels of DHEA alters the body–brain dialogue. Instead of receiving "over-the-hill" messages, the brain hears that muscle mass is increasing, activity levels are up, immunity is gaining strength and stress levels are down.
2. The brain concludes that the body is growing younger, and responds accordingly. It sends anabolic instructions throughout the body to repair, rebuild and restore. The message is, "Hey body, we're not over the hill after all. In fact, according to my calculations, we're about 29 years old! So hang on; I'm going to turn up metabolic efficiency, immunity, energy production, muscle building, fat burning, learning ability, bone density and [you never know] sex drive."

There's not space in this chapter to catalog all the benefits associated with optimal levels of DHEA. Documented effects include the entire range of immune, energy, body composition, mood, memory and longevity benefits. Researchers at the National Institute of Mental Health even used DHEA to treat what they termed *midlife dysthymia*, otherwise known as the "blahs." They concluded:

"A robust effect of dehydroepiandrosterone on mood was observed. . . . The symptoms that improved most significantly were anhedonia [lack of pleasure], loss of energy, lack of motivation, emotional 'numbness,' sadness, inability to cope, and worry."

In 1999, Etienne-Emile Baulieu, perhaps the world's foremost hormone biochemist, decided to conduct the definitive human trial with DHEA. He called it the DHEAge Study. This year-long trial included nearly 300 men and women ranging in age from 60 to 79. For the undertaking, Baulieu assembled a team of 22 researchers that reads like a *Who's Who* in European endocrinology, geriatrics, immunology and human performance. The study was double-blind and placebo-controlled (the gold standard of scientific methodology) to eliminate any conceivable bias in observations or effects. The initial results, published in the prestigious *Proceedings of the National Academy of Science,* were dramatic. The benefits? Increased bone density in women, improved libido and marked improvements in skin tone, hydration thickness and color.

THE DHEA DILEMMA

Dr. Sam Yen, a leading DHEA researcher at the University of California at San Diego, concluded that "DHEA in *appropriate replacement doses* appears to have remedial effects with respect to its ability to induce an anabolic growth factor, increase muscle strength and lean body mass, activate immune function, and enhance quality of life in aging men and women."

But although Baulieu, Yen and many others have proven that DHEA is a safe and effective metabolic enhancer, one has to admit that well-controlled scientific studies are one thing, and unbridled use by the North American public ("If a little is good, a lot is better") is something altogether different.

DHEA is a powerful hormone. As I've mentioned, it influences more than 150 biochemicals throughout the human body. It's not like vitamin C, which is easily excreted in the urine. If you take too much DHEA, you can experience adverse effects. That's because the body converts some DHEA to testosterone and estrogen, two powerful sex steroids. Thus one must be careful—something that is rather difficult to get across in a health food store when the product is right next to the corn chips. I spelled out the appropriate cautions quite clearly in my book *DHEA Breakthrough*, but still received reports of overdose symptoms related to elevated sex hormones, even in people who were taking a reasonable (25–50 mg) dose. Well, I have good news.

THE 7-KETO BREAKTHROUGH

About the time that American pharmaceutical companies were pulling out their hair at the Food and Drug Administration's decision to release DHEA as a nutritional supplement, Dr. Henry Lardy and his research group at the University of Wisconsin were finalizing work on what was to be the most important DHEA analog of all, 3-acetyl-7-keto DHEA or 7-Keto™ for short.

Dr. Lardy determined that 7-Keto™ was a natural metabolite of DHEA, produced by the body as part of the cascade of DHEA metabolism. Importantly, it was "downstream" from the sex steroids and therefore could not be converted to testosterone or estrogen. When he went shopping for an interested pharmaceutical company, however, he got no offers.

Consumer Education

1. Some people should not take DHEA. This includes people under age 35 (unless following the advice of their physician), men with prostate cancer, pregnant or nursing women, and women with a tendency to grow facial hair (indicates high testosterone).

2. Easy does it. We live in an instant-results society. The benefits of DHEA and 7-Keto™, however, tend to be experienced *gradually* as tissue levels are optimized. In fact, full benefits will be enjoyed only by those following a comprehensive program of diet, exercise and stress management. Unfortunately, the hype surrounding DHEA has set up an expectation that you can take it and instantly feel 20 years younger. When this does not occur, people often assume that they just need to take more. Remember that the human body, even at age 25, produces only 40–60 mg of DHEA per day. A sensible replacement dose therefore should be well below that level, and my research suggests that 10 mg of DHEA and 25 mg of 7-Keto™ will be sufficient for most people.

3. Purity and potency. Every day I receive calls from people offering me 100% pure DHEA for unbelievably low prices. I simply ask them to fax me an independent lab assay that I can verify, and I never hear from them again. But someone is buying this raw material, and spot checks are turning up purity levels of 90–95%.

   Now you might think that's fine, but a chemist will have one question about 95% purity: "What's the other 5%?" In other words, these people are not saying the material is 95% DHEA and the rest is starch. They're saying the 5% is unknown, and that is an unacceptable risk. Don't accept anything less than 99.5% pure.

   It gets worse. If you are a manufacturer, you can take low-grade DHEA, press it into tablet form, label the product 100% DHEA and get away with it. How? By claiming that because the product contains only DHEA, it is in effect 100% DHEA.

   What's a consumer to do? Request a certificate of analysis (C of A) for the raw material in your product. This certificate should specify the batch numbers that were produced from the tested material. Do not accept general C of As. You want to know the purity of the product you are ingesting, not what was produced last year.

4. DHEA hype. I have seen ads for micronized, soy-based, emulsified, activated and potentiated DHEA. This was bound to happen as manufacturers strive to create product differentiation, but does any of this make sense?

Micronized and Emulsified

These terms refer to the reduction of the DHEA particle size, the claim being for enhanced absorption. There is no data to support that claim, but I see no disadvantage in this process. One clinical study showed that women taking high doses of DHEA (200–300 mg per day) as a treatment for lupus might benefit from a micronized preparation because there was less conversion to testosterone.

Soy-based

A few manufacturers are claiming that DHEA derived from soy oil is superior to that obtained from the dioscorea barbasco yam. There is absolutely no science to support this. A DHEA molecule is a DHEA molecule, whether it comes from soy or Mexican yam. All that matters is the purity of the final compound. As I have said, I would not accept anything less than 99.5%.

Potentiated

This is a term used in homeopathy, and some manufacturers are combining homeopathic substances with DHEA. Because no one making this claim has produced a shred of scientific support, I would not put much credence in potentiated DHEA.

That's because Big Pharma still did not understand DHEA, but a small research and development company known as Humanetics saw the light. They realized that conversion to testosterone and estrogen was only a minor effect of DHEA. Far more important was the anabolic signal that it sent throughout the body—the message that the body was getting younger.

Remember, aging is fundamentally a metabolic shift from youthful, high-energy rebuild-repair-restore activity (anabolic metabolism) to a progressively more catabolic state characterized by low energy, degeneration, and eventual decrepitude. We knew that DHEA could restore youthful anabolic metabolism, but could the same results be obtained with 7-Keto™? If so, given 7-Keto's™ enormous safety profile, we would have a formula safe for over-the-counter sale.

In 1999, a joint research project was launched by Univera Pharmaceuticals and Humanetics to evaluate the effects of DHEA, 7-Keto™ and their combination on the anabolic metabolism of 76 volunteers. In a double-blind, placebo-controlled study, the combination of a small daily amount of 10 mg of DHEA and 25 mg of 7-Keto™ produced dramatic improvements in anabolic metabolism. A separate lab, measuring a different anabolic biomarker known as IGF-1, was used to confirm the results. Here also the treatment group experienced remarkable improvements, whereas the placebo group experienced "normal" aging and declining anabolic drive.

Today, there is a great deal of confusion regarding hormone therapy. Baby boomers are seeing a steady stream of articles and TV programs about estrogen, progesterone, DHEA, testosterone, androstenedione and pregnenolone. The Internet is filled with anti-aging miracle pills and potions, yet their doctors are saying, "Wait." The relevant question in response is, "How long?" For people over 40, waiting even a few years may be costly, especially because the data is now conclusive regarding the proven benefits of this powerful anabolic combination of DHEA and 7-Keto™.

A LOOK AT HEALTH SCIENCE ADVANCES

To get a clear idea of the importance of the metabolic model of aging, consider the advances in health science that have occurred in the last century. These can be divided into four distinct waves.

1. **Wave One:** Improved sanitation, the development of vaccines, antibiotics and rapid response medical care.

   Result: This increased life expectancy (LE) from 45 (at the beginning of the 20th century) to 76.7 (today). Interestingly, however, LE hasn't budged in more than 20 years. In other words, we've squeezed everything we could out of Wave One advances.

2. **Wave Two: Dietary Improvements.** In response to the deterioration of the North American diet with widespread use of white flour, sugar, highly processed and chemicalized foods, the health food "movement" grew from a small group of health nuts to a $35 billion industry.

   Hallmarks: Increased fiber, increased intake of fruits and vegetables, decreased consumption of red meat, wide variety of whole-grain products.

   Results: Improved quality of life due to reduced risk for age-related disease. Interestingly, Wave Two advances did not extend longevity.

3. **Wave Three: Nutritional Supplements.** Wave Three started out with pioneers like Linus Pauling and vitamin C, One-a-Day™ vitamins, etc. Last year, more than $9 billion in nutritional products were sold in the U.S. alone.

Hallmarks: The achievement of nutritional improvements that could not be obtained from diet alone, for example, antioxidants. To obtain the equivalent of a single 300 mg capsule of vitamin E, one would have to eat .5 kg of wheat germ or 1.5 L of unprocessed olive oil.

Result: Dramatic reduction in risk for age-related disease, e.g., high antioxidant intake has been shown to reduce heart disease mortality by 42% in women and 36% in men. Interestingly, Wave Three advances *still* did not extend life. Scientific studies have confirmed that people who take large numbers of vitamins, minerals, herbs and amino acids still die at around the same age as people who take no supplements whatsoever.

4. **Wave Four: Metabolic Intervention.** We now know that the ana-bolic-to-catabolic shift results in the myriad *symptoms* of aging, including loss of muscle, accumulation of fat, declining immunity (lower resistance, delayed wound healing, increased risk for autoim-mune diseases such as multiple sclerosis, rheumatoid arthritis, fibromyalgia, lupus), decreased emotional and mental resilience, declining bone density, degeneration of brain (memory loss, decreased motor skills, Alzheimer's disease and other dementias), etc.

You can deal with each of these symptoms one by one as they arise (which will *still* not restore robust health and may or may not reduce suffering) OR you can deal with the underlying *cause* of these symp-toms, which is metabolism.

For the first time, we now have the ability to restore youthful ana-bolic metabolism. This is not wishful thinking or science fiction.

SUMMARY

1. Aging is fundamentally a metabolic process.
2. Youthful anabolic metabolism can be restored.
3. This has been documented in human clinical trials, published in peer-reviewed biomedical literature.

Here is the critical point: *This strategy does not simply optimize your current metabolic status.* Good diet, nutritional supplements, stress management and exercise can do that. In other words, if you're 50, Waves One, Two and Three advances will enable you to look, feel and perform like a very healthy 50-year-old.

Metabolic intervention, or Wave Four in health science, can actually *restore a more youthful metabolic state*, enabling people to look, feel and perform as they did 10, 15 or 20 years earlier. Thus, the restoration of youthful anabolic metabolism should be at the core of any effective anti-aging program.

9

Cellular Insurance

Sam Graci, M.A.

THE POWER OF PHYTONUTRIENTS

The human body was designed for wellness, not illness. Every single one of your 100 trillion cells is made to function extremely well and cohesively to give you dynamic mental and physical vitality and well-being.

Plants capture the life force of the sun. This process of photosynthesis allows plants to manufacture oxygen, protein, vitamins, minerals, fiber, cell salts, essential fatty acids and energy. When you eat plants, these very same biodynamic disease-protective elements, which researchers now call phytonutrients, skillfully, predictably and measurably protect your bloodstream, cells, tissues, membranes, mitochondria, skin, organs and immune functions from the onslaught of chemicals, toxins, automobile or factory emissions, chemical intruders, bacteria, pesticides, viruses, fungi, yeast, microbes, mutagens, food additives, free radical assaults and carcinogens. This has brought the plant-disease prevention connection to the present forefront of serious worldwide nutritional research.

"Phyto" is a Greek derivative meaning "from plants." Phytonutrients are powerful protective elements from plants that are neither vitamin nor mineral. Phytonutrients defend and protect your 100 trillion cells (molecular motors) from excessive wear and tear and the onslaught of degenerative diseases, such as cancer, heart disease, cataracts, arteriosclerosis and arthritis.

Before we explain how the 30,000–50,000 plant phytonutrients protect you, let us examine how plants benefit the human life cycle. Your body has the innate ability to properly self-diagnose and self-heal. It only requires the powerful biodynamic phytonutrients from colorful plant-based foods. The latest discoveries in plant research give undeniable support to why you should return to the base of the food chain to experience optimal emotional, mental and physical well-being.

Let me not get ahead of myself. The story of the disease-preventing effects of phytonutrients is so compelling and critical to your health, well-being and longevity that I want to explain it in some detail, so you can fully appreciate the power and healing capacity in plants. However, it is important to introduce you first to a rich and informative array of research and ideas that will serve as a comprehensive background from which the full impact and importance of phytonutrients will emerge fresh and clear.

BIOENERGETIC FOOD
Researchers refer to natural, whole plant-based foods as bioenergetic, or as energy-rich: nuts, seeds, legumes, vegetables, herbs, grasses, sea vegetables and fruits. These plants nourish you with protein, vitamins, minerals, organic water, fiber, cell salts, essential fatty acids and those powerful toxic garbage cops called phytonutrients. These essential parts, in whole foods, affect your health, vitality and well-being. Refined foods are not considered whole foods, as many of their essential nutritional elements and components have been removed or damaged through processing.

When you use plants for your food and energy source, you directly eat foods alive with energy. If you use animals as a food source, then you eat the energy of plants indirectly, since the plants are converted by the animals; the animals' energy is then converted into the tissues, cells, atoms and sub-atomic particles of your body.

Energy cannot be created or destroyed, but it can be stored. If we eat more food than our body's energy requirements for that particular day, then that excess energy must be stored. The body stores energy as fat. As a survival mechanism during our forefathers' and foremothers' hunting and gathering days, the human body developed an almost infinite capacity to store fat. The body developed an enzyme called lipoprotein lipase to collect digested fat in your bloodstream and then stuff it into cells. This enzyme keeps storing extra calories, especially fat calories, as excess body fat.

We can utilize the sunlight's energy (through plants' photosynthesis) to maintain good physical health and mental acuity. Also, this process of replenishing the human body with an energy environment fueled by the light of the sun is critical to your body's ability to self-diagnose and self-heal on a daily basis. In short, the body will operate on optimum.

The plant kingdom captures the life force of the sun. When you consume plant-based foods, supported by rich soils and water, they help you to slow down the effects of entropy, the breakdown of your energy system.

If you are slowing down entropy, your body is in a restorative, replenishing and rejuvenating state called the anabolic drive. If you are knowingly or unknowingly speeding up entropy, your body is in a self-exhausting state called a catabolic drive.

An anabolic state is synonymous with anti-aging, at any age, and a catabolic state is pro-aging at any age.

Food Is Energy

Bioenergetic foods, as I mentioned earlier, are the natural high-octane fuels the human body requires to support an anabolic drive. They convert their energy fuel (energetic) to the efficient and effective biological (bio) rejuvenation and revitalization of every cell in your body.

Food is energy. Your body is an energy system. Every single one of the 100 trillion cells in your body (little molecular motors) requires energy to work. Digestion, respiration, talking, seeing, hearing, circulation, thinking, metabolism—all require energy. When your body's energy is low, it just does not have the resources to run well, and that is when illness begins to dominate. When your energy is high, your peak performance and health are optimal. Food is the source of energy your body needs most.

Food can either give you dynamic energy or rob you of it. What you eat on a daily basis either nourishes your anabolic state and health or it diminishes the healthy balance into a declining catabolic state. If your last meal or snack did not promote your anabolic drive, then it accelerated your aging.

If you are always tired mid-morning or mid-afternoon, if you feel sluggish throughout the day or find it difficult to get out of bed, this is an indication that your energy is drained and you are running on empty. This is serious!

Bioenergetic whole plant-based foods are pure life energy. Grown in sunlight and infused with the energy of the soil and water, they can increase your energy, moods and motivation. They can bring you back to an energetic anabolic drive. You only have to eat them. It is that simple!

Much of the foods the average person eats today are processed in factories to look good, smell good and taste good. These processed foods are no longer bioenergetic whole foods. Part of them is removed, and unnatural, chemical preservatives, pesticides, colorings and flavorings are added. These foods are devoid of the sun's energy and are really "dead" foods. The addition of the artificial additives makes these foods toxic. They quickly hurl you into a catabolic drive and hasten entropy and cellular dysfunction.

Choose your foods well. The more you consume the high-energy, life-sustaining bioenergetic foods, the more your body will be in a biologically dynamic balance—an anabolic drive.

ADVANTAGES OF BIOENERGETIC FOODS

Researchers are attributing powerful disease-preventive capabilities to plants. For many years, researchers have recognized that diets high in fruits, vegetables, herbs, grains, seeds, nuts and legumes reduce the risk of a number of diseases, including cancer, heart disease, diabetes, and high blood pressure, when compared with diets high in meat. Originally it was thought that the malnutrition- and disease-preventing effects of these foods were partly due to their vitamin, mineral and enzyme contents that helped prevent cancer and other disorders. Researchers worldwide have recently discovered that fruits, vegetables, grains, herbs, grasses, legumes, nuts, seeds and sea vegetables contain phytonutrients.

Progressive researcher Dr. Gladys Block and colleagues at the University of California, Berkeley, analyzed all of the 170 controlled studies to date on the effects of fruit and vegetables on cancer. Some examples of their analysis are:

Types of Cancer	Number of Studies Showing Protection
Lung cancer	24
Colorectal cancer	20
Stomach cancer	17
Esophageal cancer	15
Oral cancer	9
Cervical cancer	7

Researchers are now certain that bioenergetic phytonutrients obtained by eating large amounts of produce can reduce your risk of developing all types of cancer.

It appears that some of these previously unknown bioenergetic phytonutrient compounds will fight not only deficiency-type diseases such as anemia but also elusive, age-related illnesses such as heart disease and cancer.

Life energy from bioenergetic whole foods not only gives you energy, but keeps you in healthful balance (anabolic capacity) by preventing either the initiation or promotion of degenerative diseases. It is vitally important to note that approximately 75% of North Americans die from either heart-related disease or cancer, so the humble salad on your plate, or lentils in your bowl, or red peppers diced on your asparagus, or the pumpkin seeds in your oatmeal are offering you biodynamic compounds that protect you from infection, pain, degenerative heart disease, cancer and even premature aging itself.

When you eat the fresh, colorful fruits and vegetables teeming with bioenergetic phytonutrients, you are also protected by these powerful compounds. Nature wonderfully recycles her resources so that these disease-preventing and health-promoting plant phytonutrients prevent and fight every disease known. Yes, it is absolutely true.

To understand how phytonutrients protect the body from cancer, it is important to understand that cancer formation is a multistep process. Bioenergetic phytonutrients, formed during photosynthesis, block one or even more of the steps that lead to cancer. For instance, cancer can begin (initiate) when a carcinogenic molecule from the food you eat, or air you breathe, invades a cell. If sulforaphane—a phytonutrient found in broccoli, cauliflower, cabbage, broccoli sprouts or brussels sprouts—also reaches the cell at the same time, it quickly activates a group of enzymes that whisks the carcinogen out of the cell before it can cause serious harm.

WHICH PHYTONUTRIENTS FIGHT CANCER?

There are some phytonutrients known to prevent cancer in other ways. Flavonoids, found in citrus fruits and berries, keep cancer-causing hormones from latching onto cells (initiation) in the first place. Genistein and daidzein, found in non-genetically modified soybeans, kill tumors by preventing the formation (promotion) of the capillaries needed to nourish them. Indoles, found in cruciferous vegetables like broccoli and cauliflower, cabbage, turnips and brussels sprouts, boost immune activity and make it easier for the body to excrete toxins or chemical intruders. Saponins, as found in lentils and red kidney beans, prevent the promotion of cancer cells from multiplying. P-coumaric acid, chlorogenic acid and lycopene, found in tomatoes, interfere with and prevent certain chemical unions that can create malignant tumors.

The list of these protective, bioenergetic phytonutrients goes on and on and on. A tomato is believed to contain an estimated 1000 different phytonutrients. Fortunately, it is very easy and vitally important to get a healthy dose of phytonutrients at every meal. Every fruit, grain, legume, seed, nut, grass, sea veggie and colorful vegetable tested has been found to be a veritable warehouse, jam-packed with these disease-preventive compounds.

Moreover, unlike most vitamins, these phytonutrients do not appear to be destroyed by cooking or other processing. As a matter of fact, lycopene in a healthy red tomato sauce may be made more bioavailable by the cooking process. Genistein, the powerful phytonutrient found in soybeans, is also found in soybean products that are cooked, such as miso, tempeh and tofu. Similarly, the phytonutrient sulforaphane, found in cabbage, remains intact even when the cabbage is made into coleslaw or sauerkraut. The potent sulfur compounds from garlic and onions become activated only when they are chopped or chewed.

Of course, by eating most of your vegetables and fruit raw or lightly cooked "crunchy-tender," you will be able to enjoy the benefits not just of the many bioenergetic phytonutrients, but of all the bountiful vitamins, minerals, protein, fiber and other nutrients that fresh whole foods have to offer.

HOW PHYTONUTRIENTS FIGHT CANCER

As mentioned earlier, phytonutrients block the *initiation* of the cancer process and suppress the *promotion* of cells already initiated into the cancer growth process.

Stop It Before It Starts

The following are three brief explanations of phytonutrient cancer initiator-blocking mechanisms.

1. The sulfur compounds from garlic and onions, the dithiothiones and isothiocyanates from cruciferous vegetables, phenols in blueberries or raspberries or other fruits, green tea, plus several carotenoids such as alpha- and beta-carotene or lycopene, vitamin E or vitamin C in many fruits and vegetables, have strong antioxidant activity that scavenge and neutralize free radicals and other electrophilic molecules before they can attack your cellular membranes and expose your DNA or mitochondria to severe damage that is pro-aging. This free radical attack, left unchecked, leads to a spiraling catabolic decline and degenerative disease.

    The mitochondria are your little energy furnaces in cells that combine glucose (fuel) with oxygen (igniter) in a biochemical process called cellular respiration, which produces energy as adenosine triphosphate. The natural by-products or "smoke" from this biochemical process are corrosive little "free radicals" that literally smash into fine cell walls and eventually weaken and destroy them, leaving the cellular material open for further destruction. Cell walls can be "hit" by these free radicals up to 100,000 times a day.

Furthermore, free radicals are quickly formed through stress, excess sunlight, a hard workout or exercise regime, water or airborne pollution, veterinary residue from antibiotics or bovine growth hormones in animal products, pesticides, herbicides, late nights, lack of deep rejuvenating sleep, factory or car emissions and the natural process of cellular respiration. You cannot avoid the formation of free radicals, but you can minimize their destructive potential. Here is the clue! Just eat abundantly from nature's naturally low-calorie bioenergetic whole foods at each and every meal or snack, but practice portion control. The fewer calories you consume, the less energy is required to process the incoming food and the fewer free radicals you make. The fewer free radicals you make, the longer you live.

2. A large number of different phytonutrients interfere with the metabolism and activation of carcinogenic compounds. Indoles and dithiothiones from cruciferous vegetables; flavonoids in berries, squash, parsley or tomatoes; catechins in green tea; carotenoids in spinach, kale, Swiss chard, yams and sweet potatoes; sulfur compounds in garlic or scallions; protease inhibitors in soy sprouts; the omega-3 polyunsaturated fatty acids in flaxseeds or walnuts; the plant sterols in wheat grass or barley grass; polyacetylenes or flavonoids in ginkgo biloba, bilberry, green tea, grape seed or skin, milk thistle and Siberian ginseng extracts—*all* stimulate enzymes that deactivate precarcinogenic compounds and prevent their transformation into a more dangerous form.

3. Soluble and insoluble fiber—from all fruit, veggies, legumes, whole grains, herbs, seeds and nuts—in the intestines and stomach inhibit the uptake of pathogens and carcinogens from the gut into the circulatory system by absorbing them and excreting them harmlessly, preventing your body from being exposed to dangerous carcinogenic substances.

Sam Graci's Six Favorite Anti-Cancer Initiator Whole Food Groups

1. Garlic, onions, leeks, shallots, scallions
2. Blueberries, strawberries, blackberries, raspberries
3. Tomatoes, sweet potatoes, squashes, colorful peppers, yams (also a glass of fresh vegetable juice each day)
4. Broccoli sprouts, broccoli, cauliflower, horseradish, radishes

5. A high-quality "green drink" for cellular insurance
6. Green tea

HOW PHYTONUTRIENTS CAN HELP IF CARCINOGENIC PROCESSES HAVE BEGUN

If cancer has already begun, phytonutrients have many channels through which they can suppress the process and inhibit the *promotion* of a precancerous cell to a malignant state. These bioenergetic phytonutrient compounds stimulate enzymes that convert the cell to a non-cancerous form.

Examples of disease-preventing and cancer promotion-inhibiting phytonutrients are as follows:

1. Some carotenoids such as alpha- or beta-carotene, lycopene and lutein, liminoids in citrus fruits and quercetin from onions help a precancerous cell to be transformed into a non-malignant form, or actually cause it to age quickly and become inactivated.
2. Vitamin E in vegetable oils, nuts, seeds, protease inhibitors in soybeans or soybean products, isothiocyanates from cruciferous vegetables, phenolic acids from whole grains, or isoflavones from legumes, peas and beans reduce the growth and inhibit the proliferation of initiated, precancerous cells in experimental laboratory work.
3. Vitamin C, vitamin E, zinc, selenium, alpha-lipoic acid, coenzyme Q10 (CoQ10), the amino acid cysteine and carotenoids neutralize or scavenge and absorb corrosive free radicals before they damage tissues or cells. This scavenging or neutralizing activity inhibits tumor promotion by reducing the turnover of pre-cancerous cells and preventing them from rapid cell division.

   Each of these powerful antioxidants works as a *network*, so the synergistic effect is greater than the antioxidant ability of any one of them acting singularly. These antioxidants also network with a remarkable flavonoid-glutathione sub-network made up of water-extracted, high-quality extracts of ginkgo biloba, European bilberry, green tea, milk thistle, full-spectrum grape seed and grape skin and Siberian ginseng to (a) "regenerate" each other once they expend their electrons as an antioxidant and themselves become a free radical; (b) all work together as a network to produce glutathione and the antioxidant enzyme glutathione peroxidase, which are the most important antioxidants inside your 100 trillion cells. Glutathione binds to toxic, cancer-causing chemical invaders from the environment, making them harmless and escorting them out of cells and tissues. Glutathione maintains immuno-competence by stimulating the proliferation of lymphocytes, white blood cells that are responsible for the body's immune reactions and the production of antibodies. Glutathione, among its many other functions, primes DNA synthesis for cell division and switches on the enzymes that repair DNA.

Sam Graci's 6 Favorite Cancer Promoter-Inhibiting Whole Foods

1. Undenatured whey protein isolate powder (high in alphalactalbumin)
2. Organic citrus fruits, including some of the pulp and rind
3. Non-GMO organic soy sprouts and fermented soy products such as miso, tempeh, extra-firm tofu and soy protein isolates (non-GMO)
4. Seeds, nuts, legumes, peas, beans and whole grains
5. High-"lignan" flaxseed oil taken with sulfur-bearing amino acids as found in organic fat-free yogurt, quark cheese or cottage cheese
6. Cherries, grapes, apples, prunes, pears, plums

Bioenergetic Phytonutrients Reduce Cancer Risks at Every Meal

It is the intake of bioenergetic phytonutrients that helps explain why a diet high in fruits and vegetables is associated with lower rates of all types of cancer.

Canada's Food Guide to Healthy Eating has upgraded its recommendations of daily servings of colorful fruits and vegetables because of all the published research we have discussed.

The Canadian food guide and American Food Pyramid both recommend a minimum of five to ten servings of fruit and vegetables a day and ten servings of whole grains every day. (A serving is half a cup.) Remember, lightly cooking or heating does not destroy phytonutrients but it will destroy some vitamins. Try a glass of fresh vegetable juice each day for a glass full of phytonutrients.

MY FAVORITE JUICE RECIPE

3 medium-size carrots (no more than three because of their high sugar content)
1 medium beet
1 heaping tbsp fresh ginger, chopped
1 stalk celery
6 stems watercress
6 stems parsley
1/2 yellow or orange pepper
1/2 red tomato

Optional additions:
1 level tbsp of a high-quality "green drink"
1/2–1 tbsp of lemon juice
dash of cayenne pepper, or curry or turmeric (curcumin)
1 tsp of any salt-free, non-irradiated herbal seasoning

Sip and enjoy!

PHYTONUTRIENTS ELIMINATE TOXIC WASTE

Another avenue through which bioenergetic phytonutrients keep you healthy is by neutralizing and quickly flushing toxic chemicals from your body before you even know they are there. They act as toxic garbage cops, always on tireless patrol looking for chemical intruders.

Dr. Gary Stoner, director of the cancer chemoprevention program at the Ohio State University Comprehensive Cancer Center in Columbus, Ohio, and other researchers demonstrate that bioenergetic phytonutrients boost the production of phase-1 and phase-2 enzymes.

1. A toxin enters your body as a chemical intruder.
2. Your body, under the direction of a phase-1 enzyme, attaches an oxygen molecule to the toxin in your liver.
3. Oxygen is very reactive to oxidation and this combination can create a more active and dangerous toxin than the original toxin.
4. If you eat sufficient bioenergetic phytonutrients such as sulphoraphane from broccoli, they promote or boost the production of phase-2 enzymes, which attach themselves to the oxygen/toxin compound, neutralizing and making it stable.
5. If you eat specific bioenergetic phytonutrients to raise your glutathione levels, glutathione acts as a carrier molecule to whisk the chemical intruder out of your bloodstream or cell and excrete it from the body.

Foods that Raise Cellular Glutathione Levels

Network Veggies and Nuts

Avocados, walnuts, peanuts, almonds, sesame seeds, asparagus, okra, watercress, leafy greens, lettuces and tomatoes.

Network Fruits

Watermelon, grapefruit, strawberries, canteloupe, oranges and acerola berries.

Network Protein

Undenatured whey protein isolates with all the subfractions intact, such as alpha-lactalbumin, serum albumin, beta-lactoglobulin and immunoglobulins with high amounts of the amino acids trytophan and cysteine. Whey protein powders that are 99% undenatured, and over 90% bioavailable protein, give you world-class protein and all the immune support that colostrum does.

Network Herbs

The critical flavonoid-glutathione subnetwork herbal extracts derived from a water-extracted method using no biotoxic solvents synergistically work well. They are ginkgo biloba, European bilberry, milk thistle, full-spectrum grape seed and grape skin extract, Japanese green tea and Siberian ginseng that must be consumed together with other vitamins, minerals and antioxidants in your body as a network to produce elevated endogenous glutathione levels in your cells, tissues and liver.

Network Supplemental Antioxidants

- vitamin C as a mixed group of ascorbates, comprising calcium ascorbate, magnesium ascorbate and potassium ascorbate, mixed with bioflavonoids
- CoQ10 with tocotrienols (Tocotrienols are like the vitamin E tocopherols except they disperse themselves in tissues more uniformly for antioxidant protection than do tocopherols, which tend to clump together. Tocotrienols are derived from red palm and rice bran oils.)
- vitamin E as mixed tocopherols, or tocopheryls, with abundant amounts of gamma, delta and beta tocopherols
- zinc
- selenium (Combined with organic selenomethionine, inorganic sodium selenate and, if available, selenodiglutathione.)
- full spectrum grape seed and skin extract
- alpha-lipoic acid (Use twice a day spread out as it is water soluble.) If you use more than 100 mg daily, also supplement with 100 mg of the B vitamin, biotin.
- N-acetyl cysteine is a precursor to glutathione. It contains volatile sulfur that can be dangerous, but if used simultaneously with all the other supplemental antioxidants, they protect the sulfur from becoming oxidized and volatile in the acidic stomach.

PHYTONUTRIENTS REGULATE ESTROGEN

Another known way phytonutrients ward off disease is by regulating hormones—most notably the female sex hormone, estrogen. They balance the amount of estrogens in a female body.

When estrogen levels rise, they can stimulate hormone-related cancers like those of the breast and ovaries, says Dr. Leon Bradlow, director of biochemical and endocrinology at the Strang Cancer Research Laboratory in New York City.

One group of bioenergetic phytonutrients called isoflavones are very similar to natural estrogen and are called phytoestrogens. When women eat non-

GMO soy sprouts, soybeans or soy products such as miso, tempeh and extra-firm tofu or water-extracted soy isolate protein powder, they are receiving the phytoestrogens genistein and daidzein. These phytoestrogens bind to the body's estrogen receptor sites. In PMS when there is too much estrogen, these weak phytoestrogens block the escalation of the real estrogen hormones. In perimenopause or in menopause, when there is not enough estrogen being produced, these plant-derived phytoestrogens increase a beneficial estrogen, 2-hydroxyestrone, and decrease the levels of the dangerous 16-alpha-hydrox-yestrone hormone. (See Chapter 12 for an in-depth discussion of this process.)

ELEMENTS IN FOODS THAT PREVENT OR FIGHT CANCER

Allicin and allyl sulfides in garlic, onions, leeks, chives and shallots reduce the risk of stomach and colon cancer and are broad-spectrum antioxidants in the gastrointestinal tract and bloodstream.

Anthocyanidins are the red pigments in red grape skins, citrus, berries and yams functioning as potent antioxidants and anti-inflammatory agents.

Catechins found in green tea, black tea and berries dismantle pathogens in the gastrointestinal tract.

Ellagic Acid, abundant in apples, berries, cherries, grapes and all nuts, stop the initiation of cancer cells and dismantle mutagens.

Indoles are present in broccoli, brussels sprouts, cabbage, turnips, kale, Swiss chard, watercress and lettuces; indole-3-carbinol (I3C) as DIM appears to protect against breast cancer and has anticarcinogenic properties.

Isoflavonoids (genistein and daidzein) from soybeans deactivate excess estrogen (in PMS) and thereby lower the risk of hormone-like cancers of the breast, cervix and uterus. They add phytoestrogens to the estrogen pool in menopause to greatly reduce its severity and symptoms.

Lignans in flaxseeds and whole grains appear to block excess estrogen and dihydrotestosterone from the inflammation stage and the initiation stage of cancer.

Lycopenes are powerful reddish carotenoids that reduce the risk of prostate cancer—tomatoes, red grapefruit, watermelon and apricots are the main sources.

Monoterpenes increase liver enzymes that detoxify carcinogenic compounds—all citrus fruits are good sources; eat some of the pulp and skin.

P-coumaric acid and chlorogenic acid in pineapples, strawberries, peppers and tomatoes detoxify carcinogens and absorb oxygen free radicals effectively.

Phthalides are anticancer compounds found in carrots, celery, parsley, dill, coriander and fennel.

Polyphenols in green tea dismantle pathogens in the stomach and gastrointestinal tract.

Protease inhibitors in legumes, rice and eggplant stop the promotion of cancer cells and are free radical scavengers.

Sulforaphane is abundant in cruciferous veggies like broccoli sprouts, broccoli and cauliflower; they boost phase-2 enzymes to whisk away chemical intruders from the body.

Triterpenoids in citrus and soybeans greatly reduce both the initiation and promotion of cancer.

YOUR PERSONAL GUIDE TO OPTIMUM HEALTH

To be successful you don't need to be obsessive with your new dietary strategy. You can be consistent and deliberate in incorporating the following dietary strategies one week at a time, then one day at a time, then one meal and snack at a time. It is all that easy! It is a conscientious return to the base of the food chain so that you can eat high-octane fuels that are in harmony with your long-standing genetic predisposition to bioenergetic, low-calorie, whole foods.

You can modify and tailor these suggestions to your own special needs and time limits. But it is important that you make an effort to plan your weekly and daily menu on paper. When you put something down on paper, you have demonstrated your commitment. This will encourage you to make a basic shift in progressively monitoring and purchasing your food supplies from nature's bioenergetic whole foods. Never impulse buy! High-tech synthetic food manufacturers know how to package foods for irresistible eye appeal and make their products look good, smell good and taste good. Don't be fooled!

The foods you fuel your body with today will dictate your peak performance level and optimum self-healing capability tomorrow. The bioenergetic whole foods you eat today that give you vitality and mental acuity—or the processed, chemically treated partial foods you eat today that rob you of vitality and mental acuity—will show up on the balance sheets of your wellness and health for the rest of your life. It is never too late to begin. The time to begin is *now*. Be wise for your own sake!

EPILOGUE

When you follow healthy dietary and lifestyle strategies diligently, you will gain the zest, robust energy, mental acuity and fine sense of well-being you were created for. Illness is always multifactorial—and to prevent it, you must not place lopsided emphasis on the physical body and ignore the mind and spirit. You do have the ability to control the outcome.

I sincerely wish you abundant good health.

10

Running on Empty

Edward J. Conley, M.D.

HOW IS ENERGY PRODUCED IN THE BODY?

Millions of people do not understand how we actually make energy, and without understanding the process, it is impossible for you to know how to maximize your energy.

We produce energy, of course, from food, but how we produce this energy is not some mysterious event. It is through a defined process that happens inside the mitochondria, which are inside nearly every cell of your body. (There are some cells that do not have mitochondria and therefore cannot make their own energy.) The mitochondria are small power plants located inside each cell, some cells containing several thousand power plants. Believe it or not, your average heart cell contains 5000 mitochondria (power plants) inside each cell. The more active the cell, the more power plants the cell needs to generate energy. The mitochondria is the area within the cell where this energy production takes place through something we call the Krebs cycle.

The Krebs cycle is how we convert our food, which is basically protein, carbohydrates and fat, into a form of chemical energy called adenosine triphosphate (ATP). ATP runs everything in the body. We make this conversion through chemical reactions. These are defined chemical steps where we convert our food to energy. It is very complicated, and indeed, we do not fully understand nor can we recreate exactly how the body makes chemical energy using a form of electron transfer. Be that as it may, you can think of this as an energy assembly line that processes the raw materials (our food). The raw materials are proteins, fats and carbohydrates. After going through this assembly line, the raw materials are converted via these chemical reactions, eventually becoming ATP—our finished product that is shipped out the back door of the factory.

ATP AND HEAT

As we mentioned earlier, ATP is needed for everything we do, from making our muscles move to brain function, which requires a large amount of ATP. (Our heart uses huge amounts of energy every day, as it is a muscle that is constantly functioning.) Every cell in your body requires ATP to pump waste products out of the cell, pump nutrients into the cell and maintain electrical chemical gradients. These gradients function somewhat like a battery, with positive and negative ions on certain sides of the cell that create the appropriate electrochemical charge to allow for proper functioning.

During the average day we burn a tremendous amount of ATP. Eighty percent of the ATP we generate goes for heat. We pay a tremendous price for being warm-blooded animals. The other 20% is all we have available to do everything else we need to do. Obviously, the more ATP you can generate, the more energy you have for all normal functions. Prior to working with people with fatigue and fibromyalgia, I worked with athletes to improve the amount of energy (i.e., ATP) that they had available. If we could improve how they generated their ATP, we could improve their athletic performance and, hopefully, enable them to win gold medals at the Olympics. As I will discuss later in this chapter, there are ways to improve and maximize your energy production so that you can produce more energy and function at a higher capacity. We may have drops of anywhere between 1 and 5% in our total energy production because of damage to our energy-producing machinery (see next section). As I said earlier, 80% of our energy goes to heat. If you have a 5% drop, it comes out of that 20% that we have for everything else, which is effectively a 25% decrease in the amount of energy that you have available to expend. To put things in perspective, if you reduce your energy production even by 1% that will be enough to reduce your immunity, cause some significant problems with thinking and make you feel general mild fatigue.

AGING IN THE MITOCHONDRIA

To a great degree, aging is the process of damage to your energy-producing machinery, the mitochondria. One of the things that always impresses me when I visit my father, who winters in Florida, are automobiles from the 1960s that have over 400,000 km on them, yet they look fabulous. We have all seen automobiles with only 40,000 km on them and they look terrible. The reason for this is that it is not necessarily the age of the automobile, but the care that has gone into its maintenance. So it is with you and me.

We all know people in their eighties who seem to have the energy production and vitality of a person much younger. We also know many people in their twenties, thirties and forties who have the energy production of an 80-year-old. To a large degree, they have the function of someone much older although their chronological age may be only 40. Why is that? How does that happen? It is not just your age that counts, but the amount of damage you have sustained to your energy-producing machinery that to a great extent determines how old you are.

How Does Our Energy-Producing Machinery (the Mitochondria) Get Damaged?

The free radical theory of aging states that our energy-producing machinery is damaged through the production of free radicals, loose ions that cause damage to cells and other structures, much like meteors plunging into the moon or the earth. Fortunately, the earth has an atmosphere that protects it from meteors and protects us from catastrophic damage. Still, over the course of millions of years the earth has been struck by many thousands of meteors, causing significant damage. So it is with our bodies. These free radicals slam into various tissues—either the cell wall, internal organs or even the nucleus of cells—causing damage. We can protect ourselves from this damage, of course, and I will discuss that in the next part of this chapter. Antioxidants absorb these free radicals before they are able to damage more important structures such as your genes. We produce free radicals every minute we are alive. It is part and parcel of using oxygen to make energy. Inside the mitochondria we must have oxygen to produce energy via the Krebs cycle.

Unfortunately, as we use oxygen it can degenerate into a free radical, so oxygen, that life-giving substance that we all must have to stay alive, can also damage us. A good analogy of this is the automobile. Even if you take excellent care of your car and follow all the maintenance recommendations, you nevertheless cause a small amount of damage every day just through normal driving at regular speeds. That is why cars do not last forever. Eventually, even if you take wonderful care of your car, it will wear out either through rust or damage to the engine. So it is with us. Even if we take wonderful care of ourselves and have the proper amount of antioxidants, eventually we will become so damaged that we die. Unfortunately, for most of us, we will not die at our normal life span, which for a human should be in the neighborhood of 120–150 years. Most of us will die premature deaths because we damage ourselves to a greater degree by free radical production.

DAMAGING OUR ENERGY-PRODUCING MACHINERY

What are some of the things we do to ourselves to increase the damage to our energy-producing machinery? Perhaps the greatest damage is the adrenal glands' production of adrenaline through stress. Adrenaline has an evolutionary advantage. It improves your strength, your vision, allows you to run faster, and increases your heart rate and the amount of blood that you pump with each beat of your heart. As was discussed in Chapter 4, if you come face to face with a tiger, you want to produce enough adrenaline to either fight off the tiger or run away quickly. Early *Homo sapians* who produced adrenaline to a greater degree lived longer than those who did not, so that is why we all produce adrenaline today.

Even though adrenaline has survival advantages, it damages us by producing large amounts of free radicals. It was important in the past to be able to make adrenaline on demand very quickly. Nature felt that we could later repair the damage that was generated through the production of adrenaline. We now have job stresses, lawsuits, traffic jams and divorces, among other long-term stresses. No longer do we produce adrenaline just for a few seconds or minutes once or twice a month. We now produce adrenaline daily for weeks, months and even years on end. I routinely see people in the clinic who have been under tremendous stress because of their jobs or families. These people have been producing adrenaline day in and day out for years, slowly but surely damaging their energy-producing machinery.

Over the course of months and years, we become low in antioxidants as we use up our antioxidant reserves. We continue to produce this adrenaline because of the stresses that we are under and we damage that energy-producing machinery within the cells. Our energy-producing machinery is built to handle certain amounts of damage. It can repair itself and continue to function, but the genes within the mitochondria are 200 times more susceptible to damage than the genes within the nucleus of the cell, which are much better protected because they are coiled.

A Vicious Cycle

Unfortunately, nutrient deficiencies and the wearing down of the adrenal system lead to a vicious circle in which stressors that might have been only moderate now feel severe and stressors that were severe now feel overwhelming, so of course we produce more and more adrenaline. Fortunately or unfortunately, depending on how you look at it, the adrenaline-producing part of our adrenals seems to be resistant to wearing down. Therefore, we continue to make adrenaline even when we are not able to make other hormones such as DHEA or cortisone from other parts of our adrenals. For example, you can still startle someone who is 80 or 90 years old and he or she will still produce adrenaline. The body will not be able to respond the way it did when the person was 20 years old, but the body will still respond to that adrenaline challenge by increasing the heart rate, the blood flow to the muscles and all the survival advantages that I explained earlier. What other things may be a problem?

Cigarettes

One of the ways that cigarettes damage us is by producing free radicals. Over the course of years, cigarettes will produce enough free radicals to eventually damage the nucleus within the cells, causing the cells' reproduction systems to run amok. This is essentially what cancer is. Cancer happens when damage to the nucleus has become so severe, and the cell's ability to repair that damage has been so impeded, that eventually the cell loses control and starts reproducing wildly. Its turn-off mechanism is now no longer working and the cells start to reproduce madly, piling up upon each other, eventually causing what we know as cancer. But long before that happens, the free radicals damage our energy production.

Recall that our energy-producing machinery is 200 times more susceptible to damage than our genes inside the nucleus of the cell. Therefore, years before people develop cancer they will start to damage their energy-production through smoking. Unfortunately, this becomes a vicious cycle because most people use nicotine to control stress and to help give them a boost. Nicotine is a very unusual drug because it is the only drug I am aware of that both calms and stimulates at the same time. The longer you smoke, however, the more damage you sustain to your energy-producing machinery. The worse your energy level, the more you have to smoke. Also, of course, smoking over the course of years starts to damage our ability to assimilate oxygen, and without proper oxygen assimilation, we cannot produce energy efficiently. So over time, long-term smoking has a double whammy on energy production. First, it slowly damages the energy-producing machinery, and second, it impedes our assimilation and absorption of oxygen, which also impedes energy production. As a result, people will feel more and more fatigued, so they will smoke more heavily.

Chemical or Heavy Metal Exposure.

There are 30,000 chemicals that have been produced since the 1930s, some 12,000 of which we are exposed to on a regular basis. Many of them have been designed to damage the energy-producing machinery of insects. These, of course, are pesticides, which usually kill insects either by damaging their nervous system or by interfering with their energy-producing machinery. Humans and insects produce energy in exactly the same way by using the Krebs cycle inside the mitochondria. Pesticides are supposed to kill insects without damaging us. However, I've seen thousands of people who have been injured by pesticide exposure.

One possible mechanism is through direct exposure. That usually happens, for example, when the person is home and the exterminator comes and sprays the house for ants, termites, cockroaches or whatever and the person has direct exposure to the pesticide. Exterminators are supposed to spray at doses that do not directly damage human beings. However, our homes are becoming more and more airtight as we try to achieve energy efficiency, so any chemicals sprayed within the home cannot escape through normal air exchange. Exterminators, unfortunately, use extremely strong doses of pesticides to ensure that they get rid of the problem the first time. Indeed, I see many advertisements stating that they pride themselves on having to spray only once. Many of the products that have been used in the past and that are still being used have been demonstrated to damage energy production and the nervous system in human beings at much lower levels than previously thought, which are easily achieved in a home that has been fumigated.

Pesticide exposure can also happen over time. All of us are exposed to pesticides on a regular basis through their use on lawns or gardens or on commercially grown produce. Some of these pesticides are quite dangerous. Fortunately, we have banned several of them in the United States. Regrettably, we have not banned their production, so many chemical companies in the United States still produce them and ship them to foreign countries, where much of our produce is grown. Then the produce is shipped back to us containing residues of those pesticides. So over time we accumulate small amounts of pesticides, damaging our energy production. Most of these substances are fat soluble, so even though the body has a detoxification system in which we are able to conjugate and eliminate certain amounts of these substances over time, they permeate our fat, slowly collect within our systems and may become a source of damage to our mitochondria.

There are many other chemicals that may exert influence on the energy-producing machinery; for example, substances that mimic hormones. Many of the chemicals produced in the 20th century resemble estrogens and may trick the body into thinking that it has more estrogen than it actually does. The proper balance of hormones, DHEA, testosterone and cortisone, among others, is absolutely essentially in the adequate production of energy. (For a more detailed discussion, see Chapters 14 and 15 in *America Exhausted*, entitled "DHEA" and "Adrenal Fatigue.")

To summarize, mitochondrial damage is essentially mitochondrial aging. Through our normal everyday life, we damage ourselves a little year in and year out. This damage is inevitable and is from the use of oxygen to produce energy. This is why none of us will live forever. Eventually our mitochondria become so damaged that we must die. We have also reviewed, however, how we hasten that process by increasing the production of damaging free radicals through stress and therefore adrenaline; cigarettes; alcohol and other drug use; chronic infections including chronic bowel infections with yeast, abnormal bacterias or bacterial infections anywhere in the body; and allergies, especially allergens we are exposed to on a daily basis such as dust, mold and foods including milk, eggs, wheat, corn and citrus.

How can we protect our energy-producing machinery, the mitochondria, so that we can maintain our energy as long as possible? As we have just discussed, it makes sense to reduce stress and therefore adrenaline. If you smoke cigarettes, reduce smoking and eventually quit. If you overuse alcohol or other drugs, reduce your intake. If you have any signs of chronic infection or chronic bowel abnormalities such as irritable bowel, get appropriate diagnosis and treatment. (For a complete discussion of diagnosis and therapy see Chapter 9, "The Bowel: The Most Important Body Organ," in *America Exhausted*.) Reduce your exposure to allergens, especially food allergens. (For a complete discussion of food allergens, see Chapter 13 in *America Exhausted*, "Allergies: Why Is Allergy Important in Fatigue?") And lastly, reduce your chemical pesticide and herbicide exposure. If you have had significant solvent or heavy metal exposures, see a physician who can properly diagnose and treat you. Beyond that, how do we protect our energy-producing machinery? Certainly, one of the most important ways is by making sure we have proper levels of antioxidants.

Antioxidants

What are antioxidants? As discussed throughout *Bio-Age*, they are substances that absorb free radicals before they can cause damage to our structures. Foods that are high in antioxidants are any fruits and vegetables that are highly colored. This includes blue, red, orange and yellow. Antioxidants evolved within these fruits and vegetables to protect them from oxidated damage. One of the strongest oxidizing agents is the sun. For example, a piece of carpet or furniture exposed to sunlight over time will fade because it has been oxidized by the sun. Plants have built-in substances that help protect them from sun damage. Also, because the plants are generating energy (photosynthesis) from the sun, they develop free radicals from that system of energy production and must have built-in protective mechanisms, otherwise their energy production will become damaged. Therefore, plant food is designed to give us large amounts of varied antioxidants.

Unfortunately, the average North American diet includes mostly highly refined foods. Most of our foods no longer contain color (or if they have color it is from artificial coloration). The intake of fruits and vegetables for the average person in North America has dropped dramatically over the past 100 years. In the United States, nutritionists now recommend five fruit and vegetable servings per day, but the average American eats 1.5 servings per day and there are some who eat far below that. Over time these people are not getting the antioxidants they need in their diet. Often this is combined with increased free radical damage through smoking, stress and chemical exposure. The result of this is an overall deficiency in antioxidants that are needed to protect their energy system. They are not getting the intake of antioxidants they need, and their outflow of antioxidants is high to try to protect them from the damage they are sustaining from stress and cigarettes, etc., which in turn leads to an overall depletion of antioxidants. When this happens, they are like a fighter who has his gloves down. The various oxidative processes (free radicals) now bombard their energy-producing system and pummel it. Over time this can cause significant damage to the mitochondria and the enzymes that allow the mitochondria to function properly. This will advance the aging of your energy-producing system and in essence is one of the major factors that will cause overall aging of your body.

What can you do to prevent this? First, of course, make sure you are getting adequate antioxidants in your diet. Eat as many colorful vegetables as possible—tomatoes, broccoli, carrots, squash and sweet potatoes, just to name a few. Make sure you have a serving of these at each meal. If possible, I recommend organic vegetables. Include adequate amounts of fresh fruit in your diet, such as blueberries, cherries and strawberries, among others. Any fruit with color will contain important antioxidants. Indeed, many studies now suggest that blueberries and other berries have very high levels of antioxidants. Again, make sure that the fruit is organic whenever possible.

A Word of Caution

If you have diabetes or if you have significant yeast problems, you may have to keep the amounts of fresh fruit lower than the average person. You should also be aware that unsweetened blueberries or cherries, though higher in sugar than vegetables, are not as high in sugar as most of our refined foods. I usually allow patients with yeast problems or diabetes to have small amounts of fresh fruit. You can also take antioxidant supplements, such as glutathione; coenzyme Q10; lipoic acid; NADH, vitamins E, A, and C; and selenium. This by no means is a complete list of antioxidants that are needed for proper function of the energy system, but these are several of the most important antioxidants. (See page 274 in Appendix II for more information.) You must maintain proper levels of these antioxidants.

Glutathione

Glutathione is essential in nearly every cell of the body for prevention of free radical damage. We make glutathione in the body from three amino acids: cysteine, glutamic acid and glysine. You should have high levels of glutathione. It helps detoxify heavy metals such as mercury, lead and nickel. It is required in the enzyme formaldehyde dehydrogenase in metabolizing formaldehyde in the body. It is essential in liver detoxification of multiple substances, including organic compounds, pesticides and medications. Glutathione also produces a sparing effect for both vitamin E and vitamin C by reducing the oxidized forms of those antioxidants.

In essence, glutathione can help recharge vitamin E and vitamin C so that they can continue to work for you to improve glutathione levels if they are low. Increase those foods that are high in glutathione and cysteine, such as cold processed whey. Whey is a protein found in milk. Cold processed whey is one of the best sources of the compound gamma glutamylcysteine, which increases glutathione levels in the body. Cysteine is an amino acid that is important for making glutathione. Cysteine-rich foods include meats, yogurt, wheat germ and eggs. (Remember that milk, eggs and wheat are the three most common food allergens in North America, so make sure you are not allergic to them prior to increasing the amount.)

You can also take glutathione supplements. It should be noted, however, that glutathione is not well absorbed orally, so we usually use N-acetyl cysteine (NAC), which is the rate-limiting amino acid in the production of glutathione. By increasing NAC, we are able to improve glutathione production. Always consult your health care provider about all the amino acids that are important for glutathione production. Glutathione can also be given intramuscularly or intravenously, which is a more advanced therapy usually used for diseased processes. (Note: Do not use L-cysteine.)

Coenzyme Q10

This is a very important nutrient in the production of energy. CoQ10 is vital for stage III, the electron transport of the Krebs cycle, to function properly. It also serves as an important antioxidant for the entire Krebs cycle. CoQ10 is a potent free radical scavenger in the mitochondria and other areas of a cell, absorbing free radicals and therefore preventing damage to your energy-producing system. CoQ10 is obtained through foods high in CoQ10 such as beef, pork, sardines, anchovies, mackerel, salmon, broccoli, spinach and nuts; and through synthesis of CoQ10 in the body. The synthesis of CoQ10 requires the amino acid tyrosine, vitamins and several trace minerals. The manufacture of CoQ10 takes place in the liver.

If you have significant nutritional deficiencies, are low in the amino acid tyrosine, or if you have injured your liver in some way, you may not be able to manufacture CoQ10 as well as you should. People who are vegetarian routinely are low in CoQ10 since they are not able to obtain it through their food sources. Anyone taking the cholesterol-lowering medications, the HMG co-A reductase inhibitors (lovastatin™, sinvastatin™, pravastatin™, etc.), may also be low in CoQ10. These substances reduce coenzyme Q10 production in the body because they block the conversion of cholesterol to CoQ10. Anyone who is on these cholesterol-lowering medications should also have CoQ10 supplementation. Other studies report that in reasonable use there are no known side effects for CoQ10. If you take CoQ10 orally, make sure that you take it with meals that include a small amount of fat or take it in gel caps. Generally, we recommend 100 mg daily to patients at the Fatigue and Fibromyalgia Clinic of Michigan (FFCM), although obviously the amount will vary depending on your individual needs. Remember to always coordinate any supplementation program with your health care provider. All recommendations I make in this chapter should only be used with the permission of your health care provider.

Lipoic Acid

Lipoic acid converts carbohydrates to energy in the Krebs cycle. This antioxidant is needed as a cofactor for two enzymes that are absolutely necessary for proper energy production, acetyl-coA and alpha-ketoacid hydrogenase. Lipoic acid also works as an antioxidant for the entire energy-producing system. It is both fat- and water-soluble, which means it can go everywhere. Antioxidants such as vitamins C and E, lipoic acid and glutathione may have synergistic actions.

We obtain lipoic acid from substances that contain mitochondria, such as meat (all animal muscle contains mitochondria). In addition, some plants contain small amounts of lipoic acid, mainly in non-photosynthetic tissues like potatoes. However, most vegetarians may be low in lipoic acid and should strongly consider supplementation. At the FFCM we use doses between 50–100 mg one to three times daily. In the literature there have been no reports of side effects in over three decades of use in the treatment of diabetic neuropathy. Therefore, this substance appears to be extremely safe. There are also no known drug interactions and no known interactions with other nutrients. (As always, you must check with your health care practitioner prior to proceeding with any of the recommendations I outline in this chapter.)

In summary, lipoic acid is an important antioxidant for controlling damage within the mitochondrial structures. It appears to be very low in toxicity and therefore supplementation should be considered, especially for those people who have a vegetarian diet or who have had significant mitochondrial damage due to the factors that we have discussed earlier in this chapter.

Nicotinamide Adenine Dinucleotide with Hydrogen

NADH is commonly referred to as coenzyme 1 and is found in all natural living cells. It is absolutely necessary in energy production, as it occurs at the beginning of electron transport in stage three of the Krebs cycle. If you are low in NADH, it may short-circuit that phase of the Krebs cycle, which means you will not produce energy as well as you should. The more NADH you have available, the better you will be able to produce energy. Muscle and brain cells contain high levels of NADH because energy production is so essential for those tissues.

NADH also appears to be a very potent antioxidant within the mitochondria itself, helping to protect your energy-producing machinery against the damage caused by free radicals. The more effectively the mitochondria quenches the free radicals, the less the damage and more effective and better your energy production will be. NADH has been studied at Georgetown University Medical Center in a double-blind study of patients with chronic fatigue syndrome. Eight of the 11 (73%) of patients enrolled in the longer, open-labeled follow-up study showed significant improvement in clinical symptomatology and energy levels. No side effects were reported during the course of the study. (See *America Exhausted*, page 215.) Unfortunately, there is no commercially available test for determining your level of NADH. Therefore, we usually prescribe NADH as a clinical trial for 90 days at 5–10 mg every morning on an empty stomach.

If a patient has significant improvement in energy, we assume the level of NADH is low, so we continue the NADH supplement. If there is no improvement in energy, generally we discontinue it because of the cost of the nutrient. There are no known side effects or interactions with NADH, making it appear to be an extremely safe substance. Therefore, a clinical trial for those patients with fatigue or other symptomatology of low energy and mitochondrial dysfunction may be appropriate.

Vitamins E, C, and A and Selenium

We should not overlook these very important vitamins in controlling damage to the energy-producing system. Vitamin E is very important. It is generally obtained through unprocessed grains, including wheat germ and the germ of other grains. Unfortunately, most of our grain products are processed and most of the vitamin E has been removed to help improve the storage of bread. However, this removal of vitamin E also significantly affects our ability to prevent antioxidant damage. Recent studies have also shown that vitamin E (d-alpha tocopherol) and multiple tocopherols may be important in preventing damage to the energy-production system. Therefore, when we recommend vitamin E, we usually recommend a mixed tocopherol supplement, which is available at most health food stores. Generally we are conservative with vitamin E supplementation; the maximum I recommend is 1200 mg daily. (You must get approval from your health care practitioner prior to starting vitamin E supplementation.) It is more important to take smaller amounts of multiple antioxidant substances than it is to take large amounts of a single antioxidant. Some studies show that large amounts of antioxidants given as a single entity may not be as beneficial as once thought.

A good example of this is vitamin C, which is a very important water-soluble antioxidant that we should obtain in proper amounts. What is the proper amount? No one knows. There have been guesstimates ranging anywhere from 60 mg to 6000 mg. I recommend vitamin C supplementation to most patients at 2000–4000 mg daily. You must make sure that it is buffered so that it does not contribute to stone formation, and you must realize that most vitamin C is made from corn. Therefore, if you have a corn allergy, you should use vitamin C that is made from beets or from sago palm.

Vitamin A is an antioxidant that has been overshadowed by beta-carotene Indeed, vitamin A is an often overlooked antioxidant. We convert beta-carotene, which is obtained in our food, into vitamin A within the body. We also obtain vitamin A through fish oils and deep-ocean fish such as mackerel, sardines and salmon. I see many patients who have difficulty converting beta-carotene to vitamin A. Their beta-carotene levels are normal, but their vitamin A levels are low. Vitamin A is a fat-soluble antioxidant, which means it helps control free radical damage within the fatty portions of the body. As it is fat-soluble, you can overdose on vitamin A, so generally we are very conservative with vitamin A supplementation, generally staying at 10,000 IU daily. (Please consult your health care practitioner and do not take fat-soluble antioxidants without his or her express permission.)

Selenium is a mineral that is important for the production of SOD. SOD is an important antioxidant in the body. Millions of people in North America are low in selenium because our soil is now depleted in trace minerals. Therefore, our food no longer contains the selenium that it should. On top of that, processing further removes trace minerals from our food. You should consult your health care practitioner prior to proceeding with any supplementation program and discuss your individual risks versus benefits.

IN CONCLUSION

There are many other substances that help with mitochondrial function and energy production, such as the hormones testosterone, progesterone, DHEA and other nutrients not discussed in this chapter. For more detailed information on how we damage our energy production and other factors that may play a part in the reduction of our energy and the aging of our mitochondria, see *America Exhausted: Breakthrough Treatments of Fatigue and Fibromyalgia,* published by Vitality Press (1998). In addition, I also refer you to our upcoming book called *Super Metabolism,* which should be available through Vitality Press in the spring of 2001.

11

Drying Up

F. Batmanghelidj, M.D.

The greatest tragedy in medical history is the assumption that a dry mouth is the only sign that a body is dehydrated. The whole structure of modern medicine is built on this pitifully flawed assumption that brings about painful, premature death to many millions of people. They suffer because they do not know they are only thirsty.

The human body uses a different logic from the basic "dry mouth" premise that is the cornerstone of modern medical science. Ample saliva is produced in order to facilitate and lubricate chewing and swallowing—a basic human function. Water is too important to the body for its shortage to be signaled only by a dry mouth. This mistake in medical thinking has given birth to the self-expanding sick-care system that survives and fraudulently thrives on people remaining sick.

It is now clinically and scientifically clear that the human body has many other distinct ways of showing its general or local water needs. Depending on where there is water shortage, many localized complications are produced. In this chapter, I will present an overview of chronic, unintentional dehydration and the many ways the human body can manifest its internal drought, causing an increased rate of biological aging and the complications that come with it.

Naturally, to understand dehydration, we need to become alert to the early indicators of water shortages in different parts of the body. One thing must be made clear. In dehydration, 66% of the water loss is from inside the cells in the drought-stricken area, 26% is from the environment outside and around the cells, and only 8% is lost from blood circulation. Since the blood vessels are made of soft and muscular tissues, they constrict and tighten on the empty space and correct for the 8% shortage.

THE INADEQUACY OF BLOOD TESTS IN DETECTING DEHYDRATION

This is why routine blood tests do not show any abnormality, yet the patient develops sufficiently severe discomfort to seek professional advice. Their blood tests did not reveal the underlying damages of dehydration. You see, by and large, the blood that is circulating is pretty well standardized by the liver. Function-reducing dehydration in an outlying area of the body that might even be shut off by decreased circulation to the area will not show itself in the routine blood tests that are now used for dehydration. The blood tests will show some markers when tissue damage and severe complication of water shortage in the body have been established for some time. Unfortunately, by this point, the body has undergone sometimes irreversible damage and premature aging.

To understand dehydration, we need to recognize the vital functions of water and recognize dehydration by the missing signs of what water would normally do in the symptom-producing areas of the body. I have used this approach toward the understanding of disease for the past 20 years and have developed an insight into the body's markers of dehydration.

It is my researched opinion that the human body has three categories of indicators that signal dehydration in parts of the body. They include perceptive indicators, crisis calls of the body for water, and adaptive drought management and water rationing programs. They are distinct and recognizable, and all are preventable.

THE PERCEPTIVE INDICATORS OF DROUGHT IN THE BODY

1. Feeling tired when it is not the result of strenuous work; in its extreme form, chronic fatigue syndrome.
2. Feeling flushed.
3. Feeling irritable and angered over the slightest provocation.
4. Feeling anxious without a justified cause of anxiety, neurosis, panic disorder and agoraphobia.
5. Feeling dejected and inadequate.
6. Feeling depressed; in its extreme form, depression and suicidal tendencies.

As we age, we experience a decline in cognitive function. This may in part be due to the loss of water from certain areas in the brain. In fact, there are indicators that dehydration is affecting some aspects of the functions of the brain, the wet part of which is over 80% water. Shortage of water in the brain can cause the loss of certain functions and result in the conditions described above. The extreme complications of dehydration in the brain tissue are neurological disorders that devastate life in the later years.

The body's 9 trillion brain cells are alert at all times and they consume vast amounts of energy in their constant intercellular chatter. The energy they consume is provided by a molecule called adenosine triphosphate (ATP). ATP has to be broken down by water to generate energy. The process is called hydrolysis, meaning water-broken. The same process of energy release takes place in all the active cells of the body, and water is instrumental in this energy liberation. In fact, water generates the primary hydroelectric energy that is stored in the ATP molecules when the cell is inactive and becoming hydrated. When water turns electricity-generating turbines, called the cation pumps (cat-ion), the voltage gradient reconstructs the ATP molecule from its primary ingredients within the cell membranes and builds up the energy stores for future use. When the cells become activated, water hydrolyzes ATP and releases energy for cell functions.

The units of energy are measured in Kilojoules (energy required to raise the temperature of one pound of water through one degree Fahrenheit = one Joule). Water is actually more important as a source of energy to the cells of the human body than any kind of food, including sugar. Therefore, low water intake causes low energy output and decreased brain function, which is what tiredness is all about when no hard work or exercise has been performed.

THE CRISIS CALLS OF THE BODY FOR WATER

Among the second group of crisis symptoms and signs of dehydration of the body are the different localized chronic pains. Much of the list reads like a *Who's Who* of advanced aging. They include:

1. heartburn
2. dyspepsia
3. rheumatoid joint pain
4. back pain
5. migraine headaches
6. leg pain on walking
7. fibromyalgic pain
8. colitis pain and its associated constipation
9. anginal pain, a sign of advanced water shortage in the heart and lung axis

10. early morning sickness of pregnancy, indicating thirst of the fetus and the mother

11. bad breath is also an indication of water shortage in the body; it is produced by fermentation of food that has not been washed away from inside the stomach

What these pains and symptoms mean is simple. When there is water shortage in a part of the body that is actively being used, the toxic waste produced as a result of tissue metabolism is not cleared away and this causes acid buildup in the area. Nerve endings register the environmental change of chemistry with the brain. By producing these pains, the brain tries to let the conscious mind know of the impending problems that will be caused by the local drought. This is because, if the drought continues in an area of the body that is being made to work, permanent tissue damage will ensue, such as colon cancer, which is associated with long-term constipation.

The Significance of Pain

This is why the body signals local drought by producing pain. This pain is similar to the whistle of the smoke detectors to warn of a fire that would burn a house down with its unsuspecting inhabitants. Pain is supposed to tell our conscious but preoccupied and forgetful minds that the acid buildup in the area will soon set the local cells on fire and cause acid burns. Pain is the local resident genes' cry of anguish before their impending death. Normally, it is water that washes the acid away, preventing its accumulation and damage to the area, in the same way it extinguishes fires.

In short, pain means water shortage in the area of pain registration. It is a crisis call of the body for the water that is needed to wash away the toxic waste from the drought-stricken area. The basic problem in the presently practiced form of medicine is the lack of knowledge about the significance and importance of pain as a thirst signal of the body.

When the body is calling for water, the medical profession has been duped into prescribing chemical poisons such as pain-killers that painfully and prematurely kill people. The tragedy is that we in medicine have become accustomed to thinking that we are doing our patients good by continuously prescribing these expensive and slow-acting poisons.

ADAPTIVE DROUGHT-MANAGEMENT PROGRAMS OF THE BODY

The third category of conditions that denote dehydration is the body's drought-management programs, some of which have been labeled as diseases. They are:

1. asthma and allergies

2. hypertension
3. old-age diabetes
4. constipation and colitis pain
5. dry, creased and furrowed skin condition that turns into eczema
6. autoimmune diseases, such as lupus and insulin-dependent diabetes
7. cholesterol buildup in the lining of the arteries of the heart, brain and kidneys

Anginal pain is a component of asthma in older people. It means they experience the characteristic heart pain that is also associated with asthmatics' reduced lung capacity and difficulty in breathing. They may also have increased mucus production.

These conditions are major health problems produced by persistent water shortage of the human body. Could it be that we will one day wake up and realize that aging in a sense is a disease of drying up? For more information on the other aspects of persistent water shortage in the body you should read the books *Your Body's Many Cries for Water* and *ABC of Asthma, Allergies and Lupus*, or listen to my taped seminar, "Water: Rx for a Healthier Pain-Free Life." In *ABC of Asthma, Allergies and Lupus* the life-saving roles of cholesterol in the body are discussed extensively.

CHRONIC, UNINTENTIONAL DEHYDRATION

Chronic, unintentional dehydration in the body, which produces as many health problems as we in medicine have invented diseases, is produced by two main factors:

1. The loss of our perception of thirst as we grow older. We wait to get thirsty and don't voluntarily and regularly drink water. Because we drink insufficient water, this prompts our bodies to go into a strict drought-management mode that suppresses our thirst mechanisms. This suppression of thirst in early dehydration is a crisis-management effort in order to get through periods of water shortage. By this process, the body is set up to work even when it is short of water. In this way, the body will make do even if you give it no more than two or three glasses of water daily when it actually needs eight or ten.
2. Substituting manufactured beverages that do more harm than good in place of the water that the body should receive when we get thirsty.

Dehydration and Acid/Alkali Balance

Three main mechanisms regulate the acidity of the body:
1. Water intake and production of adequate urine.
2. Proper breathing and expulsion of carbon dioxide from the body through the lungs.

3. Sacrificing some of the most essential amino acids as antioxidants, including tryptophan, tyrosine, phenylalanine and cysteine, as an all-out effort to stop further disease production and metabolic deficiency disorders.

What is the ideal acid/alkali (pH) balance and how is it achieved? A pH of 7.4 inside the cells and 7.2–7.3 in the blood is an ideal reading. These numbers are the readings from a scale designed to measure the degree of acidity in the body. From 1 to 7 is the acid range, with 1 being more acid than 7. From 7 to 14 on the scale is the alkaline range, with 7 being less alkaline than 14. On the pH scale, 7 is neutral. The health-ensuring functions of the body in its internal and external cellular environment must remain within the above-mentioned exact range. If the blood begins to become acidic, the body begins to produce drastic symptoms. If the pH of blood reached about 6.9, death would be imminent! Similarly, a drastic shift toward an alkaline range would be detrimental to one's health. People who market pH-altering filters and tell people to drink strong alkaline water should be cautious with their statements and advice. They can very easily hurt their unsuspecting customers.

Gas exchanges in the lungs regulate the acidity of the body. Hemoglobin is a complex molecule that delivers carbon dioxide to the lung tissue to be released into the air about to be exhaled, and that collects oxygen to circulate throughout the body. Each hemoglobin molecule is made up of four iron-containing units attached to one another. Each red cell contains a certain amount of these hemoglobin molecules depending on the efficiency of the blood-forming mechanisms. As the hemoglobin unit rotates on its axis, it releases the carbon dioxide it collected from the outlying parts of the body into its water environment inside the red cell and in its place picks up four oxygen molecules that enter the red cell. As the carbon dioxide concentration inside the red cell increases, it will escape into the air in the air sacs. Hemoglobin does something else that is very important. It collects the excess hydrogen atoms, a very strong acid factor within its own protein structure, and neutralizes their damage-causing acidity. When carbon dioxide leaves the lungs, the body fluids become more alkaline, an ideal situation for a healthy body. Thus breathing normally is vital for the acid/alkali balance of the body. This is by far the most important pH-regulating mechanism the body possesses. It is also important to mention that as we age we tend to lose a significant amount of our bodies' ability to take in and utilize this oxygen, also referred to as our "vital capacity."

In asthmatics, because of the low rate of air exchange in their lungs, this acid-eliminating mechanism is inefficient and is the main source of danger to their lives. Every year, many thousands of asthmatics die from this imbalance of their body physiology. A physician who does not understand the locked-in relationship of dehydration to diseases of the body, particularly to asthma, diabetes, hypertension, and even autoimmune diseases, and refuses to learn about it, can cause more damage than good, not only to you, but to other unsuspecting and trusting patients.

SALT INTAKE IS VITAL

Salt is a vital substance for the survival of all living creatures. Water and salt regulate the water content of the body. Water itself regulates the water content of the interior of the cells by working its way into all the cells it reaches. It has to get there to cleanse and extract the toxic waste of cell metabolism. Salt forces some water to stay and keep it company outside the cells (osmotic retention of water by salt). It balances the amount of water held outside the cells. There are two oceans of water in the body: one ocean is held inside the cells of the body, and the other ocean is held outside the cells. Good health depends on a delicate balance between the volume of these two oceans, and this balance is achieved by regular intake of water and salt, preferably unrefined sea salt, which contains some of the other minerals that the body needs, and potassium, which holds water inside the cells.

When water is not available to get into the cells freely, it is filtered from the outside salty ocean and injected into the cells that are being overworked despite their water shortage. This is why, in severe dehydration, we develop an edema and retain water. The design of our bodies is such that the extent of the ocean of water outside the cells is expanded to have extra water available for filtration and emergency injection into vital cells. The brain commands an increase in salt and water retention by the kidneys, so this is how we get an edema when we don't drink enough water.

Initially, the process of water filtration and its delivery into the cells is more efficient at night when the body is horizontal. The collected water, which mostly pools in the legs, does not have to fight the force of gravity to get into the blood circulation. If reliance on this process of emergency hydration continues for long, the body continuously collects salt and retains water until even the lungs begin to get waterlogged at night and breathing becomes difficult. The person needs more pillows to sit upright to sleep. This condition is the consequence of dehydration. However, in this condition, you cannot overload the system by drinking too much water at the beginning. Increases in water intake must be slow and spaced out until urine production begins to increase at the same rate that you drink water.

When we drink enough water to pass clear urine, we also pass out a lot of the salt that was held back. This is how we can get rid of edema fluid from the body: by drinking more water—not diuretics, but more water! People who have an extensive edema, and have irregular or very rapid heartbeats with little exertion, should increase their water intake gradually and space out the intake. Naturally, salt intake should be limited for two or three days because the body is still in an overdrive mode to retain it. Once the edema has cleared, salt should not be withheld from the body.

THE FURTHER BENEFITS OF SALT

Salt has many functions other than just regulating the water content of the body. Here are some of the more vital functions of salt in the body:

- Salt is vital to the extraction of excess acidity from the cells in the body, particularly the brain cells.
- Salt is vital for balancing the sugar levels in the blood, a needed element for people with diabetes.
- Salt is vital for the generation of hydroelectric energy in all the cells in the body.
- Salt is vital to the nerve cells, communication and information processing.
- Salt is vital for the absorption of food particles through the intestinal tract.
- Salt is vital for clearing the lungs of mucus plugs and sticky phlegm, particularly in asthma and cystic fibrosis.
- Salt is vital for clearing up catarrh and congestion of the sinuses.
- Salt is a strong natural antihistamine. It can be used to relieve asthma symptoms by putting it on the tongue after drinking a glass or two of water. It is as effective as an inhaler without an inhaler's toxicity.
- Salt is essential for preventing muscle cramps.
- Salt is vital to prevent excess saliva production to the point that it flows out of the mouth during sleep. Drooling indicates salt shortage.
- Salt is absolutely vital to making the structure of bones firm. Osteoporosis, in a major way, is the result of salt and water shortage in the body.
- Salt is vital for those who have weak bladders and are at times incontinent. Salt strengthens the smooth muscles in the bladder.
- Salt is an effective "medication" against spider veins. It strengthens veins that have become varicose and leaky.
- Salt is vital to keep skin hydrated and moist by expanding the volume of blood in circulation to reach the blood vessels of the skin, which would otherwise be shut down to prevent water from evaporating from the skin surface, resulting in furrowed, scaly and lusterless dried skin. The impact of dehydration on the skin texture and color is what we notice as we age, hence the title of this chapter.

WHAT YOUR BODY NEEDS

If you begin to drink water according to my protocol, you might also benefit by taking a daily multivitamin tablet, particularly if you do not exercise and do not eat hearty portions of vegetables and fruits. Meat and fish proteins are good sources of selenium and zinc. If you are under stress, you might consider adding some vitamin B6 and zinc to your diet, in addition to what is available in the vitamin tablet, until the stressful period is over.

If you suffer from cold sores (herpes simplex virus on the lips and even in the eyes) or genital herpes, make sure you add zinc and vitamin B6 to your diet. Your viral sores might well be the result of zinc deficiency and its associated complications.

The body also needs fruits and a fairly high quantity of green vegetables daily. Fruits and vegetables are ideal sources of the natural vitamins and essential minerals we need. Green vegetables also contain a great deal of beta-carotene, and even some DHA fatty acid, an essential substance needed by the brain. Fruits and vegetables are important for maintaining the pH balance of the body. Chlorophyll contains a very high quantity of magnesium. Magnesium is to chlorophyll what iron is to hemoglobin in the blood, an oxygen carrier. In the human body, magnesium is the bonding anchor to the energy-storing unit within all the cell membranes in the body. The unit is called magnesium adenosine triphosphate (MgATP). If water reaches the MgATP pool and is enzymatically positioned to break it down, lots of energy will be released.

If you drink adequate amounts of water every day, take the required amount of salt and exercise regularly, your body will begin to adjust its own intake of proteins and carbohydrates, as well as its fat requirements to use for energy. Your need for proteins will increase, your need for carbohydrates will decrease, and your fat-burning enzymes will consume more fat than is in the average diet. Contrary to the belief that cholesterol cannot be metabolized once it is deposited, that too will be cleared. The cholesterol deposits may take longer to disappear than you might wish, but the body has all the chemical know-how to clear cholesterol plaques.

DRINK PURE WATER

Naturally, the quality of drinking water is most important to health. Water should be water and not any other drink! Water should be free of chemicals, particularly caffeine and alcohol.

Please bear in mind that caffeine and alcohol are toxic chemicals; they are addictive drugs as far as the cells of the human body are concerned. It is true that the manufacturers of these agents have unrestricted permission to contaminate good drinking water with these toxic chemicals and sell them to the public, but, sooner or later, their detrimental impact on society will, like the tobacco industry, become a focus of attention.

Caffeine Will Exhaust the Brain

Caffeine is a natural diuretic. It forces more water out of the body than one consumes in the beverage! Alcohol also dehydrates the body; the brain is particularly sensitive, hence hangover headaches. Caffeine also acts on the brain cells directly and forces them to use some of their critical energy reserves on trivial actions and whims (in other words, wasting energy). It lowers the threshold for triggering an action from cells that would otherwise remain inactive until a more serious engagement is deemed necessary. The effect of caffeine on the brain is energy depletion. If taken repeatedly, caffeine eventually exhausts the brain. When the brain needs energy reserves to cope with a crisis, it will be less than effective because it is depressed. The energy reserve–depleting effect of caffeine on the brain is one of the primary causes of attention-deficit disorder.

Caffeine not only depletes the stored energy pools in the brain, it also inhibits the enzyme system initiated by phospho-diesterase (PD). PD activity is a vital step in the direction of memory-making by the brain cells. Caffeine is naturally designed to cause stupefaction of the brain. Caffeine is used by the coffee plant as a nerve warfare chemical against its predators. Caffeine inhibits the nervous system and the memory mechanisms of its food chain predators so that they lose their art of camouflage and become less alert and less able to protect themselves. They thus become much easier prey for their own predators.

We humans take the same caffeine-containing coffee beans, brew them to our desired concentration and consume the plant's chemical poison as a pleasure-inducing beverage. Over-consumption of sodas and other caffeine-containing beverages is largely why many children in the United States have reading and learning problems. Despite all the money that is being spent on their education, U.S. children's grade average standard is far below that of children in less-privileged societies who do not have the same access to caffeine-containing beverages. For the same reason, more American children develop health problems such as allergies and asthma.

CONCLUSION

The major disease conditions that humans have to cope with today are produced by prolonged water shortage in the body. This information has been available to scientists for some time. When the information and the changes it can bring about become common knowledge, the major disease problems of humankind will disappear. Our approach to medicine will become physiological and nature-based instead of pharmacological and toxic to the body. It will become gentle instead of invasive. The vast financial resources of the older and more vulnerable members of society will be freed from fear-driven insurance policies and health expenditures. These people will be able to spend their hard-earned money on more useful and rewarding purposes. Younger people will remain healthy and more productive during a longer life span. In short, the life of the individual will become more pleasant and less threatening.

By correcting the current medical misconceptions on water and salt, leaps of progress in the science of medicine and a more accurate knowledge of the human body will be its natural rewards, allowing you to not only perhaps live a longer life, but live a healthier one, full of the vital energy you were designed to have right until the end.

12

A New Approach to Female Transition from PMS to Menopause

Michael A. Zeligs, M.D.

A MAJOR TURNING POINT

Menopause and perimenopause, the 10–15 years before menopause, are unique turning points for women. New discoveries are creating innovative, personalized approaches that make perimenopause and associated symptoms of premenstrual syndrome (PMS) a manageable and optimistic time. While some women treat menopause as an affliction that will make them unattractive, lonely, helpless and useless, informed women discover something else. Menopause, when approached with the help of nutrition and hormonal balance, can give women a new lease on life physically, emotionally, sexually and spiritually. Women can be enthusiastic about becoming free of concerns about pregnancy and premenstrual syndrome. For the modern woman who will spend half her life involved in the perimenopausal and menopausal transitions, there is nothing more important than developing a successful approach to these turning points.

This chapter is dedicated to natural breakthrough discoveries that can help ease the transitions in a woman's life. Whether you experience perimenopausal symptoms, PMS or menopause, this chapter will shed new light on why women experience these symptoms as they make their transitions through life. A new appreciation for the effect of diet, exercise and nutritional supplements on hormonal balance provide important new options for every woman. Most importantly, though, this chapter will bring to light a whole new perspective on dealing with female transitions, allowing women everywhere to enjoy and embrace their transitions with optimum health.

PLANT-POWERED AGING INTERVENTION: USING DIINDOLYLMETHANE TO PROMOTE HEALTHIER METABOLISM

I. Introduction

What is phytonutrition and how does it contribute to aging intervention?

Phytonutrition is the study of unique substances in plants that are useful as natural medicines. Phytonutrients are plant substances that interact with human enzyme systems responsible for energy and hormone metabolism. Researchers in phytonutrition are discovering a basis for the dietary prevention of cancer, resulting in a new era of dietary supplementation for aging intervention and cancer control.

Adequate intake of specific phytonutrients can regulate hormone metabolism and cell behavior. These natural substances are effective regulators of specific enzyme targets for health promotion. Cruciferous vegetables, such as cabbage, cauliflower and broccoli, possess unique constituents able to modify the metabolism of estrogen. The most active of these phytonutrients is the dietary indole, diindolylmethane. Supplemental use of diindolylmethane provides the basis for nutritional support to enhance estrogen's beneficial metabolism and safe action. Optimal estrogen metabolism has implications for cancer prevention and successful aging in both women and men.

New discoveries are revealing exactly how phytonutrients interact with cellular metabolism to provide these remarkable health benefits. Initially considered "non-essential" by the scientific community, many phytonutrients are proving to be important health promoters and active regulators of human metabolism. The long-held notion that metabolism is fixed by inheritance has been shattered by the finding that women at risk for breast cancer can reduce their risk status by including diindolylmethane in their diet.

An Italian study confirms discoveries made in the 1980s that men and women with cancer, together with their first-degree family members, possess a deficient metabolism of estrogen. Dietary supplementation with diindolylmethane improves metabolism of estrogen in "at risk" women and provides a simple and practical approach to cancer-risk reduction.

Phytonutrition can benefit a spectrum of aging-related conditions, including heart disease, obesity and cancer. This chapter will focus on the actions and uses of diindolylmethane from cruciferous vegetables. An increasing scientific consensus supports the use of diindolylmethane and other phytonutrients as effective agents in preventive nutrition and aging intervention.

II. Diindolylmethane: The Phytonutrient Connection to Healthy Estrogen Metabolism

What Is Diindolylmethane and How Does It Promote Health?

As mentioned, diindolylmethane is an indole phytonutrient found only in cruciferous vegetables: cabbage, broccoli, bok choy, brussels sprouts, cauliflower, kale, kohlrabi, mustard rutabaga and turnip. These plants, cultivated for thousands of years, were initially used as medicinal plants. As sources of diindolylmethane, these vegetables supply a phytonutrient whose metabolism precisely overlaps with the pathway needed for healthy estrogen metabolism. Stated simply, supplementing the diet with absorbable diindolylmethane promotes beneficial estrogen metabolism and helps to restore a healthy hormonal balance.

Though discovered over 10 years ago, the connection between phytonutrients and estrogen is just beginning to be appreciated. This connection explains why people in developed nations who eat fewer phytonutrient-rich plants suffer disproportionately from the major hormone-dependent cancers, colon cancer and coronary disease. Dr. H. Leon Bradlow and his group in New York were the first to establish the link between phytonutrients from cruciferous vegetables and estrogen metabolism. They showed that supplemental use of particular cruciferous phytochemicals can promote a dramatic and beneficial change in the metabolism of estrogen, which can greatly reduce estrogen exposure as a risk for cancer.

This discovery proved that the metabolism and growth-promoting activity of estrogen is modified by the intake of milligram amounts of dietary indoles from crucifers. When these cruciferous phytochemicals are added to the diet, estrogen action is regulated and its metabolism is shifted. This produces a predominance of active metabolites called good estrogens. They function as antioxidants and have the power to eliminate damaged or cancerous cells throughout the body. Without these phytonutrients in the diet, there is increased production of a different, undesirable group of estrogen metabolites. These so-called bad estrogens act negatively to allow oxidation to damage DNA and promote cancer.

A diet-derived imbalance in estrogen metabolism explains population studies showing a high prevalence of estrogen-related disease, especially breast cancer, in societies consuming a diet low in total vegetable content. Supplemental use of diindolylmethane, the most active cruciferous indole, can restore and maintain a favorable balance of estrogen metabolites. Supplementation with diindolylmethane provides an innovative approach to reducing the estrogen-related risk of breast cancer. Diindolylmethane supplementation can also increase the safety of estrogen replacement therapy in postmenopausal women. Premenopausal women also suffer from estrogen imbalance in the form of excessive estrogen. This is a factor in premenstrual syndrome, endometriosis and cervical dysplasia.

Why Not Just Eat More Cruciferous Vegetables?

Recent reports, like one from the Fred Hutchison Cancer Center in Seattle, indicate that higher intake of cruciferous vegetables is associated with a lower risk of prostate cancer. A similar study showed that women eating more cruciferous vegetables were protected from lymphoma. In these studies, those who ate three servings of cruciferous vegetables per week had a lessened risk of getting cancer. These studies are further evidence indicating that cruciferous vegetables provide protection from hormone-sensitive cancer. However, direct measurements of upward, beneficial shifts in estrogen metabolism indicate that you would have to eat at least 2 lbs. per day of raw or lightly cooked vegetables to derive the same benefit as you would from one or two capsules of specially formulated diindolylmethane. Taking formulated supplements is by far the preferable way to increase diindolylmethane. Plain diindolylmethane in its crystalline form is just not absorbed due to its poor solubility in water and oil, so it requires an absorption-enhancing delivery system for use in dietary supplements. Formulated diindolylmethane provides the phytochemical in a consistent, absorbable form that mimics the intake of diindolylmethane from the diet. These amounts of diindolylmethane are similar to that found in large portions of brussels sprouts or broccoli, but exceed amounts conveniently absorbed from diet alone.

When taken as a supplement complexed with absorption-enhancing ingredients, diindolylmethane is absorbed well because of its increased solubility. In this delivery system, diindolylmethane is used at about twice the amount you might derive from 2 lbs. of vegetables. Due to the large amounts of cruciferous vegetables needed to deliver adequate amounts of diindolylmethane, consistently obtaining diindolylmethane from diet alone is not practical.

Supplemental use of absorbable diindolylmethane has proven to be successful in improving estrogen metabolism. Diindolylmethane supplementation in perimenopausal women has been found to benefit PMS, recurrent premenstrual breast pain and ease painful menstruation. Its use also facilitates easier weight loss in both women and men.

What Is Estrogen Dominance?

A new study of midlife aging reveals that patterns of hormone metabolism change with age. Slower hormone metabolism in midlife can mean higher than normal levels of estrogen and a deficiency in its beneficial 2-hydroxy metabolites. Faltering estrogen metabolism often occurs in women during perimenopause (the 10–15 years before menopause), and is characterized by higher monthly estrogen levels in the years before estrogen's dramatic fall at menopause. Also, during perimenopause progesterone levels begin to fall, resulting in a rising estrogen-to-progesterone ratio. This is one form of estrogen dominance. This reduction in progesterone output during the second half or luteal phase of the menstrual cycle can cause irregular periods and contribute to premenstrual mood disorders. The good estrogen metabolites, 2-hydroxy and 2-methoxy estrogen, stimulate increased progesterone production from ovarian cells. By promoting 2-hydroxy production, diindolylmethane supplementation may help support progesterone production and maintain progesterone levels throughout the perimenopausal years. This balancing effect can benefit disorders associated with estrogen–progesterone imbalance, including chronic breast pain, fibrocystic breast disease and endometriosis.

Another important variety of estrogen dominance relates directly to cancer. This has to do with how estrogen is metabolized. Women with breast and uterine cancer make too little of the 2-hydroxy or good metabolite of estrogen and too much of the 16-hydroxy or bad variety. Since 16-hydroxy is an unregulated form of estrogen that behaves like "super estrogen," higher levels create a particularly unhealthy form of estrogen dominance. The 16-hydroxy estrogens and related 4-hydroxy estrogens can result in mutations, abnormal growth, as in cervical dysplasia, and an increased risk of future breast cancer. Overproduction of 16-hydroxy estrogen is also seen in obesity, high-fat diet and exposure to a host of "estrogenic" environmental chemicals. Therefore, this form of estrogen dominance, resulting from inheritance or environmental exposure, is a pervasive issue in preventive medicine. Apart from preventive use of the drug Nolvadex® (Tamoxifen), diindolylmethane supplementation is the first natural approach to intervene in estrogen dominance. Reducing estrogen dominance with phytonutrition is a breakthrough in aging intervention.

III. New Uses for Supplemental Diindolylmethane

How Does Diindolylmethane Specifically Benefit Premenstrual Syndrome?

Premenstrual syndrome (PMS)—defined as typical monthly symptoms of irritability, aggression, tension, depression, mood swings, bloating, breast pain or breast swelling—is frequently seen in adolescent girls and peri-menopausal women. While PMS severity can be reduced with nutritional intervention—including lower-fat diets, supplementation with minerals, vitamin D and herbal extracts from *Vitex* agnus-castus (Chasteberry), full resolution of PMS has been elusive.

Improvements in PMS symptoms have been noted since beginning dietary supplementation with absorbable diindolylmethane. These results suggest that diindolylmethane is able to correct the estrogen imbalance in PMS. Dr. Torbjorn Backstrom, an eminent researcher in the field, and others have documented that estradiol, the primary active form of estrogen, is elevated in PMS. Backstrom has also shown that the degree of elevation of estradiol correlates with the severity of the symptoms. Also encouraging is the observation that the enzyme pathways promoted by diindolylmethane also help to metabolize pregnenolone sulfate, a brain hormone. Like estrogen, pregnenolone sulfate is elevated in PMS. Its healthy metabolism produces beneficial, immune-stimulating metabolites and may help relieve anxiety. Therefore, absorbable diindolylmethane supplementation promotes healthier metabolism of both estrogen and pregnenolone in PMS.

A strong nutritional approach to PMS that includes bioavailable diindolylmethane has now been developed. This approach is the first to help normalize metabolism and the balance of mood-altering hormones. This contrasts with the use of anti-depressant drugs, which can mask the imbalance of estrogen and coexisting cancer risk. The use of absorbable diindolylmethane for PMS clearly offers a safer and more physiologic approach to this common adolescent and midlife disorder of hormonal balance.

Using Diindolylmethane to Resist Cancer

The most exciting discovery relating to diindolylmethane concerns its beneficial impact on cervical health. Cervical cancer in its early stages is of growing concern since its occurrence is closely linked to infection with the human papilloma virus (HPV). HPV infection is the most common sexually transmitted viral disease in the United States. Epidemic spread of this virus threatens a rising tide of cervical cancer in younger, sexually active women.

Dr. Maria Bell, a cervical cancer specialist, made the dramatic report that almost half of a group of women with cervical cancer had complete disappearance of their disease after 12 weeks of supplementation with the diindolylmethane precursor, indole-3-carbinol (I3-C). There was no response in the placebo group. I3C is converted in the stomach to diindolylmethane. Since this study, further comparable cases of cervical cancer regression have been observed during supplementation with absorbable diindolylmethane, which increased 2-hydroxy estrogen production.

Diindolylmethane induces the programmed death of cancer cells while not affecting normal cells. Such programmed cell death, known as "apoptosis," is now recognized as the most basic defense against cancer. Each removal by apoptosis of a cell damaged by viral infection or overstimulation from unmetabolized estrogen prevents the survival of a first cancer cell and a subsequent tumor. The combined contribution of 2-hydroxy estrogen metabolites and diindolylmethane may be the essential interaction explaining the cancer-preventative action of phytonutrients. Both diindolylmethane and 2-hydroxy estrogens are known to independently support apoptosis.

Can Diindolylmethane Help Improve the Safety of Hormone-Replacement Therapy (HRT)?

Despite a growing list of benefits clearly related to estrogen replacement, including younger-looking skin, stronger bones, more comfortable sex and better memory, women often view its potential side effects—the risk of breast and uterine cancer—as unacceptable. Other concerns include an increase in risk of life-threatening blood clots, especially after fracture. Most recently, the nationwide Heart and Estrogen Replacement Study (HERS) reported that women with a history of heart disease had an increased risk of heart attack in the first year after starting estrogen.

Many of these risks can be related to a lack of estrogen's beneficial metabolites. It is now known that higher 2-hydroxy estrogen levels lower the risk of future breast cancer. Supplementation with bioavailable diindolylmethane increases protective 2-hydroxy estrogen and therefore may reduce the risk of HRT-related cancer. Reduction in the risk of abnormal blood clot formation related to HRT estrogen would benefit women who suffer fractures while on HRT but may also benefit women with early heart disease. It has been known since the Framingham study in Massachusetts that men with the highest estradiol levels had the worst risk of early heart attack. Diindolylmethane may help normalize the estrogen-related cardiac risk in both men and women. Also, the beneficial

2-hydroxy metabolites have been shown to be powerful antioxidants, which may contribute to protecting against the early stages of atherosclerosis, which leads to heart attacks.

In postmenopausal women, about 20–30% of eligible women participate in long-term use of supplemental estrogen, including supplemental dehydroepiandrosterone (DHEA), the natural source of estrogen in postmenopausal women. DHEA, sold as an over-the-counter dietary supplement in the U.S., has been shown in long-term clinical studies to promote immunity and bone mineralization without uterine stimulation. Supplementation with diindolylmethane can decrease estrogen-related breast cancer risk in all women taking HRT. This includes women taking estrogen, DHEA or phytoestrogen supplements.

Diindolylmethane supplementation balances estrogen by reducing undesirable metabolites now known to be responsible for the cancer-initiating and cancer-promoting effects of estrogen. Supplemental diindolylmethane produces desirable metabolites associated with a lower risk of breast cancer and other estrogen-related disorders. The risk of breast cancer from HRT can be significantly reduced by the complementary steps of adding supplemental diindolylmethane and reducing alcohol consumption. Alcohol raises circulating levels of estrogen from all sources by interfering with its metabolism. If coupled with a tendency to produce dangerous estrogen metabolites, like 16-hydroxyestrone, alcohol can promote cancer whether or not supplemental estrogen is used. Diindolylmethane supplementation is an effective means to ensure a favorable estrogen metabolism. With its estrogen-balancing effects, diindolylmethane provides a margin of safety and reduces the negative consequences of estrogen associated with HRT and alcohol use.

In addition to a decrease in overall premature mortality, estrogen replacement supports better memory, lowers the risk of Alzheimer's dementia, strengthens bones by reducing fractures and, most importantly, decreases cardiovascular disease by 50%. In addition, estrogen may be important in preventing osteoarthritis and reducing the occurrence of colon cancer. There are also the benefits of more youthful skin, less vaginal dryness, increased libido, and less urinary incontinence. Following a long history of postmenopausal use of DHEA in Europe, its addition to regimens of hormonal supplementation is now advocated as an advantageous source of estrogen for women.

Applications of phytonutrition can now be combined with HRT to provide protection from estrogen's risks while still taking advantage of estrogen's many benefits.

IV. Conclusion

Plant-Powered Hormonal Balance for Healthy Aging

Diindolylmethane is a valuable addition to anti-aging dietary supplements. Diindolylmethane supplementation is a nutritional approach to achieving a safer and healthier estrogen metabolism. This benefits PMS, cervical dysplasia, breast health and improves hormone replacement. These and other important benefits for women's successful aging all relate to the promotion of a safer and more optimal hormonal metabolism with phytonutrition.

13

Mom's Best-Kept Secret, Colostrum: The Perfect Anti-aging Food

Donald Henderson, M.D.

AN INTRODUCTION TO BOVINE COLOSTRUM

Colostrum is a natural food, and is the first substance that a mother's breast produces during the first 72 hours after giving birth. It has also been described as a "pre-milk fluid." Colostrum contains powerful growth and immune factors that ensure the health and vitality of the newborn, be it animal or human. Hundreds of medical and clinical studies conducted worldwide conclude that bovine (cow) colostrum may be one of the most important substances we can take to support our health.

Colostrum is a complex fluid rich in nutrients, antibodies and growth factors. Colostrum contains vitamins, minerals, antioxidants and proteins that we can still find useful as adults. It also contains ingredients that are designed specifically to protect us from the bacteria, viruses and toxins we face each day. Research has shown that bovine colostrum and human colostrum are nearly identical.

THE BENEFITS OF COLOSTRUM

Mammals produce colostrum for only a short period of time after birth. After those first 72 hours, the mother produces milk rather than colostrum for the duration of nursing. However, the benefits of the colostrum should last a lifetime. Unlike humans, cows produce up to 34 L of colostrum in the first two or three days after birth. Researchers of colostrum's miraculous properties are excited about the fact that bovine colostrum is in such abundance. They are also excited that the quality of bovine colostrum can be controlled, thereby ensuring an optimal and effective product. Even more exciting is the medical evidence indicating the benefits of bovine colostrum for adult humans. The use of bovine colostrum is becoming an important part of health maintenance.

Colostrum contains important bioactive substances, such as:

- immunoglobulins, which help build our resistance to disease-causing organisms, as well as protect the body against bacterial and viral infections
- cytokines, lactoferrin and interleukins, which help maintain healthy immune system functions
- growth factors, which rejuvenate and maintain every cell in our body (giving it anti-aging properties)

THE VARIOUS STUDIES AND USES OF COLOSTRUM

For thousands of years in India, Ayurvedic physicians have used and documented the health benefits of bovine colostrum. In the U.S. and worldwide, colostrum has been studied for decades and recognized for many of its beneficial properties. In the 1950s colostrum was used to treat rheumatoid arthritis. Shortly thereafter, Albert Sabin, the physician who developed the polio vaccine, created that vaccine by using antibodies found in bovine colostrum. There have been other notable uses as well. These include using bovine colostrum to:

- *Promote athletic performance* by increasing an insulin-growth factor (IGF-1) in athletes during speed- and strength-training sessions. IGF-1, a component of bovine colostrum, acts as a hormone and stimulates cell growth. It also improves the intestine's ability to use food and protein more effectively by repairing the intestinal wall in order to make absorption of vitamins and minerals more efficient.
- *Enhance the immune system* by successfully decreasing the frequency of diarrhea in patients who have compromised immune systems. It has also been used to decrease diarrhea in children with rotavirus and those with acquired immunodeficiency syndrome (AIDS).
- *Protect against infections*, including: infectious diarrhea, cryptosporidiosis, caused by the Cryptosporidium parasite, a common cause of diarrhea in children in particular; shigellosis, a type of bacillary dysentery caused by shigella bacteria occurring mostly in children; a variety of microor-

ganisms, including *Helicobacter pylori* in adults, which is a proven precursor to stomach ulcers.

- *Promote health at a cellular level* by effectively interfering with the herpes virus mechanism of action, leading to necrosis or apoptosis of the infected cell.

Clearly, there are many factors in colostrum that help protect us. Bovine colostrum can be safely used by any mammal, including humans, because most of its constituents have a molecular structure similar to our own. This means bovine colostrum contains virtually the same ingredients as human colostrum, although some are at greater levels.

The importance of colostrum to our immune system cannot be overstated. In an era when resistance to antibiotics has reached alarming proportions, and we are assaulted daily by environmental toxins, it is essential that our immune systems work efficiently. Colostrum provides us with the elements needed to maintain a healthy immune system. It has been shown to increase and repair cells, which makes it useful in creating a healthier gastrointestinal tract. It protects against infectious agents that enter our body through the gastrointestinal wall and promotes the general health and healing of our body. Colostrum strengthens and improves the way our bodies work in addition to providing many anti-aging benefits.

THE AGING PROCESS

The Fountain of Youth Rediscovered

The search for youth started long before Spanish explorer Ponce de León roamed the New World seeking the fountain of youth. Much of that search, then and now, has focused on the superficial effects of aging—graying hair, wrinkles and reduced endurance. However, aging is far more than the physical changes in our body's appearance.

While "feeling old" may be a state of mind, the aging process itself is a biological one. Thus, no matter how young we feel, our body goes through physiological changes. These changes bring about a decline in our ability to fight disease and infection. They also affect our central nervous system and alter our cellular structures, which, in turn, affect our muscles, skin and skeletal form.

However, it is possible that the fountain of youth—or a part of it, anyway—has been found in colostrum. For the 63% of American adults who report they are concerned about the effects of aging, and the 19 million people expected to be over age 85 by 2050, this is great news.

But just how is colostrum able to do all this? To understand better how colostrum works and how it can help slow down the aging process, it will help to understand what happens biologically as we grow older.

OUR CELLS AND TISSUES

When we are young, our cells duplicate, but as we age, something scientists call a senescent factor (SF) comes into play. The SF causes the cell duplication to slow down or even stop. Part of the slowdown factor, or the SF, is due to free radicals, which are those internal agents that have an extra electron and thus damage our healthy cells.

Our cells also become larger as we age and this, too, impedes the process of the necessary division and reproduction. Pigments and fatty substances (lipids) inside the cell increase and many cells stop functioning or function incorrectly. The cell membranes change too, making it more difficult for them to get the oxygen and nutrients they need. Our connective tissues change and become stiff. This makes the organs, blood vessels and airways more rigid. Because our cells and tissues change, our organs begin to lose their ability to work properly.

The growth factors found in bovine colostrum contain important ingredients that can stimulate new cell growth, thus increasing elasticity and potentially improving oxygenation.

Our Muscles

Between the ages of 50 and 70, we lose about 15% of our muscles each decade. When we hit 80, we've lost about 30% of our muscle strength. This loss in muscle strength can contribute to problems in walking and cause falls, hip fractures, herniated disks and back pain. The decline in muscle strength stems, in part, from a decrease in skeletal muscle fiber that comes with aging and disease. Colostrum provides our bodies with the necessary factors to maintain more muscle mass and bone density as we age.

Our Immune System

If our immune system is not armed and working well, we become increasingly at risk for many life-threatening illnesses. Allergies, viruses, autoimmune diseases such as HIV and cancers are all evidence that the immune system has been compromised and may not be functioning as it should.

Our immune system protects us from damage from free radicals, infections from injuries and burns, and aging prematurely. Immunity is a state of heightened resistance or accelerated reactivity toward microbes or foreign organisms that enter our body. It is the job of the immune system, which comprises millions of cells, numerous chemicals, glands and organs, all of which work together via a complex communication system. Some of the more significant components of the immune system are the immunoglobulins. Significant amounts of immunoglobulins IgG, IgA and IgM are found in bovine colostrum. They circulate in the body fluids and attack bacteria, viruses and toxins that enter the body.

There are two subsystems of the immune system: the humoral and the cell-mediated. Each part is necessary and must function properly in order for the body to produce the best response to invading pathogens. B-cells and T-cells, both of which are white blood cells, recognize foreign organisms and control the attack against them. B-cells, located in our bone marrow, make antibodies. T-cells, which are manufactured in the thymus gland, move through our system and kill the invading organisms. These cells can be thought of as the master planners in the immune network. B-cells are used in the humoral system while T-cells are part of the cell-mediated system. In fact, B-cells will react more quickly and proliferate more efficiently in the presence of a T-cell response.

The immune system is more than white blood cells and antibodies. Other cells and tissues are involved too. Our skin acts as a shield against invading microorganisms and it, along with the mucus linings of our respiratory and digestive tracts, contains antibodies. For that reason, these mucus linings are very important, for without them, our ability to fight off infection would be severely compromised and the aging process would be accelerated.

We also have proteins that circulate within our system to assist the humoral and cell-mediated immune factors. Some of the important circulating proteins are lactoferrin, lysozymes, cytokines and lactoperoxidase. They attach themselves to the bacteria and viruses and destroy them by activating the killing functions of the immune system.

Aging and the Immune System

As we age, however, some of our immune responses lag. While we may maintain some of our immunity, new toxins become more prevalent. Bacteria is becoming increasingly resistant to available antibiotics, further impeding our ability to stay healthy and young

In addition, our T-cell response may decrease. This is the crux of the problem. As we age, our T-cells and B-cells can no longer undergo rapid cell division. As a result, the immune system can't keep up with the rate at which the bacterial or viral cells divide and spread. So as we age, we tend to be ill more often and more seriously. The end result of these changes in immune function is our body's vulnerability to infectious diseases, cancers and general lethargy and malaise. Nutritional deficiencies can also compromise the immune system and accelerate aging.

There are simply too many factors that adversely affect our immune system. To help fight disease, we need to help the immune system return to its original order. We can do this by enhancing the way it responds. The key to anti-aging is the maintenance of a properly functioning immune system. Colostrum can help.

COLOSTRUM: THE ANTI-AGING CONNECTION

While the changes to our cells, muscles and immune system sound like a series of irreversible processes, they can be slowed with colostrum because of the growth factors it contains. Among its myriad ingredients, colostrum contains natural antibiotic factors:

- immunoglobulins, substances that neutralize toxins, viruses and bacteria, particularly in the digestive and respiratory systems
- cytokines, small proteins that affect the behavior of other cells
- antibodies (IgG, IgA, IgD, IgE and IgM), substances that aid in cellular, muscular and skeletal growth
- lactoferrin, a substance that neutralizes bacteria and helps release cytokines

Immunoglobulins

Immunoglobulins, or antibodies, specifically recognize any foreign compound that enters the body. When one enters, various antibodies direct themselves to different areas of the invader and attack it, wherever it is in the body.

During our lives, we are exposed to a variety of foreign substances and rely on a vast array of antibody-producing lymphocytes (more than 100 million by some estimates) that we build over time and that persist at low levels for years. Their goal is to surface again if we are exposed to the same substance. The immune system is able to remember what we have been infected with and often can prevent us from being infected again, which is the premise on which vaccines work.

The most abundant antibodies in the bloodstream are of the immunoglobulin G class, IgG, but there are also IgA, IgD, IgE and IgM classes. These antibodies have similar structures but different functional properties. For example, immunoglobulin A, or IgA, plays a key role in mucosal immunity, which is of particular importance in maintenance of mucosal health and avoidance of infection, while IgG neutralizes toxins and microbes in the lymph and circulatory system.

Antibodies carry out two basic functions. First, they bind specifically to molecules from the foreign substance that caused the immune system to respond. Second, they recruit other cells and molecules to destroy the substance once the antibody is bound to it. Antibodies can also block receptors on cells and prevent viruses from entering cells.

When we think our antibodies are not responding well enough to something like an infection, we may take a series of antibiotics, but, by doing so, we reduce the body's active immune response to that organism, whatever it may be. In essence, this means that the next time we face the same organism, our own immune response will likely be less effective than it otherwise would have been. Even when an antibiotic is properly prescribed and works as it should, it does not just kill the offending organism. It also kills others that perform important functions, such as bacteria that aid in the breakdown and digestion of food.

Any process that can replenish our natural antibodies and keep them strong has massive potential, and also has many implications. Imagine a natural food or supplement, such as colostrum, that provides a natural immunity against bacteria and viruses, allowing us to rely less on antibiotics. Using colostrum can assist our immune system.

GROWTH FACTORS

Although there are clearly many ingredients in colostrum that are of utmost importance, perhaps it is the growth factors that hold the most promise in slowing the aging process. Growth factors stimulate our skeletal and muscle growth on a cellular level while regulating our metabolism. The growth factors contained in colostrum include:

- epithelial growth factor (EGF)
- insulin-like growth factor-I and II (IGF-1 and IGF-2)
- fibroblast growth factor (FGF)
- platelet-derived growth factor (PDGF)
- transforming growth factors A and B (TGA and TGB)

Children need these growth factors to flourish. If they are absent, then growth hormone therapy is prescribed. But such replacement therapy is not often done for adults, even though data indicate that adults who have abnormal body composition can benefit from growth hormone replacement. Specifically, the researchers found that GH replacement in adults with growth hormone deficiencies resulted in marked alterations in body composition, fat distribution, bone-mineral density.

Growth hormone helps our long bones, joints and muscles grow. As we age, we create less GH and we tend to experience osteoporosis and less lean muscle mass. Yet several studies done in the 1990s indicate that—at least in older men—the administration of GH can slow this aging process by lowering body fat content, increasing lean muscle mass, increasing bone-mineral density and improving skin moisture and elasticity.

A study published in the *New England Journal of Medicine* concluded that GH treatment could prevent some signs of aging. Dr. Daniel Rudman treated 26 men between the ages of 61–80 with GH. He documented that his patients experienced a decrease in overall body fat, as well as an increase in bone density and lean muscle mass. He also reported an increase in skin thickness and elasticity in these patients.

Another study found that long-term, low-dose growth hormone treatment in mice significantly prolonged their life expectancy. Similar data even suggest that those without the needed levels of growth hormones have a much higher mortality rate!

In my mind, this is certainly one of the top benefits of colostrum. Taking colostrum provides us with essential growth factors, immune factors, antibiotic factors, vitamins, minerals and antioxidants. It is a whole and complete food and/or supplement.

Colostrum's Package of Growth Hormones

Each of the growth factors in colostrum helps stimulate cell and tissue growth by activating DNA formation. In fact, epithelial growth factor (EGF) demonstrates the highest ability to stimulate epithelial (skin) regeneration on wounds.

EGF is a protein that helps protect and maintain the skin. When it is combined with insulin-like growth factors, it works even better—and this is what happens with colostrum. Unlike other supplements that provide only single growth factors, colostrum combines a complete package of growth factors that work together synergistically, as nature intended.

Most of the anti-aging effects of GH therapy are a result of increasing the body's concentration of IGF-1 and IGF-2. IGF-1 and IGF-2 are the most active ingredients found in bovine colostrum. They tell the body how to use the fat, sugar and protein that it gets from food. They also control how cells grow and repair themselves. The fact that colostrum contains these growth factors, and that aging is a result of low levels of growth factors, suggests that colostrum could help counteract the biological aging process. Studies have shown that taking bovine colostrum by mouth can increase the body's IGF-1 levels.

IGF-1 can also stimulate the growth and repair of DNA and RNA, the two most important ingredients in a cell. DNA contains all our genetic information and RNA controls how we synthesize protein.

Bovine colostrum is the only natural source for IGF-1. IGF-1 accelerates our healing process; balances our blood glucose and reduces the need for insulin; increases muscle mass and strength; and assists in bone growth and repair. In addition, IGF-1 is capable of increasing T-cell production. And T-cells, the ones that help control our immune reactions, also release cytokines, which activate the immune system.

CYTOKINES

The benefits of using cytokines for the treatment of cancer were first made known by the book *Quiet Strides in the War on Cancer*, written by Steven Rosenberg in 1985. Since then, cytokines found in colostrum have been one of the most researched protocols in the cure for cancer. Cytokines act as anti-inflammatories and help boost the production of other immun-oglobulins. As we grow older, however, our cytokine production is reduced by a significant extent. It also seems that cytokines might be responsible for regulating our immunological and metabolic responses.

Thus, as we age, we produce and have access to fewer of the essential substances that we need to maintain our health. It is estimated that colostrum triggers at least 50 processes in breast-fed infants. In adulthood, we should try to maintain that same level of nutrition through whole-food nutrition and dietary supplements. For this, colostrum is the natural choice.

THE IMPORTANCE OF A HEALTHY DIGESTIVE ENVIRONMENT

The digestive tract is the source of a vast majority of our body's immunity. As infants take colostrum from their mothers' breasts, the cells of the digestive organ begin to develop. Too often we forget the relationship between what we eat and how the food is processed. If the cells and organs are not healthy, then even the best diet will be of no benefit. Simply stated, if our intestine is unusually permeable, then bacteria, viruses and other toxins may enter the bloodstream. This can lead to inflammation, food allergies, and a malabsorption of minerals. Some of the more common culprits that cause a leaky gut include the use of non-steroidal anti-inflammatories (NSAIDs), antibiotics, birth control pills, caffeine and alcohol. The result of a leaky gut is a compromised immune system.

Research has shown that colostrum can help maintain a healthy digestive environment and prevent the development of a leaky gut. Moreover, the growth factors in colostrum play a key role by keeping the intestinal mucosa sealed and impermeable to toxins. Colostrum has been shown to prevent gastrointestinal tract injury caused by NSAIDs. It has been shown to provide the ingredients we need to help with nutrient absorption. In essence, colostrum's anti-inflammatory factors help repair the damaged intestinal walls.

WHAT WE CAN LOOK FOR IN THE FUTURE

While the idea of replacing our dwindling immune system with human colostrum may be appealing, it cannot happen. There just isn't enough of it. However, that is not the case with bovine colostrum. In fact, bovine colostrum offers greater amounts of immunoglobulins than does human colostrum, and the benefits of bovine colostrum are biologically transferable to all mammals, including human. Also, bovine colostrum is much higher in immune factors than a human mother's colostrum, and it is in plentiful supply.

When choosing a colostrum, we must pay close attention to how the colostrum is processed. The effectiveness of the colostrum (as with any whole food) will be reduced if it isn't processed properly. Excessive heat is particularly bad. Also, if colostrum is frozen, as is most colostrum, the resultant substance is not water-soluble and is thus very difficult for humans to assimilate, as it doesn't readily disperse in the intestinal tract.

More importantly, excessive heat and cold can destroy the beneficial, bioactive ingredients found in bovine colostrum. However, as more people become aware of this substance—one of nature's great miracles—we hopefully will see fewer poorly processed and poorly packaged colostrum products. Make it your priority to become informed and purchase only the highest quality and properly processed colostrum to ensure maximum effectiveness.

More research is being conducted. Here is just a partial list of the ways bovine colostrum can potentially help us:

- rheumatoid arthritis: colostrum can reduce inflammation
- osteoarthritis and osteoporosis
- colostrum can build bone density
- transplantation: the immunoglobulins could help reduce infection with fungus and bacteria
- cancer fighters: the cytokines in colostrum include the powerful interleukins
- a slowing of the HIV virus: colostrum can reduce the infectious pathogens that cause related conditions
- reduction in obesity: colostrum can help your body better utilize the food it eats
- wrinkles and aging: colostrum cream can moisturize skin to help reduce the effects and appearance of aging

CONCLUSION

Bovine colostrum is one of nature's greatest miracles. Its nutritional properties alone are of tremendous value to us. The highly beneficial immune and growth factors present in bovine colostrum offer considerable possibilities for the prevention and recovery of illnesses and diseases. Colostrum also offers doctors, researchers and the general population great hope in the quest for treatments that will help reverse the aging process.

There have already been many reported studies and uses for colostrum to date, and this is just the beginning. Based on the current popularity of natural substances and whole-food supplements, we should continue to witness a substantial increase in the amount of public interest, scientific research and studies and the number of uses for bovine colostrum worldwide. Remember to stay informed.

14

Waking Up Younger

GERRY'S STORY

Gerry (a pseudonym) had been feeling under the weather for some time. She had consulted me for problems that might be labeled non-specific organic dysfunction. The term really means nothing, except that Gerry was just feeling bad all over. Her immune system didn't seem to respond as well as she would have liked, but there were no clinical or laboratory signs of immune dysfunction. She had the impression that her energy was far from being the level it was a year or so ago. Worst of all for Gerry, her mental clarity and focus were impaired. Here again, there were no objective signs of dysfunction. There were also monthly bouts with depression and anxiety that seemed to be related to her menstrual cycle, but laboratory assessments of hormone function also came back as normal.

We worked on improving Gerry's diet, eliminating any possible foods to which she might be intolerant, and suggested a comprehensive nutritional supplement program. Gerry improved. After about one month she felt she was 40% better. This, however, was not enough according to her. Gerry was a single mother of three small children and had recently returned to private practice as a lawyer, so, like many of you reading this book, Gerry just couldn't afford to have less than exuberant energy.

After further reviewing Gerry's lifestyle, we decided to work on a very simple but often forgotten health factor—her sleep. Her sleep wasn't that bad, but it wasn't that good either. Gerry finally realized that the only infallible way of treating her fatigue was to rest. After three weeks of an improved sleep pattern, Gerry was feeling 90% better. Both she and I were surprised at the positive effects improved sleep had on her energy, immunity, hormonal balance and, yes, even her skin and hair.

Gerry's incredible recovery from a systemic dysfunction was improved with dietary and lifestyle changes. However, significant improvement was precipitated by an improvement in her sleep habits and patterns. Understanding the effects of sleep on health and well-being will help us understand the vital importance of this non-activity on recuperation and healing, adaptation to stress and longevity.

WHAT IS SLEEP?

One definition states that sleep is "a state of unconsciousness from which a person can be aroused by appropriate sensory or other stimuli" (Arthur Gyton, *Medical Physiology*).

Of course, we know that we need sleep. Although a considerable amount of research has been done on sleep, it remains largely a mystery. Within the last two decades more than 15,000 scientific articles have been published on sleep in an attempt to explain its effects and understand its secrets.

What Happens During Sleep?

First of all, there is a relative unconsciousness in sleep. When you are awake, you know what's going on around you. You can see, feel, hear and respond with thoughts and actions. When you are asleep, your senses—most of them anyway—have become temporarily dormant. They still function, but most of their messages are not reaching your brain. In deep sleep you are not conscious of anything in your environment, at least you don't remember it.

Sleep, of course, is more than just unconsciousness. It is a very complex phenomenon and is controlled by a variety of actions within the brain itself and by certain environmental influences.

The human brain is a masterpiece. It is encased in a solid frame of bone and further protected by the spinal fluid in which it floats and a fibrous sling, called tentorium, in which it is cradled and held in place by ligaments.

Although it is one of the most powerful of our biological organs—and the only one we can't replace—it is one of the most vulnerable. In order to function, the brain must have at least minimum levels of oxygen, glucose, hydration, amino acids and fatty acids. If these are not available in the required amounts, the brain dies. Depriving the brain of oxygen for just 8 minutes, for example, produces irreversible damage to the brain cells.

One of the most important functions of the brain is its attention response, which results in consciousness or awareness. This awareness gives us the ability to take action, either to supply our needs (such as eating when we are hungry) or to conceptualize and be creative. Furthermore, it gives us our special individual and personal identity, our capacity to love and make intelligent choices.

In order to find out where this awareness function originates in the brain, technology was developed in the 1950s for measuring the electrical discharges in brain cells. Using animal models, one attention response center was found by stimulating a certain area in the cortex of the parietal lobes.

A further breakthrough came when a plant enzyme, horseradish peroxidase, was used as a chemical tag to trace nerve connections within the brain. Researchers discovered that these parietal cells had a two-way communication with such areas as the emotional control of the limbic system, the reticular network of the brain stem and certain motor areas such as the muscles that control eye movement, the hypothalamus and the pituitary gland.

The messages of the brain are carried within the nerve cell by an electric current. At the point where one nerve cell connects with another is a tiny gap called a synapse. The electric current cannot jump across this gap. Here transmission is achieved by certain chemical messengers that we refer to as neurotransmitters. Once the message reaches the membrane of the other cell, it is again converted into an electrical signal. Proper functioning of this mechanism is essential to mental health.

Neurotransmitters are related to the mechanism of sleep because they may either increase or reduce consciousness. The neurotransmitter acetylcholine, for example, stimulates certain hormones that aid memory and awareness. It keeps you awake. On the other hand, the neurotransmitter serotonin inhibits awareness and helps initiate sleep. Serotonin is made from the amino acid tryptophan. In combination with vitamins C and B6, tryptophan taken just before bedtime can promote sleep by increasing the amount of serotonin in the brain. When tryptophan is unavailable without a prescription, as is the case in Canada, a plant called *Griffonia* is an excellent source of hydroxy tryptophan, the active form of this nutrient.

So the internal workings of the brain with its electrical currents and chemical messengers have much to do with our state of consciousness and our sleep cycles.

The Role of Neurotransmitters

Neurotransmitters have many other functions. The catacholamine neuro-transmitters, norepinephrine and dopamine, are chemically related to each other and can be interchanged by simple chemical reconstruction. Both have different and specific functions, but in general they maintain alertness and are involved in movement, sexual function, behavior and memory. Dopamine causes the release of the growth hormone from the pituitary, which occurs mainly during sleep. The growth hormone is very important in the aging process. This hormone has a role to play in protein synthesis involved in muscle and bone production, and if its production is reduced, by lack of sleep, for example, there may be less repair after the wear and tear. Less repair means accelerated aging. One study, published in the prestigious *Journal of the American Medical Association*, confirmed the idea that reduced sleep did indeed affect growth hormone as well as cortisol levels. Researchers from the Université de Liège in Belgium found that even these effects on hormones may in turn affect the body's capacity to regulate blood sugar levels. This might be an interesting avenue to follow in treating people with diabetes or hypoglycemics.

The neurotransmitter acetylcholine stimulates the production of the hormone vasopressin, which helps memory control and regulates urine volume and, to a lesser extent, blood pressure.

THE MYSTERIES OF OUR CIRCADIAN RHYTHM

Along with these internal chemical and electrical events, environmental factors also influence our state of consciousness. The rotation of the earth on its axis, producing night and day, and the yearly circling of the earth in an elliptical path around the sun, producing the seasons of the year, bring into play gravitational forces that affect our bodies' rhythms.

Sleep, the most profound reduction of consciousness that we usually experience, occurs every 24 hours and is part of our circadian or daily rhythm. There appears to be no single master clock to control all of our body rhythms, yet our bodies enjoy the synchronization of all these rhythms. How this is done is not fully understood. Probably several different clocks in the brain carry out this function. A recent study by Sancar and Miyamoto, published in the *Proceedings of the National Academy of Sciences*, discovered that light affects two proteins, cryptochrome 1 and 2. These two proteins are involved in controlling the circadian rhythm. They are affected by light flashed on the skin, not necessarily in the eyes. Light, therefore, could affect our sleeping patterns, even when our eyes are closed or when we sleep. Our ancestors, who had the advantage of sleeping in an environment where there was little ambient light (like our street lights, night-lights, alarm clock light, etc.), slept much better than we do.

TYPES OF SLEEP

As any anesthesiologist will tell you, when the patient under anesthesia first starts to go to sleep, the eyes move rapidly and in many directions. As the patient goes deeper into unconsciousness, these eye movements stop. This phenomenon also happens in normal sleep. In 1953, two medical researchers studied sleep in infants at Children's Hospital in Hollywood. They noticed periodic, jerky movements in the eyes of sleeping babies. When the researchers studied adults, they found that these eye movements occurred during light sleep for a period of 10–12 minutes. At the end of this time the eye movements disappeared and sleep appeared to enter a deeper state. These researchers further discovered that people sleep in cycles. They move back and forth between light sleep and deep sleep four or five times in an 8-hour period. Since these observations, sleep has been classified into two main categories, REM (rapid eye movements) and NREM (no rapid eye movements). Some prefer the classification of desynchronized and synchronized sleep.

Remember Gerry? Well, she was typical of many patients I have seen who couldn't sleep. Even with seven hours of sleep, she never really felt rested. She continued to be tired and irritable, and complained of problems with her memory. The reason was simple—she was not getting enough REM sleep.

During REM sleep muscles relax and the electromyograph shows little activity except for eye movements. During this stage our dreams seem more vivid and there is better dream recall. REM sleep should make up 20–25% of our total sleep time if we want to get the restorative, healing and anti-aging benefits of sleep.

Alcohol and certain drugs, including most sedatives, actually work against this type of sleep. We may sleep soundly through the night, but usually we will not feel as refreshed as we would have been if our sleep came naturally. This is one difference between plant sedatives and pharmaceutical sedatives. Most plant sedatives actually increase REM—quality—sleep whereas most drugs actually interfere with it.

If you do not get enough REM sleep during one night, you will try to make up for this when you can. During the next sleep period there will be a REM rebound. You will spend more time in the REM stage to make up for the loss.

One of the laboratory experiments illustrates this rebound. A sleeping subject was awakened whenever the rapid eye movements were present.

During the first night he had to be awakened only five times. But on following nights he had to be awakened more and more frequently. His body was simply trying to make up for the loss of REM sleep. One night he had to be awakened 200 times!

NOT ENOUGH SLEEP?

When I was teaching, certain students were notorious for their "all-nighters." When the final exams came around, their final grades, all other factors being equal, were not that good. What they may have gained from their last-minute cramming, they lost in memory, concentration and inefficiency—all from lack of sleep. Though there are several studies on the subject, I'll mention just one, published in *Brain Research*. Researchers concluded that REM sleep may be associated with factors that contribute to memory functions. As a matter of fact, one study demonstrated that moderate sleep deprivation led to cognitive impairments equal to those caused by alcohol intoxication.

As you can see, depriving yourself of sleep will interfere with all your body functions. It will reduce the growth and repair process of every tissue while affecting memory and learning capacity. It will seriously restrict your efficiency. Losing too much sleep can even cause depression, paranoid delusions and hallucinations.

How Much Sleep Do We Need?

Research hasn't given us a definitive answer as to how much sleep we really need or how much sleep we can do without. According to the 1984 edition of the *Guinness Book of World Records,* the record for going without sleep under medical supervision was set in 1968 by a 52-year-old woman in Capetown, South Africa, who remained sleepless for 11 days, 18 hours and 55 minutes. Other people have come close to that record but their experiments had to be terminated because of paranoid delusions and hallucinations.

Of course, some people have claimed to be able to go on without sleep for years! Thomas Edison and Napoleon Bonaparte both thought they went without sleep. Observers, however, reported that both men catnapped; it is estimated that each of these men got approximately 4 hours' sleep in short naps over a 24-hour period.

The amount of sleep needed for good health differs with age. Newborn babies may sleep 16–20 hours a day. Young children need 10–12 hours of sleep daily. By age 40 most adults need six to seven hours of sleep a day. The amount of sleep seems to be associated with the need to grow. Or, is the growth potential affected by the amount of sleep?

After 40 there is a slight increase in the amount of sleep needed. This continues until about age 70 when the need declines again. This increase and decrease of sleep needed may be related to brain metabolism, including the production of chemicals like melatonin. The more active the brain, the more sleep needed. Very young children have almost twice the brain activity of young people, so they require twice the amount of sleep.

One study on sleep involved 1 million men and women between 45 and 85 or more years of age. It showed that those who had seven hours of sleep per night had the lowest death rates. Those who had more or less than seven hours had death rates that increased in proportion to the difference.

It might be well for all of us to experiment a little with our sleeping habits if we haven't done so already. See how well you get along on seven hours of sleep each night. Don't stay in bed for nine hours if you can function on seven. This is the principle of effective economy. Sleep as much as you need to without sleeping more than you have to.

How About Lost Sleep?
As I work on this chapter, my workload is heavier than usual, so I have also had to cut down on my sleep. I know, however, that lost sleep can never be completely recovered, yet there seems to be no permanent ill effect from occasional losses.

One who goes for two days without sleep, if given the opportunity, will sleep 12 hours, not 16. Studies indicate we need about 75% of the sleep lost in order to recuperate, not the entire 100%.

The best sleep comes from an uninterrupted period of six or seven hours. Short naps and even a 30-minute siesta can be very relaxing and restful because it may break up the stress and monotony of a long day's work. These, however, don't replace sufficient sleep during a single stretch of time.

Sleep Disturbances
Even normal sleep will have its disturbances. Few of them are really serious, and most of them will respond to treatment and proper management.

One of the most common sleep disturbances is the irritable leg syndrome. It is characterized by rhythmic jerks or muscle twitching that occurs just when one wants to drop off to a restful sleep. This condition can rob us of sleep and may even be a bit frightening.

Occasionally the muscle twitching is caused by muscle fatigue. Perhaps overworked legs are complaining. Hot applications, massage and rest will usually handle this problem. In many cases, this is a sign of calcium deficiency. Calcium is not only involved in bone formation, but is also a muscle and nerve relaxant. Calcium supplementation can therefore be helpful in many cases. It is preferable to use a form of calcium that is well absorbed, such as calcium citrate. Certain herbs, such as scullcap and passionflower, may also help relieve the twitching if it is not calcium related.

Sometimes the cause of the twitching is neurological, in which motor signals are sent to the nerve-end plates producing segmental muscular contractions. At other times impaired circulation may be a factor. Circulation can be improved with vitamin E as well as with herbs such as aged garlic extract, ginkgo biloba and hawthorn. Of course, if the symptoms are debilitating or if they do not respond to nutrient or herbal treatment, it is important to get a diagnosis from a health professional. Holistic MDs, chiropractors and naturopathic physicians are most indicated when it comes to this type of sleep disorder.

Most people have experienced the sensation of a sudden jerk just as they are going to sleep. This is usually a psychophysiological phenomenon caused by the sensation of falling as they pass the threshold of consciousness. I've certainly experienced this a few times. Anyone falling instinctively tries to grab for support. Don't worry about this experience. It is perfectly benign! One of the best remedies for this problem is quite simple. Take a brief walk before bedtime. A footbath may also help! The *Journal of Physiology, Anthropology and Applied Human Sciences* published research by Japanese scientists who found that a bath, or foot bath, helped facilitate earlier sleep onset.

Some people have an overwhelming urge to fall asleep during waking hours, even when they have had plenty of sleep the night before. This happens more often during periods of decreased activity or boredom. This sleep problem is called narcolepsy. These sleep periods are usually brief, lasting no more than 10 or 15 minutes. It often occurs after meals because of improper liver function or blood sugar regulation. Herbal formulas such as Liv-Tone™ can help support liver function. Reducing the amount of refined sugars in the diet and supporting adrenal (stress glands) function with adrena+ can also be very helpful. Exercise and vigorous walking are also helpful.

Sleepwalking? This is a less common sleep disturbance. Sleepwalking occurs during the deep stage of sleep. It is very likely that increased mental activity and unpleasant dreams are factors in this subconscious activity. There is no specific treatment for sleepwalking, but anything that relaxes you before going to bed will help, such as a quiet time, a short walk, meditation, a warm shower or a bath with relaxing essential oils such as lavender. Kava kava is a herb that helps relieve anxiety and may be useful here.

Insomnia

Insomnia is the most common of all sleep disorders. It consists of either difficulty in falling asleep or staying asleep. Insomnia may be caused by emotional disturbances such as anxiety or depression, by recounting the day's events, or even by anticipating and worrying about what will happen tomorrow.

However, there are often physical reasons for insomnia as well. These include pain, hunger, being too cold or hot, persistent cough, congestion or an overactive thyroid. Anything that makes one uncomfortable obviously interferes with the ability to fall asleep or to stay asleep.

Sometimes the fear of insomnia itself keeps one awake. Prescription drugs are not the answer for the majority of insomniacs. It is true that some of the tranquilizers such as lormetazapam and flurazepam can be used for short periods without interfering with REM sleep. But sedative drugs can also be a cause of insomnia. The most widely used drug that contributes to insomnia is caffeine. This drug is found in coffee, tea, cola drinks, kola nut and guarana as well as other drinks where caffeine is added. Several weight-loss formulas that act on the body's capacity to burn fat will contain caffeine. Caffeine consumption is probably the most unsuspected cause of insomnia in North America. If you drink coffee or caffeinated beverages, try to avoid doing so after midday.

How to Handle Insomnia

I've briefly touched on some of the causes of insomnia. And, although insomnia is one type of disorder for which drugs are prescribed the most, I am convinced that this leads nowhere. It treats the symptom, rather than the cause, of the problem. As I mentioned earlier, most sedatives reduce REM sleep, whereas most herbs actually improve it.

On page 231 in Part III, you will find a list of suggestions that have proven very helpful. They are at least worth trying out.

CONCLUSION

As we have seen, sleep has a major role to play in lessening symptoms associated with aging or premature aging. Symptoms such as reduced muscle tone or growth, blood sugar abnormalities, reduced memory and cognitive capacity affect the quality as much as the quantity of our lives. It is therefore vital, within a comprehensive life-extension program, to maintain or acquire proper sleep patterns to offset the premature aging most North Americans are plagued with. Aging could very well be something we can sleep away. Not convinced yet? Maybe you'll want to sleep on it!

15

The Aging Process: How to Slow or Reverse It with Albumin

Kenneth E. Seaton, D.Sc.

WHAT IS ALBUMIN?

Albumin is the most studied yet least understood of all proteins. It serves as the body's carrier for vitamins, minerals, fatty acids and hormones. One of the reasons albumin is needed is that the transport ability of the blood is critical to health and cells must receive nutrients, hormones and electrolytes in the correct amount and at the right time. Albumin is also needed for cell growth, stability and long life. This was dramatically demonstrated in experiments where cells lasted 10 times longer, grew stronger and none converted to cancer lines when the medium contained the optimal quantity and quality of albumin. This study showed a profound benefit of increasing the quantity of highly purified albumin in the medium. Human cells continued to grow equivalent to over 150 years, and none converted to cancer lines. Why? It appears to be the life factor, with albumin probably delivering and collecting electrons from cells, perhaps via nitric oxide, which it transports.

An example of albumin is the white of eggs or an important protein in milk. Unfortunately, high-protein diets will not raise albumin levels while there is stress on the immune system. Infusion of albumin in hospitals to save lives following severe trauma may be warranted; however, the outcome is often negative, and this approach does not address the stress and globulin levels.

Importance of Albumin

Albumin is the most abundant, dominant, versatile and complex protein in the body fluids, averaging a total of around 350 g. Sixty percent of the serum proteins are albumin, with a mean level in the U.S. of around 42 g/L (4.2 g/dL). Optimal serum albumin levels for maximum life span are around 52–56 g/L. Long regarded as the "bellwether" of health, its many roles are just beginning to be understood.

Albumin easily answers the waste theory of aging, the free radical theory, the autoimmune theory, the cross-linking theory, the protein synthesis theory, ionizing theory, and the results achieved with calorie restriction. In summary, the multifactorial evidence in aging is answered by maintaining albumin levels around 50 g/L, with an A/G ratio of 2.0.

All eggs, seeds, fetuses and brains are surrounded with a generous supply of albumin. At commencement of lactation, milk contains especially high albumin levels. Cell growth requires optimal albumin. No other substance has so many roles or could possibly be the "life factor." The major role of the liver is manufacturing albumin (a half-ton in a lifetime), and it also serves as a packet of perfect amino acids, controlling the entire protein synthesis. Maintaining optimal albumin profiles can only be achieved by advanced hygiene techniques. Attempts to raise albumin by high-protein diets, vitamins, minerals, herbs, supplements and infusion is the ultimate in metabolic misunderstanding.

HYGIENE AND THE AGING PROCESS

Overactivation of the immune system may result in elevated inflammatory and immune proteins potentially leading to reduced carrier proteins—particularly albumin—setting a biochemical environment associated with suboptimal aging. Advanced personal hygiene may be an effective way to reduce this stress on the immune system/biochemistry and physiology. Cleanliness may be next to godliness (scientifically) after all!

Hippocrates (400 B.C.) presented a very astute description of the aging process when he noted, "Old humans suffer difficulty of breathing, catarrh, coughing, strangury, passing urine, pain of joints, kidney disease, dizziness, stroke, ill health with wasting, itchiness, sleeplessness, water discharge from bowels, nose and eyes, cataracts and hardness of hearing."

An answer to all these problems may simply be better hygiene. Better hygiene may slow and, to some degree, reverse the aging process and many of its physical problems.

It may also be possible to reduce wrinkling of the skin, loss of hair, dimming of the vision, dementia, wasting, changes in the biochemistry and loss of immunological performance that were once considered a fundamental part of aging.

Many species of fish, dolphins, whales, seabirds and other creatures reach their maximum life span looking much as they did when they were younger, avoiding to an amazing degree many of the physical problems that we humans think is normal in aging. Because of their life in the water, is the secret simple hygiene?

STRESS

A paradox is the extreme rapid aging of the Pacific salmon after spawning, which is equivalent to the last 40 years of our lives but which occurs in the fish in only a few days. Rapid aging in the salmon is caused by a massive production of the stress hormone cortisol; at the same time, there is a major reduction in albumin and cortisol-binding globulin. This biochemical stress process also is associated with the rapid aging of the marsupial mouse, octopus and several other creatures, including humans.

How is this stress linked to hygiene? The buffer against damaging cortisol is the concentration of albumin in body fluids. Albumin can bind over 1000 times the capacity of the cortisol-binding globulin (CBG); thus, the higher the concentration of albumin, which is also accompanied by a rise in CBG, the better buffered the animal is against stress and aging. The stress on the immune system reduces carrier protein levels because it elevates defense/inflammatory proteins.

The carrying capacity of serum appears to be a fundamental factor in aging. Osmotic pressure (which refers to the pressure exerted by the concentration of both water and dissolved substances inside and outside a membrane or cell) determines that when defense/inflammatory proteins are reduced naturally and safely, carrier proteins are raised. Albumin is the major carrier; a remarkable universal mother ship. But is albumin the "aging factor" or the "life factor"? And are albumin levels determined by hygiene standards more than any other factor?

Data supplied by Jim McBain, veterinary scientist from Sea World, shows that there is no decline of albumin concentration in their aged dolphins, which are perhaps equivalent to 100-year-old humans. The level of albumin normally falls in all aging animals. The level at Sea World over the decades appears to be increasing in accordance with better techniques of cleaning the water environment. The dolphins with higher albumin levels are also living longer and showing minimal signs of aging.

Edward Masoro, a distinguished researcher on aging, presents the case that long-term, low-level and acute stresses play a role in the basis of aging. Masoro identifies that the exact levels of cortisol are important—without it we would not be able to survive being late for work. Yet excess of this stress hormone damages the thymus and the immune system, prevents repair and unbalances the entire homeostasis. Again, the answer may be better hygiene to maintain very high albumin levels to ensure precise cortisol homeostasis despite the multitude of stresses encountered during the human life span. Accordingly, maintaining higher albumin levels may increase the life span.

Disease and Stress

Illness is the most damaging form of stress. There is epidemiological evidence that low serum albumin levels are associated with increased risk of cancer and other diseases. There is a fine line, almost indistinguishable, between aging and disease. That fine line appears to be the reduction in albumin, as it is the common denominator in both disease and aging.

No breakthrough in anti-aging strategies may occur until we maintain the entire homeostasis of the biochemistry and physiology. Claude Bernard, the renowned physiologist, who taught at the Sorbonne and Collège de France, summed up his research with his famous concept of homeostasis, which he called "milieu interieur" (perfect interior environment). In addition, cells kept in a maximum life span experiment must have a perfect medium in the culture dish. The most important substance in the medium is the quality and quantity of albumin.

You may swim, run, ski, work, make love and sleep, all in conditions that vary dramatically. Yet all the trillions of cells in your body must remain at very precise conditions of temperature, pH and chemical and water balance. Minute changes can cause damage, confusion, even death. Maintaining this dynamic feedback and regulation between all the organs, blood, tissues and cells is homeostasis. Again, the concentration of albumin in the blood and interstitial fluids is a remarkable buffer against dramatic and sudden changes. The answer to maintaining homeostasis is hygiene. Homeostasis may be maintained by special ion baths every night.

SENILE DEMENTIA

No scourge is more feared and no threat to independence is greater than the loss of mental competence that often accompanies aging. Any attempt to solve the problems associated with aging must include preventing senile dementia.

High concentrations of albumin in the serum are needed to ensure optimal levels in the brain and cerebral spinal fluid (CSF), vital for the security and performance of the CSF. Only one in 200 albumin molecules are specially selected to enter the CSF. Albumin is also the amyloid-degrading enzyme and the purifier. This may account for the relationship between intellectual standards and the standard of hygiene/albumin levels in civilizations. Long-term stress, particularly chronic infection, is linked to senile dementia.

THE BASIC TRIANGLE

Three areas have been outlined for maintaining good health during the aging process: diet, exercise and hygiene. Each one of these supports and reinforces the other.

Diet

Repeated studies by labs and zoos around the world over the last 50 years have consistently shown that the aging process can be slowed dramatically by restricting dietary calories. The religious concept of fasting has a sound scientific basis. Unfortunately, dietary restriction is difficult to implement, and it is unlikely to be a popular anti-aging practice, thus placing greater emphasis on hygiene and exercise. Dietary restriction and hygiene appear to function in the same way by reducing the stress on the serum to transport nutrients and wastes. Dietary restriction reduces the food molecules' need to be carried. Hygiene reduces immune/inflammatory proteins, making more room for carrier proteins.

There is increasing evidence linking infections to a tendency to overeat. In addition, it takes lots of calories to run an overloaded immune system. Diabetes may even have a link to lower albumin and an over-stressed immune system.

Exercise

Exercise is valuable biochemically because it pumps and restores the connective tissue, ensuring that nutrients reach cells and waste products return to the blood. Exercise also ensures that serum proteins leave the blood and surround cells and finally neutralize and transport toxic wastes through the lymphatic system. Serum proteins like albumin, besides transporting nutrients and wastes, are also used as a vital packet of amino acids for the rebuilding and repair of the body that proceeds every day. The ability to repair correctly is a fundamental basis of optimal aging. The wasting in disease and aging is caused by insufficient albumin.

Exercise in the presence of disease and stress on the immune system can have negative benefits. The combination of better hygiene and moderate exercise may provide the answer to how we achieve optimal health.

Hygiene

Hygiene is the newest discovery of the three basics. Only 150 years ago, Semmelweis in Europe and Oliver Wendell Holmes Sr. in the United States were ridiculed for educating doctors in the importance of handwashing before coming to the pregnancy ward. In those days, it was acceptable for one in four women to die in childbirth. Today, because of the first steps in handwashing, it is one in 100,000.

Certainly, improvements in personal hygiene and living standards have been at the forefront of extending the average life expectancy from around 38 years in 1850 to 85 years in Japan and Australia today.

SUPER GERMS

We are just beginning to understand that germs live in colonies, like cities, perceive their environment and adjust in a way to benefit them. Many produce toxins (venoms) far more powerful than any snake or spider, more than a match for any immune system. These clever germs are often "immunologically invisible" with proteins and sugars on their surface, identical to many of our own organ tissues. Infections with these common microbes regularly generate antibodies and T-cells that cross-react and attack our own healthy tissues. This "autoimmunity" plays a major role in aging and stress on the immune system.

Over the years of testing, it has become clear that germs from under and around the fingernails, inside the nasal passage and around the eyes are far more capable of causing disease in the host, and in larger concentrations (critical infecting dose) than the germs from the air or surfaces. This is one of the reasons why advanced hygiene that ensures thumbs/fingernails are cleaned, as well as the nasal passage, eyes, teeth, skin and hair, may be effective.

Infections and Free Radicals

Reactive oxygen radical molecules that chemically bind with our tissues, aging them, are generated in large amounts mainly during infections. They overwhelm our anti-oxidant potential regardless of any amount of anti-oxidant supplements. It is a devil's circle, because over-activation of the immune system generates the damaging free radicals and reduces albumin, which is the "800-pound gorilla" of all the other antioxidants combined. Albumin concentration is 4000 times higher than all other antioxidants combined. The antioxidant potential of serum depends on the concentration of albumin, according to tests performed at Genox and Pantox laboratories. Hygiene may break this aging, mortality and morbidity devil's circle.

Prevention of infection is a basic way to stop free radical damage. Free radicals are designed to kill germs. However, white cells are damaged and free radicals released, particularly in chronic disease, just at the time when albumin, the major antioxidant, is at its lowest. This is not the time to take plenty of antioxidants, as supplements may feed the germs and overload the liver, further reducing albumin.

Wastes

An important cause of aging is the toxic wastes that are naturally produced by every cell during its metabolic cycle. These wastes must be deactivated in the connective tissue before being allowed back into the blood and then safely transported to various sites for final elimination. Overeating, infections and over-activation of the immune system increase wastes, reduce albumin and thus prevent proper neutralization and transport of wastes. Lower albumin and accumulation of waste products set the scene for instability and damage to cells leading to cancer. This may explain the mystery of why albumin is low in all cancers and why remission is associated with restoration of albumin levels above 45 grams per liter.

IMMUNE SYSTEM DECLINE

Loss of immunological performance is well-known in aging and is deeply involved with the shrinking of the thymus. This small gland above and in front of the heart has been called the pacemaker of aging. Sir McFarlane Burnett proposed the thymus as the pacemaker in the 1950s. The involution of the thymus must be arrested to prevent loss of T-cells and their performance in any successful attempt to slow the aging process. Repeated and chronic infections and over-stressing the immune system result in over-production of cortisol and lower albumin, leading to free cortisol and causing the involution of the thymus. There is a need to prevent chronic infections in order to preserve the thymus in old age. Hygiene may again be the answer.

CLUES TO PREMATURE AGING

The positive results in people following the advanced hygiene system I began in 1980 were the motivation for my search for the secret of aging. The healthiest group of elderly people possible were studied and then compared with younger control subjects to see differences in their biochemistry. Fortunately, many of these tests have been going on in laboratories devoted to the study of aging, including at the National Institute of Aging. The only real biochemical difference was a decline in albumin.

Plasma is the watery fraction of the blood including the clotting factor. Serum is the liquid without the clotting factor, and albumin is the most abundant (60%), versatile and complex soluble protein. In a healthy old person the decline in albumin may only be 0.2 of a gram per deciliter (2 grams per liter). Yet, each gram lost is trillions of albumin transport ships. Albumin fits the aging jigsaw puzzle brilliantly because it has so many important roles. Albumin is the biochemical measure of stress and homeostasis. The lower the level, the greater the stress on the physiology. Albumin levels vary over a few days or months depending on the condition of the person at the time of measurement, explaining the good and bad days. When it is high, we feel and look glowing; when it is low, the opposite is true. Albumin concentration has emerged in all studies as the most powerful indicator of all causes of mortality and morbidity.

CONCLUSION

Basic hygiene practices only became widespread with the additions of bathrooms and soap in mid-1900. Hygiene increased life span from approximately 39 years in 1830 to over 70 years by 1980. It is reasonable to expect that advancements in hygiene will have a similar effect, resulting in 100 years as a normal life span. More important than maximum years, however, is the robust condition that ensues from raising albumin and reducing globulins. High albumin through pregnancy and childhood ensure optimal development and brain size, setting the scene for optimal aging and human development. Cleanliness is next to godliness, after all!

16

AGEing with Sugar: Browning and Stiffening from the Inside Out

Brad J. King and Michael A. Schmidt, M.D.

Sugar is one of the most vital commodities in living things. It allows an athlete to run a marathon or bicycle the grueling Tour de France. It helps generate the energy for repair following an auto accident or surgery. It fuels our brains' extraordinary complexity 24 hours a day, every day of our lives, and allows us to retain vast amounts of information. In one respect, sugar is the energy prize that allows us to move and function in the world with remarkable ease and efficiency.

Yet sugar has a dark side of which few people are aware. Indeed, sugar may be one of the most powerful *aging* substances known. In the drama of premature aging there are at least two main characters: sugar and protein. They team up to form an unruly family of compounds called AGE.

WHAT IS AGE?

AGE is an acronym for Advanced Glycation Endproducts. It is a term we will use throughout this chapter. You can think of AGE as a family of rogue molecules that develop when sugars in your body react with the different kinds of structural and functional proteins. They are like the mutants in a science fiction movie who rove the planet, creating havoc and chaos in everything they touch.

One might picture sugar molecules like the little plastic balls with Velcro® strips attached. You could picture the velvet target as a matrix of protein similar to that found in the skin, bone, muscle, brain or cartilage. When you throw a Velcro® ball at the velvet target, it sticks. Throw two or three or 50 and you begin to clog up the velvet surface with the "sticky" little balls. In the body, we can accumulate sugars that chemically bond or stick to our body proteins in a way that alters their structure and function. With more sugar, more of our proteins become "glycated" or aged.

So when you think of AGE, think of sugars that stick to your body proteins creating wrinkles, stiffness, browning and malfunction. AGE is central to the accelerated aging process. If you can slow down the formation of AGEs, you dramatically lower the stress on your system.

Browning and Stiffening from the Inside Out

As just noted, the process of glycation is a reaction between sugar molecules and protein.

Another way to view AGE is to explore the browning of a turkey. As a turkey bakes in the oven, natural sugars gradually interact with the proteins in the turkey's skin. With time, the sugars and proteins become bonded, causing a brownish hue. The longer the turkey is baked, the deeper the browning effect. The same occurrence takes place when many other foods, such as bread, are baked in the oven. The inner portion of the bread is soft and moist, while the crust is brown and hard. If we were to test the crust of these newly browned foods, we would find they contained AGEs, or modified proteins. Just as the skin of a turkey becomes brown from basting in the oven, our human interiors also "brown" from years of cooking at our natural body temperature. Just as the turkey's skin becomes more rigid and stiff, so too do our own tissues become rigid and stiff.

As glycation takes place in our bodies through the bonding of sugars with proteins, the structure of our proteins becomes modified. In some ways, they become unrecognizable. As we consume more and more sugars, we hasten the biological aging of the body by increasing these AGEs. As AGEs accumulate, they create cross-links or bridges between proteins that support our body structures. Skin, cartilage, muscle, ligaments, brain tissue, eye tissue and others begin to stiffen and wrinkle. In essence, the longer this process is left unchecked, the less mobility we have with age. This may be one of the most extraordinary discoveries yet as we try to understand the aging process.

WHY IS PROTEIN IMPORTANT?

These proteins have a full array of roles to play, and these roles are determined by the actual size and shape of the proteins themselves. Proteins are vital to every area of our being. Once a protein is modified and inactivated by the chemical process of AGEs, it can create myriad disorders. Here are just three examples of many:

Albumin. Albumin is the most abundant, versatile, soluble and remarkable of all proteins in the blood. It has been called the life factor by many top researchers because the more albumin you have, the healthier you are and the longer you will live. The shocking reality, however, is that this life-marking protein can be damaged easily by AGEs when there is too much sugar circulating in the blood. In a surprising discovery, out of hundreds of blood samples, it was shown that one third of the albumin molecules tested were damaged beyond repair by AGEs.

Hemoglobin. Another vital protein is hemoglobin, the oxygen transport protein found in our red blood cells. One molecule of hemoglobin can carry four molecules of oxygen. Whenever hemoglobin levels fall or when hemoglobin is damaged, it cannot efficiently carry oxygen to the brain, muscles and other tissue. As a consequence of this dysfunction, all tissues can suffer from a lack of vital energy and begin to age prematurely. Energy cannot be produced without sufficient oxygen, and over the last 20–30 years we have seen a large increase in energy deficit disorders (chronic fatigue, etc.).

As circulating sugars become too high over time, hemoglobin becomes damaged through AGEs. As a predictor of the oncoming damage, doctors now routinely test for glycated hemoglobin. Basically, AGE damage to our vital oxygen-carrying molecule is a scientific fact and is occurring with ever-increasing frequency.

Collagen. Collagen is the connective-tissue protein that forms the structure of our skin, bone, cartilage, ligaments and tendons. Studies have repeatedly shown that excess sugars cause the collagen tissue to cross-link in ways that make them weak, rigid and unstable. This contributes to arthritis, heart disease, neurological disease and other conditions common as we pass age 35.

A look at a short list of protein functions shows that we cannot operate without them:

1. Structure of our bones, ligaments, tendons, muscles, skin and hair.
2. Enzymes that digest our food.
3. Neurotransmitters that run the elegant network within our brain.

4. Enzymes that help manufacture a vast array of vital proteins, hormones, etc.
5. Transporters that carry vital oxygen and nutrients from place to place.

SUGAR: THE SWEET DOUBLE AGENT

Every good spy movie has a double agent, the one who is outwardly attractive, but hides a sinister side of deception and danger. In our body, sugar is the sweet double agent. It looks good and tastes good. We need it in order to generate the energy currency called ATP. With too little sugar, our cells may die. If severe enough, this would be followed by our own death. With too much sugar, our cells slowly malfunction or, in the worst case, we may die. This powerful capacity that lies within the domain of this very simple molecule has been widely appreciated for many, many years. The process of glycation is generally not so dramatic as life and death, but it is a slow, silent disabler of multiple body systems.

The Agents by Name

The sugars most commonly known to contribute to AGE are glucose, fructose and galactose. The first two are found in most of the sweeteners used throughout the food industry. High amounts of glucose are found in common table sugar in high amounts. Fructose is also found in table sugar and high-fructose corn syrup in large amounts. Galactose is found in milk products such as milk and ice cream.

The average North American consumes between 55–68 kg of sugar each year. Fructose is one of the fastest-growing sweeteners in the food industry. Fructose is a natural sugar found in fruit. It is not uncommon to find most beverages on the market laced with 20–30 g of fructose. That is equivalent to taking 20–30 vitamin capsules, only in this case, they would be filled with fructose. In fact, North Americans consume 22 kg of fructose each year.

A startling animal study published in the prestigious *Journal of Nutrition* in September 1998 compared the effects of fructose-fed groups with other sugar-fed groups. The study revealed that animals consuming fructose developed significant AGEs of the skin, which would contribute to advanced wrinkling in humans. The same animals showed AGE damage to bone as well. This is just one dramatic illustration of how a common sweetener can cause accelerated aging in the body.

Recently, galactose from milk sugar has been associated with stiffening of the heart's blood vessels and stiffening of the lens of the eye. Glucose, fructose and galactose are all dietary sugars that appear to advance the aging process in surprising ways.

Increased levels of AGE are believed to be associated with many degenerative processes. In the end, one can confidently state that as AGE levels increase, the premature aging of the human body increases right along with it. If we are to attack aging where it counts most—in the cells of the body—then we must without a doubt control the rate at which we experience AGE.

FREE RADICALS AND AGE

One of the disturbing things about AGEs is that they contribute to extraordinary amounts of free radicals in the body. They seem to participate in this in two ways. First, by one estimate, AGE proteins produce up to 50 times more free radicals than normal body proteins that have not been damaged by sugars (non-AGE proteins). Second, when the body detects AGE proteins, it attempts to remove them. One way this is accomplished is by producing free radicals. Remarkably, the body actually generates free radicals in an effort to essentially "bleach" the AGE proteins out of existence.

As AGE proteins accumulate in the body, free radicals are produced with greater frequency. This begins to tax our antioxidant defenses and may even deplete certain antioxidants. What's more, one of the key AGE-protecting enzymes is actually dependent upon a specific antioxidant called glutathione. In short, AGE proteins set up a vicious cycle of free radicals coupled with depleted antioxidants. As you might guess, proper antioxidant defenses are crucial for preventing AGE and premature aging of the body.

DISEASES OF AGE

As AGE proteins accumulate in the body, they may contribute to a wide range of disorders that are seen commonly in adults. For example, one study showed that stiffness increased in the heart chambers due to sugar–protein interactions resulting from elevated blood sugars.

Doctors studying non-diabetic people found that stiffening and glycation products (AGEs) in the skin increased by 33% from ages 30–80. In people with diabetes, glycated proteins increased by almost 100% over the same time span. Thus, AGE may be associated with aging of the skin.

Another study showed that AGE compounds found in the skin were associated with increased AGE in the blood vessels. In fact, AGE in blood vessels may be one of the key ingredients in coronary artery disease, a leading form of heart disease. AGE may also affect the brain. Recent studies have linked accumulation of AGE proteins to at least some of the damage that occurs in diseases like Alzheimer's.

AGE proteins may also impair our ability to generate energy because they can damage the mitochondria within our cells. Mitochondria are the tiny energy-generating units within every cell. They are sensitive to free radical damage. In fact, when the DNA of mitochondria is damaged, the damaged DNA can be passed on and on as mitochondria produce new mitochondria. In this way, the damage to our energy system caused by AGE can actually spread.

AGE products have been implicated in arthritis, especially rheumatoid arthritis. Scientists have recently discovered that cigarette smoke contains vast amounts of proteins that have already been glycated in the processing of tobacco. Smokers, in essence, bathe themselves in untold trillions of AGE molecules with every puff of cigarette smoke. Smokers engage in a deliberate daily ritual to coat their facial skin with layer upon layer of AGE proteins that stick to and link with the delicate collagen proteins that make up the skin. This wrinkling and leathering process that is so common in the face of smokers is a classic example of how AGE can cause wrinkling of any protein matrix within the body.

AGE can create more extensive damage to the body. Consider this list of possible consequences:
- stiffening of connective tissue (muscles, ligaments, tendons, etc.)
- stiffening of heart muscle
- stiffening and wrinkling of skin
- stiffening of joints (cartilage)
- allergic responses
- gum disease
- eye disease
- brain disorders

FOOD AND AGE

Food has a significant effect on the formation of AGE within the human body. As mentioned previously, the amount of sugar in the diet influences the amount of sugar that enters the bloodstream. Increased sugar means an increased risk of forming AGEs.

Now it appears that cooking methods influence the levels of AGE to which we are exposed through our foods. Scientists have known for many years that cooking proteins with sugars in the absence of water creates advanced glycation endproducts. The troubling new evidence is that eating foods with these advanced glycation endproducts raises blood and tissue levels of AGE and may increase nerve damage in susceptible individuals.

One group of susceptible individuals is people with diabetes, who suffer a very high incidence of nerve, artery and kidney damage because high blood sugar levels in their bodies markedly accelerate the chemical reactions that form AGEs. A presentation at a recent meeting of the American Diabetes Association in San Francisco reviewed evidence that eating foods with AGE proteins aggravated their neurological and blood vessel symptoms.

Cooking with water prevents sugars from binding to proteins to form these poisonous chemicals. Cooking without water causes sugars to combine with proteins to form AGEs, so baking, roasting, frying and broiling cause the poisonous advanced glycation products to form, while boiling and steaming prevent them.

According to these new findings, brown foods—such as brown cookies, brown bread crust, brown basted meats, brown beans and even brown coffee beans—may increase nerve damage, particularly in people with diabetes who are unusually susceptible to nerve damage. On the other hand, since steamed and boiled vegetables, whole grains, beans and fruits are made with water, they do not contain significant amounts of AGEs. This is one more reason why you should eat your fruits, vegetables, whole grains and beans fresh, boiled or steamed.

This does not mean that you give up cooking your food. It merely alerts us to the fact that cooking methods can increase AGE proteins in the body and that they may, when coupled with other factors, contribute to poor health over time. Eating more whole foods and ensuring that your protective nutrient defenses are in place is one way to minimize the AGE effect. Nutrient defenses are turning out to be a vital insurance policy.

Nutrient Defenses Against AGE

As we get older our ability to control our blood sugar slowly declines. The combination of inactivity, dietary habits, nutritional deficiency, stress and other factors contribute to a gradual malfunction of the system that regulates blood sugar. This makes AGE formation, to some degree, inevitable. Fortunately, a variety of nutrient molecules protect against the formation of AGE in our bodies. The nutrients fall into three basic categories:

1. Those that help balance blood sugar and insulin.
2. Those that protect against free radicals.
3. Those that directly influence the reaction where sugars link with proteins (forming AGE).

Some of the most important protective nutrients are listed below.

Glutathione: The Premier Protector

Glutathione is one of the body's brilliant sentinels. In protecting ourselves against AGE, glutathione is a molecule we cannot do without. Glutathione is called a tripeptide, a sort of mini-protein that is made up of three amino acids.

The amino acids are cysteine, glycine, and glutamic acid If we are low in any of these amino acids we cannot make enough glutathione to protect our bodies from a range of threatening substances. Of the three, the amino acid we are most likely to be deficient in is cysteine, a sulfur-bearing amino acid. This is one of the key points to know about protecting against AGE. If we don't have enough protective sulfur compounds, we will not be well protected against AGE.

To make glutathione in the body, we also need magnesium and potassium, two nutrients commonly low in modern humans. Scientists have discovered that an enzyme the body uses to eliminate AGE proteins must use glutathione as a cofactor. Thus, without glutathione we simply cannot get rid of two entire families of AGE proteins. Glutathione is very expensive and there is some debate as to how efficiently oral glutathione is absorbed. It is presumed to be better absorbed in those who are glutathione deficient. Doses range from 50 to 300 mg per day. People with diabetes should consult a doctor before taking glutathione. While people with diabetes commonly have low levels of glutathione, glutathione can affect insulin levels. As discussed in detail in Chapter 6, research shows that high-quality whey proteins can increase glutathione levels very effectively.

N-acetyl Cysteine

N-acetyl cysteine (NAC) is a sulfur compound that is a close relative of cysteine. We can use NAC to help manufacture our own glutathione. In experimental studies of AGE, NAC has been shown to be a very useful preventive substance. Doses commonly range from 50 to 600 mg per day.

Alpha-Lipoic Acid (ALA)

Alpha-lipoic acid (ALA) is another sulfur compound vital to the human body. ALA has a couple of key functions in protecting against AGE. First, it helps regulate blood sugar. If you can better regulate blood sugar, you lower the chance that excess sugars will be around to stick to proteins. Second, ALA appears to prevent the formation of different complicated molecules associated with AGE. Finally, ALA appears to be one of the best ways to increase the body's own production of glutathione. In this regard, ALA becomes a kind of glutathione insurance policy. Doses range from 50 to 600 mg per day. In studies of diabetic neuropathy, a condition where AGE proteins damage nerves throughout the body, 600 mg per day have been found useful. For prevention, lower doses seem reasonable.

Vitamin E: Fat-Soluble Defense

Vitamin E is one of the body's key fat-soluble nutrients. It sits nestled in the body's cell membranes to trap free radicals that may threaten the cell's health. Vitamin E also happens to be one nutrient that also influences the formation of AGE.

Chromium: The Key Trace Element in the Battle Against AGE

Chromium has been shown to inhibit the formation of AGE by virtue of its effect on insulin and blood sugar. A recent study of over 40,000 patients revealed that chromium levels decrease by nearly 50% in our bodies as we age. Surprisingly, the very mineral capable of preventing AGE and slowing the aging process is actually depleted as we age.

Numerous studies have also confirmed that eating sugar causes more chromium to be excreted in the urine. Remarkably, the sugars that contribute to AGE formation also cause us to lose the one mineral that acts as a powerful AGE protector—chromium. The daily dosage of chromium that has been shown to reduce one form of AGE protein (glycosylated hemoglobin) ranges from 600 to 1000 mcg. These levels have been used for people with diabetes and may not be necessary for everyone. A reasonable dose may be 100–400 mcg for people who do not have diabetes.

PLANT PROTECTORS

Plants contain a vast pharmacy of phytonutrients that are among the most promising protectors against AGE. As shown in Chapter 9, "Cellular Insurance," phytonutrients are potent scavengers of free radicals. This makes them among the most powerful AGE protecting substances, since, as noted earlier, AGE proteins are associated with a dramatic increase in free radical stress. Plants also contain substances that directly block the formation of AGE proteins even when there is too much sugar in the blood. A short sample of phytonutrients that prevent AGE includes:

Plant Constituent	Plant Source
Curcumin	Turmeric
Thymol	Thymus vulgaris
Quercitin	Onions (many others)
Resveratrol	Red wine, grapes (skin)

SUMMARY OF GLYCATION

Advanced Glycation Endproducts

A chemical reaction that happens when reducing sugar (such as fructose, glucose or galactose) reacts with proteins. It affects any protein structure, especially the amino acids lysine, arginine and tryptophan.

Problems Associated With Age

1. Chemical modification of these amino acids in food proteins may render these amino acids nutritionally unavailable, leading to deficiencies.
2. Chemical modification of proteins could block the activity of protein-digesting enzymes, causing incomplete digestion of these proteins and eventually leading to protein deficiency.
3. The absorption of partially digested proteins into the bloodstream could trigger allergic reactions and may cause autoimmune disorders.

Age Physiological Factors

1. The chemical modification of an enzyme could diminish or destroy the activity of that enzyme.
2. Glycation of tissue proteins might be perceived as foreign molecules (antigens) by the immune system and subjected to autoimmune attack.
3. Glycation of long-lived biological molecules leads to the formation of cross-links, increasing the aging factor.
4. It is widely accepted that glycation is behind the pathogenesis of the end organ damage in people with diabetes.

17

Biocize: Anti-aging Exercise

Brad J. King

INTRODUCTION

All of us at some time in our lives have wondered what it would be like to live forever, to never grow old. While we know this is not realistic, we would all love to at least slow the effects of aging. So we press on at all costs, looking for that fountain of youth, that one magic pill that will erase all our aging woes even though reality tells us it doesn't exist. Or does it? There is no magic pill, but we *can* slow down the effects of time with exercise—specifically, with a scientifically valid anti-aging exercise we call Biocize.

Research on the myriad benefits of exercise as it pertains to our aging bodies is now irrefutable. Proper exercise has been shown to retard aging; reduce cholesterol, high blood pressure, stress levels, insulin levels and osteoporosis risk; keep us from losing vital hormones; and increase oxygen utilization and our self-esteem, just to name a few.

In fact, masters athletes, who are a class of athletes that are still competitive in sports well past middle age, can often resemble the biological age of someone much younger. Even though a masters athlete may be 60 or older, his or her cardiovascular health, muscle strength and coordination can often be similar to someone in their twenties or thirties. So even though the vehicle may look like a collector's item, inside the engine is still purring.

Dr. Miriam E. Nelson and colleagues at The Human Nutrition Research Center on Aging at Tufts University were among the first to discover the potential of weight-resistance exercise in the elderly. These early pioneers proved that two of the top biomarkers of aging, loss of lean body mass and muscle strength, could not only be stopped, but actually reversed by performing proper resistance exercise over a relatively short period of time. In a 1990 ground-breaking study presented in the prestigious *Journal of the American Medical Association*, muscle strength was greatly improved in as little as eight weeks of resistance training, even in 90-year-old subjects, further proving Dr. Nelson's theory.

BORN TO MOVE

We were all given a body at birth, a miraculous machine capable of moving us around at peak proficiency. In youth, the human body is amazing indeed. Given the proper training and fuel, it can be programmed to achieve remarkable feats of speed, agility, flexibility and strength.

Many of us never give a second thought to the downward inevitability that a sedentary lifestyle eventually brings. We ignore the fact that by retirement age, nearly two thirds of the population will have lost at least one third of their lean body mass (muscle, bone and organs) and gained the rest in fat. Who cares how much lean body mass you lose? No one really wants to look like Arnold what's-his-name anyway. The fact is, lean body mass also brings with it confidence, health and vitality. Muscle strength and your cardio-respiratory rate become limiting factors as you age, so that simple things you take for granted when you're young, such as getting out of a chair or walking to the store and carrying a few groceries, now become a chore. Women are at more of a disadvantage than men when it comes to progressive muscular decline. Women show a continuous loss of muscular strength at an earlier age than men, which is one more reason for you ladies not to shy away from weight-training exercises.

Almost everything we do on a daily basis requires muscle strength and our vital capacity, the ability to take in and utilize oxygen from the air we breathe. Lung performance usually reaches its maximum around 16 years of age and then declines by about 1% a year thereafter, so that by the time we are around 60 years of age, we may only have two thirds to one half of the capacity we once had. Losing our vital capacity can result in much more than needing to take a few extra breaths. It can lead to serious heart conditions and a greater susceptibility to pneumonia and other kinds of infections. If you've been ignoring the facts until this point, by now you must realize the vast importance in both retaining lean body mass (muscle tissue and strength) as well as holding on to your vital capacity if your goal is health extension. Let's now take a look at the philosophy of Biocize exercise, and how this scientific approach to training can help us accomplish these goals.

THE ADVANTAGES OF BIOCIZE EXERCISE

Biocize exercise is a training concept born out of the realization that many of the changes in health status that have been deemed the normal result of aging are actually the result of a long-standing sedentary lifestyle. Research indicates that activity in the later years of life (middle age) is strongly correlated with the level of independence of a senior citizen. So if you are one of those independent types, this is one more incentive to get moving. In essence, movement, strength and flexibility are among the most powerful tools for a liberated, independent life.

Biocize exercise was developed after researching the most effective exercise strategies (including timing, duration, hormonal elevations and nutrient partitioning) for positively affecting one's Bio-Age from a hormonal perspective. After all, hormones are the key cellular messengers, and losing key messages (through the decline of certain fundamental hormones) as we age is one of the biological markers of aging itself.

Having closely observed top-level athletes and the events that help to continuously improve their performance we soon discovered that athletes are never quite happy with their performance; they are always striving to run a little faster, jump a little higher, gain a little more muscle, increase their strength and so on.

This led to the realization that the human body can only be pushed so far before it decides to fight back by shutting down. It's the body's way of saying, "If you won't let me catch up on my repair mechanisms, than I'll have no choice but to shut down the system until it is repaired properly." Remember the word "anabolic" from earlier chapters? It means to repair oneself. When athletes are succeeding at their goals they are in an anabolic environment. They are repairing their bodies faster than they are tearing them down. Anabolic metabolism spells success for any athlete as well as any other person interested in health extension. The athlete who remains anabolic also shares many similarities of youth. In youth, we are highly anabolic and able to repair ourselves at an astonishing rate. One doesn't have to look any further than how fast a child heals from a cut or an injury.

On the other side of the coin however, the athlete who pushes himself or herself even a little beyond what the body is ready for will experience "the overtraining spiral," or what sports medicine/rehabilitation physician at UCLA, Dr. Karlis Ullis calls it the "Critical Point." The Critical Point is a catabolic state (the breakdown phase) experienced by the majority of elite athletes at one time or another, which closely approximates the physiology of an aged person. Some of the traits experienced by these catabolic athletes are depressed immunity (including flu-like symptoms as well as susceptibility to viruses and infections), fatigue-related disorders (such as chronic fatigue), aches and pains accompanied by increased inflammation (not unlike fibromyalgia and arthritic conditions), depression (due to low neurotransmitter levels) and sleep disturbances (due to inadequate serotonin, melatonin and growth hormone levels). Doesn't this sound like what we have come to expect through advanced age?

Biocize is a training philosophy that incorporates the latest science on exercise and cutting-edge nutritional information to offer the average person a realistic way to increase an anabolic response. If you are going to remain sedentary and still believe that you can affect your Bio-Age in a positive manner, think again! If there is very little activity in the factory, then most (if not all) of the workers will be laid off. The human body is very much like the factory analogy—if you don't use it, you're almost guaranteed to lose it.

Biocize exercise is a scientific approach to balancing what we normally lose and in some cases gain as we age. We lose lean body mass, muscular strength, vital capacity, certain hormones, our ability to control blood sugar and our cognition, and we gain unwanted body fat, higher insulin levels and more stress hormones through normal (or abnormal) aging. Biocize exercise seems to offer us a fighting chance against this onslaught toward our overall physiology.

BOOSTING IMMUNITY THROUGH BIOCIZE

Starting in adolescence our body's internal army, the immune system, slowly begins to lose its ability to fight off invaders such as viruses and bacteria. The reason for this is believed to be the gradual shrinking of our body's primary organ of the immune system, the thymus gland, which begins to shrink around puberty and by age 60 is barely visible. It is in a sense a definitive marker of the aging process itself, making it yet another biomarker of aging referred to as immunosenescence. As the thymus gland declines through age, the rise in age-associated disease occurs.

So what does this have to do with Biocize exercise? Well for one, Biocize exercise elevates growth hormone levels, which in turn help to regulate immunity. Researchers have known for years that one of the most effective ways to invite illness into your life is to experience several bouts of mental or physical stress. But more and more research is indicating that regular exercise can help guard against the negative effects of stress on our immune systems. To experience the rewards of this immune insurance from exercise, the exercise program needs to begin before the stressful situation takes place. If you delay exercising until the day the stress begins, you will most certainly not prevent the negative effects of stress on the immune system.

Other research points to the fact that regular exercise helps to increase the numbers of internal soldiers in response to the exercise. One of our most powerful lines of defense lies in our ability to up-regulate the numbers and activity of a group of immune cells called Natural Killer cells (NK), which are able to gobble up infected cancer and virus cells. As we age, our NK numbers and activity decline, opening the door to illness and disease. Biocize exercise is one way to naturally increase the overall activity and numbers of these important allies, in young and old alike. In a 1999 study, otherwise sedentary elderly people were carefully monitored while exercising over a six-month period. At the end of the study the researchers concluded that six months of supervised exercise training could lead to nominal increases in certain measures of immune function, especially the NK cells.

GAINING MUSCLE AND LOSING FAT, THE BIOCIZE WAY

Most people think that aerobics is the best exercise for long-term fat loss. Unfortunately they're wrong in this approach. Unless you're planning on getting a flat, your main objective is to get rid of the spare tire. If you were going to commit yourself solely to aerobic training, then you will be carrying around the spare for a lot longer than you'd like. Studies show that too much cardio performed in the absence of resistance training can be detrimental to long-term fat loss. Cardio itself is not the enemy. The problem lies in the amount and intensity of the cardio activity. The truth is, too much high-intensity cardio exercise is detrimental to your metabolic engine, muscle. Research has confirmed that high-intensity cardio activity cannot maintain muscle mass on its own.

In a landmark study published in the *American Journal of Cardiology*, aerobic training was compared to aerobic with resistance (weight) training. Two groups had to complete a 10-week exercise program of 75 minutes. One group completed 75 minutes of aerobic exercise twice a week, while the other completed 40 minutes of aerobics plus 35 minutes of weight training. The time spent training was identical. At the end of the study, the aerobics group showed an 11% increase in endurance, but no increase in their strength. The group that completed the combination of aerobics plus weight training showed a massive 109% increase in their endurance, and a 21–43% increase in their overall strength. There are many other studies that further prove the theory that resistance training combined with low-impact cardio is superior to either one alone.

In order to stop our bodies from declining, we first have to engage in a progressive resistance program. A Biocize weight-training routine is changed monthly in order to keep your body from adapting to the exercises so that you keep progressing. Studies prove that our bodies can adapt to an exercise routine in as little as six sessions. For continuous results we need to keep our bodies guessing as to what is about to hit them. Weight training is the only scientific way to increase the lean muscle and strength that you lose through aging. Why is muscle so important? Because muscle is the metabolic engine of the body. The more muscle you carry on your frame, the higher your basal metabolic rate (BMR), which refers to your ability to utilize calories, and the more fat you burn, 24 hours each day.

One kilogram of active muscle burns in excess of 20 calories a day. So if you add muscle during your exercise program or at least keep the muscle you had in your youth, you will be well on your way to reversing some of the biomarkers of aging. When it comes to Biocize exercise (you're going to like this part), less (duration) can often mean more (results)—less fat and more muscle.

Fat-burning Sleep

If the above section doesn't convince you to train effectively for long-term fat loss, maybe this will. How would you like to be able to burn large amounts of fat while you sleep? Just as there is an RMR or resting metabolic rate, there is also an SMR or sleeping metabolic rate. The higher the SMR, the more calories are burned during sleep. Research has proved that exercise can raise our ability to burn fat while sleeping. Exercise can increase our SMR by as much as 18.6%. This gives us a whole new perspective on getting a good night's fat-burning sleep.

Biocize Synergy

The name of the game in Biocize exercise is to stimulate the production of the good (anti-aging) hormones, decrease the overall production of the bad (pro-aging) ones, and stimulate lean body mass development and strength, all the while reducing body fat. In order for an exercise program to be deemed Biocize exercise, it would have to incorporate a cross-training program of both anaerobic (weight training) and aerobic (walking, etc.) in the proper order to affect as many hormonal pathways as possible. The two together become the magic pill for reversing your Bio-Age.

JOIN THE RESISTANCE

Walking will do wonders for your vital capacity, but unfortunately it won't reverse the two top biomarkers of aging, loss of lean body mass and muscular strength. In order to rebuild the old muscle tissue with new stronger fibers, you must work out in an anaerobic fashion. Anaerobic exercise creates an intensity sufficient enough to ensure that the muscles cannot receive enough oxygen transfer. As the muscles strain to work in this environment, they end up producing a by-product of glucose metabolism called lactic acid. The more vigorous the exercise, the higher the lactic acid production. Newer research confirms that lactic acid benefits the heart and also helps to cleanse our systems by binding to and removing toxic metals that accumulate over time. When you feel like you can no longer perform a repetition during a weight-training session because of the intense burning sensation, you have entered what is referred to as your lactate threshold. The longer you stick with an exercise program, the higher your lactate threshold becomes, allowing you to exercise with a great deal more intensity than you previously could.

This anaerobic environment and the lactate threshold help to stimulate growth hormone and testosterone, which are needed for building new muscle mass (yes, even for you ladies). Growth hormone and testosterone are responsible for the hypertrophy (increased size and density) of muscle cells as well as the repair of micro-tears in the muscle tissue. Together they increase your anabolic metabolism (rebuild, repair and replace worn, damaged cells throughout the body). Nothing accomplishes this task better than a Biocize exercise program.

THE REAL MAGIC OF BIOCIZE EXERCISE

Another benefit of Biocize exercise lies in its ability to raise your metabolic rates (the rate at which you burn calories at rest) afterwards. A great deal of this is due to the rise in anabolic (rebuild and repair) hormones, testosterone and growth hormone, approximately 15 minutes after the exercise is completed. As long as you don't blunt this metabolic increase by consuming a high-carbohydrate energy drink (like Gatorade®) in the absence of protein, your body will have the ability to burn calories for many hours to come. As a matter of fact, in one study it was shown that over two thirds of the fat-burning activity of exercise takes place after the actual exercise sessions. This increase in fat-burning potential has been documented as lasting for over 15 hours in highly trained athletes, and is believed to be due to the increased activity of a fat-releasing enzyme called hormone-sensitive lipase.

CORE BIOCIZE EXERCISES

Normally there is no set repetition range when it comes to effective weight training. Some experts believe 4–6 reps per exercise builds the most muscle, others believe that 8–10 reps is the best way to go, and still others believe you should strive for 15 and up. All this repetition talk can become overwhelming to the novice exerciser, so let's simplify it. Your muscles come in two flavors: (1) Slow-twitch muscle fibers (best suited for endurance) with a high oxidative potential, and (2) Fast-twitch muscle fibers (best suited for size and strength) with a lower oxidative potential.

These different muscle fibers require different rep sequences to attain results. Slow-twitch requires high repetitions for maximum effect, and fast-twitch requires low to medium repetitions for best results. However, when it comes to Biocize exercise, we aren't interested in what is normally carried out during a well-designed exercise program, we are interested only in getting the best hormonal bang for your buck. It turns out that higher-intensity weight training affects growth hormone and testosterone response much better than low-intensity weight training. What does high intensity equate to? According to the latest research, approximately 70% of your maximal lifting capacity will induce a threefold increase in growth hormone levels, while lifting at 85% of your max will quadruple it. In a 1991 Pennsylvania State University study performed by Dr. William Kraemer and associates, the best rep sequence for maximum growth hormone output for both men and women was 8–10 reps with a 1-minute rest in between.

Biocize exercise follows this philosophy for maximum hormonal effect and also utilizes multijoint or compound exercises to facilitate the greatest number of muscle fibers. Compound exercises include those that target more than one muscle group, such as a bench press (upper body) or squats (lower body). More information related to Biocize exercises will be presented in Part III.

AEROBIC TRAINING THE BIOCIZE WAY

A 1994 University of Florida in Gainesville study showed that when it comes to growth hormone levels, aerobic exercise intensity and resistance training intensity are two very different things. According to the researchers, moderate-intensity rather than high-intensity aerobic training was sufficient to create a large growth hormone release and burn body fat. Now what exactly does moderate mean when it comes to aerobic training the Biocize way? The optimal intensity for sufficient growth hormone release both during and preceding aerobic activity is whatever intensity allows you to take in enough oxygen without gasping. This also happens to be the greatest way to burn fat. Brisk walks, for example, are an excellent Biocize exercise.

BIOCIZE ORDER AND TIMING

When it comes to optimum results when exercising for overall health and longevity, you must be able to decrease body fat. Increased body fat eventually leads to obesity, which eventually leads to Type 2 diabetes, which in turn accelerates the aging process by at least one third. To avoid making this a reality, both the order in which you do your Biocize exercises and the amount of time you take to perform them become very important to your success. There are two things you can do to increase your body's efficiency to burn body fat: (1) Do cardio activity longer than 20 minutes to increase the fat-burning effect, or (2) Do cardio activity *after* weight-bearing activity.

High-octane fat fuel is not the starting fuel for your cold engines. Your body usually starts warming up with a rich sugar mix instead. In order to increase the fuel mix to primarily fat, the body must first call into action a hormonal response. Once the fatty acids are in the bloodstream, they can be transported by special carrier proteins to the muscle cells and further escorted into the furnaces of those cells by specific enzymes. This entire warm-up response, depending on a host of variables (undigested food, nutrients, etc.), usually takes about 20 minutes to accomplish, so extending the cardio workout makes sense for fat burning. But why perform cardio *after* Biocize weight-bearing exercise?

If you have ever engaged in a weight-training routine and performed the exercises correctly, you are no doubt familiar with the rush at the end of the workout. This "high" feeling comes from a combination of endorphins (pain-sensitizing chemicals that are even more powerful than morphine), anabolic hormones (testosterone and growth hormone) and stress-like chemicals (norepinephrine and epinephrine). Even though you are training primarily in an anaerobic (without oxygen) fashion and therefore utilizing sugar as your main fuel source, you are still invoking a stress response that not only causes that incredible sensation after the exercise, but also frees up your fat stores.

Doing cardio right after weight training is like getting into a car that has been running for a while. Now all you have to do is turn up the heat, and you will be met with a blast of warm air. That warm air is a metaphor for your free fatty acids that are now available to be burned through the cardio activity, right from the start. Now you can complete your 20 minutes with the confidence that you have succeeded in burning body fat as your primary fuel source.

HOW MUCH IS ENOUGH?

So now you are aware of the optimum sequence of training and the duration of cardio activity needed to elicit beneficial results with Biocize exercise, but exactly how much weight training is enough?

You need a little stress to increase the levels of free fatty acids, but too much can cause a drastic increase in the muscle-wasting hormone cortisol. Dr. Barry Sears, best-selling author of *The Zone* series of books, warns against going over the 45-minute mark when it comes to weight training.

Depending on your activity level, soon after 45 minutes the levels of cortisol and free radicals rise to the point where recovery from the exercise can become blunted. Cortisol is responsible for stealing valuable nitrogen from muscle tissue and then converting that muscle into extra energy. The more cortisol produced, the harder it is to get rid of and the worse off you are for it. Talk about a waste of valuable time spent exercising! So the rule of thumb for Biocize exercise is no more than 45 minutes of the weight-training portion of your workout.

THE BEST TIME TO DO BIOCIZE

A 1998 study at the University of Liège in Belgium proved the theory that the time of day an exercise is performed can greatly influence the hormonal response to the activity. The study confirmed suspicions that the existence of circadian variations in hormonal and metabolic responses to exercise actually exist. Exercise-induced elevations of body temperature were shown to be higher in the early morning than at any other time of day, indicating that early morning exercise would be the most beneficial time for fat loss.

Growth hormone production declines by a whopping 80% by our seventies or eighties, and so we can use all the help we can get. A 1997 study in Charlottesville, Virginia, performed on healthy men, showed that by increasing testosterone levels to otherwise abnormally high levels through injections caused an elevation in growth hormone levels by 62%. This study confirms other research showing a direct correlation between elevated testosterone and GH levels.

Testosterone levels peak in the morning, and are further augmented by resistance training (weight lifting) approximately 15 minutes following the exercise routine. This further corroborates the theory that early morning exercise will induce the greatest hormonal response. By taking advantage of the testosterone elevations (post-Biocize exercise) you are also setting the stage for increased growth hormone production.

What happens if you train in the evening like the majority of exercisers? Well, let's take a look into the natural timing of our hormonal response to answer that question. Before artificial light was ever invented, our bodies developed a specialized series of timing cues. In order to deliver these cues we developed specific hormones, proteins and enzymes to tell us when to sleep and when to rise, hunt, eat and mate again. The light of day and the dark of night brought on these cues. Through the advent of artificial light, as you learned in the "Waking Up Younger" chapter, these messages became skewed.

Melatonin is a hormone that regulates our sleep/wake cycle among other things. It is also one of the most powerful antioxidants we produce internally. The production of melatonin is stimulated by darkness. Before the advent of artificial light, melatonin was in a very real sense our internal alarm clock. Through the complex cellular messages this hormone (and its allies) parlayed to our cellular structures, we were in a sense shut down for the night—a time to sleep, rebuild, renew and replace our worn-out structures for the new day ahead. When the light of day came around, our bodies picked up the photons from the sun in special proteins in our skin called cryptochromes, which parlayed the newfound energy throughout our bodies by elevating certain other messengers such as cortisol and our sex hormones (testosterone and estrogen).

Why is all of this biochemistry so important to the timing of exercise? Because exercising late into the evening throws your circadian rhythm out of balance. By exerting yourself in the evening, usually under the bright lights of a gym or community center, your body is fooled into producing more of the hormones, proteins and enzymes it usually produces in the morning. You end up increasing your stress response through the exercise by increasing cortisol and testosterone production (when both of these hormones are normally at their lowest levels, readying the body for the sleep cycle). But the worst thing of all is that cortisol can remain elevated for hours, causing sleep disturbances and interference with the body's anabolic (rebuild and repair) phase by interfering with growth hormone production, which negates the very reasons you sweated in the evening in the first place.

Through Biocize, we recommend working with the body's natural circadian response to these hormones by exercising as early as possible, and getting a good night's sleep for the anabolic process to take place efficiently (much more on this in the "Waking Up Younger" chapter).

IT'S ALL IN THE MIND

The number one Biocize rule is that you must enjoy the exercise experience. If you approach the exercise portion of the program with a negative mindset, then the experience will be less than fulfilling. Researchers now know that over half of all folks who take up exercise quit during the first six months. Why does this happen? Well, a recent study at the Washington University School of Medicine in St. Louis has shed new light on this depressing reality. Researcher Joanne Schneider, Ph.D., R.N., questioned 364 women over the age of 55 after they finished their exercise programs. She discovered that those who stayed positive by believing in the health benefits of working out tended to exercise more often, more intensely or for longer periods than those with negative mind-sets. Those who worried about how they looked while exercising reported exercising less often, less intensely or for shorter periods of time than those who didn't. This study clearly proved that if you have a positive attitude toward exercise, you will want to exercise more.

Another recent study published in the journal *Health Psychology* showed that the myriad benefits of exercise could be attributed in part to a person's self-confidence. The emotional high that people experience from physical activity depends in part on what they believe they are capable of, or what researchers call the exercise "self-efficacy." The study showed that the higher a person's self-belief, the more likely he or she is to feel emotional benefits from regular exercise. Dr. McAuley, lead researcher in the study, suggests that enhancing self-belief can improve any exercise experience, at least emotionally. People who believe they are incapable of exercising might feel themselves getting tired, reach their limit earlier or drop out of an exercise program, while those with a higher belief system would actually feel great about the experience. It all starts in your head—if you think you can, you most likely will!

EXERCISES ARE MOOD ALTERING

Proper exercises can even elicit powerful mood-lifting changes. In fact, a major study performed at Duke University Medical Center in England showed that certain exercises can be just as effective as some of the most prescribed medications when it comes to alleviating major depression. The study looked at 156 elderly patients diagnosed with major depressive disorder over a 16-week period. The participants were assigned to three separate groups: group 1 exercised but had no antidepressants; group 2 took antidepressant medication with no exercise; and group 3 took antidepressant medication and combined this with exercise. To the amazement of the researchers, all three groups showed remarkably similar improvements in their depressive states following the 16-week trial. This study, as well as numerous others, has proven that exercise should be considered a viable alternative to medication when it comes to one of our most treated disorders of aging.

Depression and a negative attitude will supress your growth hormone levels. If your goal is to stay healthy and vital for as long as possible, Biocize exercise may just be what the doctor ordered.

WHAT TO DO BEFORE AND AFTER BIOCIZE

Exercising is stressful on the body, which is why the body responds by elevating certain stress hormones. When the body is stressed, it isn't interested in digesting food. Instead, most of the blood supply is escorted to the extremities, not the stomach. This is why you should not consume a lot of solid food before exercise; it will just sit there fermenting in your gut. Instead, you should train yourself to exercise on an empty stomach, or only consume around 100 calories about 30–45 minutes before the activity. Contrary to popular belief, carbohydrates are not the best things to eat just before training; they'll raise your insulin levels, causing you to use glucose (sugar) as your primary fuel.

Instead, Biocize exercise dictates that you consume protein. Protein isolates (whey, soy or a mix) empty from the stomach quickly, but they also cause a rise in the hormone glucagon (the primary hormone for maintaining glucose levels during exercise), which allows for fat-burning activity instead of storage. So if you must eat something before exercise, make it a protein shake with water, and keep it around 100 calories (see Appendix II for recommendations).

WHAT SHOULD I EAT AFTER BIOCIZE?

After any athletic activity, especially weight training, the body requires refueling of its glycogen (stored sugar in liver and muscles) reserves. In order to ensure this happens, the body contains an enzyme called glycogen synthetase that is responsible for storing sugar for future needs. Within a two-hour window after exercise, this enzyme is extra hungry. This is the only time that you can consume larger-than-normal (and higher glycenic) amounts of carbohydrates without worrying that they'll convert to fat.

Many of us usually make the mistake of consuming only carbohydrates at this time (juice, etc.). This is wrong! Drinking carbohydrate beverages without sufficient protein after Biocize will cause a drastic increase in insulin levels, bringing the increase in growth hormone and testosterone levels to a halt. New research confirms that protein mixed with carbohydrates after training allows for faster muscle recovery and greater growth hormone and testosterone increases. Always mix protein with carbohydrates in a liquid form, as close to completing your workout as possible, to ensure rapid replacement of bodily sugars and protein for recovery. A good rule to follow is a mixture of between 2:1 to 4:1 carbohydrates to protein. The post-Biocize protein should be primarily in the form of high alpha-lactalbumin whey protein isolate for maximum timing and absorption value. The carbohydrates should come from mixed whole fruits, primarily from the berry family due to their superior antioxidant-carrying capacity.

THE IMPORTANCE OF WATER

During exercise, it's imperative to increase your water intake due to its vital role in cardiovascular function and temperature regulation. As you exercise, your body loses a great deal of water through sweating and evaporation, and your muscles create a lot of extra heat. The heat is transported through tiny blood vessels called capillaries near the surface of your skin. The release of perspiration (and its evaporation) from your sweat glands creates a cooling effect on the skin as well as the blood in the capillaries beneath it. Sweating is therefore an essential part of your body's cooling system.

If your body does not have enough water to make this system run smoothly, your blood-carrying capacity also diminishes. Don't forget, it is the blood's role to carry nutrients such as oxygen, glucose, fatty acids and proteins to the muscles to create energy. The blood must also remove the toxic elements of metabolism, such as carbon dioxide and lactic acid. Since your circulatory system is almost 70% water, the extra demand on it can be quite severe.

Intensive exercise can cause a person to lose 5–8 pounds of fluid through perspiration, evaporation and exhalation. Studies show that for every pound of fluid lost, there is a significant drop in the efficiency with which the body produces energy. In one study, a 4% loss of body weight from exercise-induced dehydration resulted in 31% shorter muscle endurance time. It's amazing to think that something as simple as water can be the determining factor in winning or losing a competition. Many studies also point out the importance of proper hydration in managing the oxidative stress load of exercise due to the overproduction of those nasty little free radicals. Still other research indicates proper hydration in protecting and modulating our immune response to exercise.

Try to Consume Clean Filtered Water Throughout the Day

Losing excess fat can also cause a release of toxins into your body, since many toxins become lodged in the fatty tissue. Water is essential in the detoxification process, and since you will be dropping fat like mad, you will need all you can drink.

As pointed out in the "Drying Up" chapter, Dr. Batmanghelidj presents an interesting theory that somewhere through our evolution the signals for thirst and hunger may have become one and the same. Dr. Batmanghelidj believes that often when we think we are hungry, we are in fact just thirsty. So in order to cut down on the urge to overeat, it is recommended that you drink a glass of water before eating. This way you will be guaranteed not to overeat to satisfy an urge for water intake. Carry your water with you in a closed container everywhere you go (I even bring my water to bed) and drink it through a straw to avoid ingesting excess air.

So there you have it, the tools necessary to reverse some of the most insidious biomarkers of aging: the rules of Biocize exercise. In Part III we will discuss a complete Biocize exercise plan. If you have never worked out in this manner before, or have never worked out period, it is highly advisable to get yourself a qualified personal trainer to show you the ropes—and don't forget to clear it with your health professional first. Welcome to the new realm of Biocize exercise; welcome to the newer, younger YOU.

18

Mind over Aging

Michael A. Schmidt, M.D.

If you could do one thing that would inspire your cells, your body and your life to wholeness, what would it be? If you pose this question to physicians, you may get one answer. Pose it to scientists and you are likely to get another answer. If you ask this question of a poet, yet another answer emerges. We have pondered this question with full knowledge that there are multiple influences on health and longevity. However, while there is likely to be disagreement, we believe that having love and intimate relationships is the answer to an inspired, healthful life.

While the scientific study of love is fraught with difficulty, any musician can quickly tell you that love is indeed the path to richness. But does science have anything to say about the matter of love and health? What are the biological and health-building effects of love? One of the most prominent researchers in this area is Dr. David McClelland, formerly of Harvard, now at Boston University. McClelland set out to unravel some of the health effects of love and intimacy through many, many years of scientific study, and has discovered that some of the effects can be quantified.

McClelland found that people who pursued relationships without excessive anxiety or fervor, something called *relaxed desire for affiliation*, had stronger immune systems. Those who prioritized relationships also suffered from fewer and less severe bouts of illness.

McClelland then studied three different groups of people looking at immune cells called natural killer cells (NK), sentinels that eliminate cancer cells and microbes. Higher NK cell activity is a desirable trait. McClelland found that people with relaxed affiliation had much higher NK cell activity compared to those for whom personal power was more important than relationships.

McClelland and his colleague, James McKay, unearthed a new force in their attempt to describe the biological effects of love: affiliative trust. Affiliative trust was defined as *the desire for positive, loving relationships based on mutual respect and trust.* Individuals with high affiliative trust were found to have higher T-helper/suppressor ratios. This, again, is a sign of a robust immune system. They also found these same people had significantly less illness.

In one of the most interesting studies, McClelland and his colleagues followed a group of adults for 10 years. Of those with affiliative *mis*trust, a striking 59% contracted a major illness over the 10-year period. Affiliative mistrust reflected a more cynical view of relationships and was common among those who preferred personal power over loving relationships. Only 30% of those with high affiliative trust contracted a major illness over the same period. In essence, McClelland found that those motivated by loving relationships had half the rate of major illness.

ADDICTED TO LOVE

To understand the power of love on the brain, one need only take a look at the addictive drug cocaine. Cocaine is taken up by an area in the brain known as the basal ganglia. When this drug is ingested, it quickly increases the brain's production of a neurotransmitter called dopamine, which is associated with pleasure and alertness. Intense, romantic love can have a cocaine-like effect on the brain by releasing great amounts of dopamine in the basal ganglia.

Psychiatrist Daniel Amen, M.D., has performed several thousand brain scans, known as SPECT scans, on patients with a range of neurological and behavioral disorders. He writes of a close friend who had recently fallen head over heels in love with a new woman. Amen says, "He was so happy he almost seemed to have a drug high." Dr. Amen already had a normal SPECT scan of Bill's brain on file and wanted to see how this "new love" had affected his brain. To Amen's amazement, the brain scan looked like a scan of someone who had just ingested cocaine. Amen commented that love has real effects on the brain, as powerful as addictive drugs.

Laurie Jackson is a clinical psychologist and addiction counselor in Denver, Colorado. She relates that during the education process of working with people addicted to cocaine and other drugs, counselors show brain scans of people kissing. Laurie notes that the close, intimate contact and the use of these drugs both generate the same brain response.

CLOSE TIES

It is clear that close personal relationships are important to good health, and even the number of relationships may bear on our health. Scientists at Carnegie-Mellon University infected 276 healthy volunteers with rhinovirus, a virus that causes the common cold. All people became infected, but not all people became sick. Those reporting the fewest types of relationships, only one to three, were more than four times as likely to develop a cold than those with six or more types of relationships.

Relationships were broken down into types: relationship with a spouse, a parent, in-laws, children, schoolmates, religious groups, etc. Having multiple relationships was more important than the actual number of people with whom an individual had a relationship.

In a now-famous Harvard study, students were asked back in the mid-1950s about how they felt about their parents. Questionnaires were scored based on a scale of 1 (strained and cold) to 4 (very close). Feelings about mother and father were considered separately and together. A startling 100% of those who rated both mother and father low in warmth were diagnosed with diseases in midlife. Of those who rated both parents high in warmth, only 47% had diagnosed disease. The researchers offered this assessment: "The perception of love itself may turn out to be a core biopsychosocial-spiritual buffer...."

Students were also asked, "What kind of person is your mother (or father)?" Ninety-five percent of those who used few positive words and rated their parents low in parental caring had diseases diagnosed in midlife. Of those who used many positive words and rated their parents high in parental caring, only 29% were diagnosed with a disease in midlife.

The powerful effect of close personal relationships on health may even be strong enough to overshadow some of the traditional disease risk factors such as high-fat diets and smoking. In the landmark Roseto study, residents of that town had strikingly lower rates of heart disease even though they shared the very same risk factors as adjacent communities. Roseto was settled in the late 1800s by Italian immigrants who retained very close social, religious and community ties. In the 1960s and 1970s, the face of the community and its cohesive social structure changed dramatically. With this shift came a significant increase in death due to heart disease, which became similar to that of neighboring towns.

LOVE AS THE UNIVERSAL COHESIVE FORCE

Some years ago, I presented a lecture on nutritional biochemistry, brain and behavior. During a question-and-answer session, one of the doctors in the audience strayed from the subject at hand and asked if I had any opinion on the fundamental force holding the universe together. I believe he expected a scientifically astute, if not clever, dissertation. Instead, I suggested that love was the primary force. I argued that love is the force that holds two people together through great joy and adversity. Love can hold entire families together. Strongly bonded families can serve to hold communities together. Love-centered communities can create societies that remain cohesive. Societies founded on principles of love and compassion can hold nations together. At the microscopic level, love appears, as shown earlier, to be a force that binds the immune system into a cohesive whole.

Dr. Linda Russek and Dr. Gary Schwartz are two former Harvard scientists who did the follow-up analysis on the Harvard mastery of stress study mentioned earlier. As I came to know them personally, I realized that they had applied rigorous scientific study to the question of love as a universal, attractive force and that they are living examples of scientists with heart and a passion for spiritual meaning. They have argued that love is the universal attractive process, a process through which we give and receive information. Love and loving are the means by which information is transferred back and forth in all systems.

They note, of course, that human love is much more complicated, but they remain so strong in their contention that their lab at the University of Arizona is focused on studying the physiology, chemistry and energetics of love as a living energy in all systems, including humans.

Hardwired for Connectedness

Could it be, then, that we are biologically programmed to form intimate relationships and that these intimate relationships are as vital to our health as food, water and oxygen? In the vast number of studies, isolation and separation from others has been found to be a significant predictor of disease susceptibility. In the view of Schwartz, Russek and others, isolation may fundamentally cut us off from the free flow of energy that feeds life. In this regard, perhaps being openhearted to all life is ultimately what fuels the human energy system and, by extension, fuels wholeness within societies.

GIVING MIRTH

Why did George Burns, Milton Berle and Red Skelton live to such ripe ages after a lifetime of making people laugh? Were humor and laughter the secret to their longevity? Did making a life out of laughter feed their energy systems in ways that were self-sustaining? Researchers have taken the question of humor and laughter quite seriously (if one can do such a thing). Many studies have pointed to one simple truth—laughter improves specific markers of body biology and chemistry. Moreover, laughter makes life a lot more fun.

We won't belabor the point that one needs to laugh and laugh well to sustain health, but at least two studies bear mention. Scientists looked at the effect of stress on secretory immunoglobulin A (S-IgA), which is the antibody that fights infections in the mouth, throat and intestinal tract. It is a vital first defense against any microbe that might threaten the body from outside. Researchers found that a higher frequency of daily hassles was significantly associated with lower levels of s-IgA. However, the effects were less severe in people who scored higher on a scale measuring sense of humor. This suggests that sense of humor can counter the negative effects of stress on the immune system.

Scientists also discovered that levels of the stress hormones adrenaline and cortisol drop significantly following a good laugh. They further noted that humor contributes to greater optimism, cooperation and socialization—all aspects of a healthy self and a healthy society. It has also been observed that intimate relationships fare better when couples experience laughter. As laughter leaves a relationship, the relationship suffers.

HOSTILITY AND ANGER: THE AGE ACCELERATORS

While love and laughter are among the delights of life that contribute to health, other states show us how emotions can harm our health. Dr. Redford Williams is noted for his study of the effect of anger and hostility on health. After gathering extensive data for two decades, he has concluded that "hostile, suspicious anger is right up there with any other health hazard we know about." It seems that the risk to disease from anger is on a par with the risk posed by smoking, obesity and high-fat diets.

Dr. Mara Julius, an epidemiologist at the University of Michigan, designed a study to assess the effects of anger on women over an 18-year period. Each woman was asked to complete a questionnaire that helped pinpoint signs of long-term, suppressed anger. Dr. Julius found that women who scored high on the anger profile "were three times more likely to have died during the study than women who did not harbor such hostile feelings."

A case report from Yokohama City University School of Medicine further illustrates the effects of emotions such as anger on physical health. A 31-year-old man suffered for many years with skin lesions of atopic dermatitis. When his anger and anxiety intensified, his skin lesions became visibly worse along with increased discomfort and itching. In addition, his natural killer cells, key immune defenders, declined right along with his angry episodes.

This notion that people with suppressed long-term anger were more likely to die echoes the title of Dr. Williams's book *Anger Kills*. Indeed, anger and hostility may be one of the best formulas in our mind–body realm to *accelerate* the aging process.

Dr. Williams gives a list of strategies we can use to work with our feelings of anger and hostility. These are useful techniques to manage these destructive feelings, but anger is really an emotion that informs us that we have been hurt in some way. By dealing with betrayal or hurt and grieving appropriately, we may be able to move deeply into the kind of healing that is transformative. This may begin with expression of feelings and forgiveness, perhaps among the most powerful means to foster true healing, to bring youthfulness to our lives.

The Power of Letting Go

One way to limit the harsh effects of difficult emotions on our health is through the expression of feelings. In fact, it may be among our most powerful tools. James W. Pennebaker, professor of psychology at Southern Methodist University in Dallas, Texas, has made a career of studying the effect of confession on health. He has shown that those who share their deepest feelings about past or present trauma are better able to cope with life and are healthier than those who do not share their feelings.

The two most common means of confession are talking and writing. In a study at SMU, Pennebaker asked students to write about their deepest anxieties and their feelings about the dramatic changes involved in being at college. Those who wrote about their current anxieties had fewer illnesses and fewer visits to the doctor in the subsequent months. Those who wrote only about trivial, superficial topics showed a gradual increase in visits to the doctor.

Pennebaker found that confession led to an increase in T-helper cells, white cells that raise our immune defenses. More recent studies on the power of confession are even more intriguing. Scientists found that confession can lessen the symptoms of arthritis and asthma. This suggests that confession may have broad benefits that lower the stress on our bodies and bolster our defenses.

While confession seems to have powerful effects on the body, our general emotional expressiveness deeply influences how we heal. Mind/body researcher Dr. Lydia Temoshok examined the psychological factors associated with the skin cancer malignant melanoma. She discovered that emotional expressiveness was directly related to the thickness of the patients' tumors as well as the course of their disease. Temoshok's research revealed that:

- Patients who were less emotionally expressive had thicker tumors and more rapidly dividing cancer cells.
- Patients who were more emotionally expressive had thinner tumors and more slowly dividing cancer cells.
- Patients who were less expressive had relatively fewer lymphocytes invading the base of the tumor (suggesting weaker defenses).
- The more emotionally expressive patients had a much higher number of lymphocytes (immune cells) invading the base of the tumor.

Scientists studying healthy men wanted to see what happened to the immune system when they deliberately tried to suppress emotions. Results showed significant decreases in white blood cells called CD3T lymphocytes, a sign that the immune system suffers when we suppress our emotions. Those who wrote about their feelings experienced an increase in CD4 cells called T-helpers.

Guidelines for Opening Up

Confession works best when you honor the process of whatever feelings may emerge. Write continuously about feelings, even if the process feels painful at first.

Don't be concerned about grammar, spelling or sentence structure. Allow the words to flow freely, without editing. By all means, do not be critical of the words that appear. Do not prejudge your thoughts even if they may seem counter to how you would like to feel or how you perceive yourself. Write about events and facts, but be certain to write about how you feel in relation to those events. Dr. Pennebaker gives some additional suggestions:

- Getting in touch with long-repressed feelings can be painful, but it is necessary in order to move fully into healing, in order to move fully into the place of freedom that occurs when repressed feelings are surrendered.
- Don't feel that your words must form a coherent story. It may ultimately evolve into a story, but let the words form as they come, even if they don't seem coherent.
- Let both feelings and thoughts flow naturally.

For verbal or spoken confessions, consider the following:

- Find a confidant whom you can trust. If you feel untrusting, do not confide in this individual.
- Find a listener who can be non-judgmental. You may wish to state before you begin, "Please do not comment or judge what I am about to say. Merely listen."

- Be certain that the person in whom you confide is truly available to concentrate on listening at this time.

FORGIVENESS: FREEDOM TO LIVE IN THE PRESENT

As adults we understand that hurt and betrayal are natural parts of life. Some of greatest works of literature, such as *Julius Caesar* and *Les Misérables*, deal with the fundamental human experience of betrayal and forgiveness.

Pro football player Mike Singletary shares a deeply moving story of betrayal and forgiveness. Mike's father abandoned his family in favor of a young woman when Mike was a young boy. Mike grew deeply angry and resentful. Having suddenly become the "man" in the family, Mike could not afford to channel his anger into destructive behavior. Fortunately, he found an outlet for his intense feelings in sports. In less than two years, his father was abandoned by his new partner, who left him with a child. Distraught and humiliated, Mike's father and new baby moved into the house next door.

Mike was now seething with anger to think that his father had abandoned them, had a child with another woman, and then had the gall to move in next door. What made matters worse, or so Mike thought at the time, was that his mother took in the child to raise, knowing that the father could not care for it. Mike was living in the most extraordinary paradox—a father for whom he felt only anger and bitterness and a mother who offered more generosity and forgiveness than seemed humanly possible.

Mike went on to win virtually every award possible and every conceivable accolade along the way, including league MVP and a Super Bowl championship with the Chicago Bears, yet he was bitter, angry and miserable. As an adult, Mike finally struggled to call his father. As the three-hour conversation unfolded, he found himself able to forgive his father. Mike was free. He had made a journey into present time where the agony of past hurt no longer formed the center of his daily life.

The phrase "holding a grudge" is often applied to those who find it difficult to let go of past hurt and betrayal. As noted earlier, holding on to any painful feelings can lead to depressed immune function and poor health. When holding contributes to a bubbling sea of anger, it can even contribute to premature death. Many people misunderstand what forgiveness really is. They believe forgiveness is somehow for the person who has committed the act that we feel hurt by. There is a misconception that forgiveness is meant to free the other person from the responsibility for the hurtful act. While forgiving another does indeed free them in some way, forgiveness is really about *you*. It is about releasing yourself from a continuous cycle of being rewounded by a past event or act.

Reasons We Forgive

How we forgive may be central to truly releasing us from the past. It may also be necessary to experience the most significant health benefits. Psychologist Mary Trainer has outlined three principal motives that people have for forgiveness based on her interviews with divorced men and women. She labeled them expedient forgiveness, role-expected forgiveness and intrinsic forgiveness.

Expedient forgiveness is forgiving in order to get something. Examples might include wanting to get healthy, wanting a better reputation, wanting to be perceived as generous.

Role-expected forgiveness is motivated by the expectations of others or God. We are told we "should" forgive. This kind of motivation is still outside ourselves, dictated by a higher authority. It is not internalized.

Intrinsic forgiveness is a free decision that flows from the heart. It is rooted in empathy—an understanding of the other person's struggles and humanity, an understanding that we too hurt others and are capable of doing what the one who has hurt us has done.

Trainer has argued that if we attempt to forgive for the first two reasons—expedient and role-expected—we will not experience the true freedom from the pain of past injury. We will not experience the health benefits or the fullness of life if our motivations are not from deep within. She may be correct.

The Health Effects of Forgiveness

Dr. Judith Strasser studied the health effects of forgiveness in 59 adults. They each described the painful hurts they had suffered in relation to a parent, a child, spouse, friend or others. She discovered that the more her participants had forgiven the people who had hurt them, the better their physical health in older adulthood. She also learned that expedient forgiveness and role-expected forgiveness were not associated with health benefits. Only intrinsic forgiveness was related to improved health.

The Templeton Foundation for Forgiveness Research has commissioned numerous studies on forgiveness and health. In one study, those who cultivated vengeful thoughts experienced increased blood pressure, muscle tension and heart rate. When they focused on forgiveness, these measures of stress decreased.

Scientists at VA Medical Center and Medical College in Tennessee found that people who suffered from chronic anxiety, depression and anger had thicker blood due to higher red blood cell counts.

In a study at the University of Tennessee, people were separated by their scores on the Forgiving Personality Inventory. Those considered low forgivers experienced higher blood pressure (diastolic) and higher mean arterial pressure. The lower forgivers were also more aggressive. High forgivers, on the other hand, more freely expressed positive emotions, were more likely to give social support and showed greater empathy.

Factors That Foster Forgiveness

Psychologist Robert Enright defines forgiveness as "giving up the resentment to which you are entitled, and offering to the person who hurt you friendlier attitudes to which they are not entitled." While we may indeed believe people who hurt us are not entitled to friendlier attitudes, the truth is that all people act in hurtful ways out of their own pain. All people deserve compassion. We may decide to no longer keep them in our daily lives or within our circle of friends, but all people, regardless of their actions, deserve compassion.

Thoughts about forgiveness:

1. It is not about condoning the actions of another.
2. Consider your role in the relationship dynamics.
3. Forgiveness does not make you weak. It empowers.
4. You may not be able to forget, but the "charge" associated with the memory may fade.
5. Forgiveness lies entirely with the injured party.
6. Attachment leads to suffering. You may need to surrender your cherished beliefs at times.
7. Recognize that you have hurt others in your life.
8. Anger is a natural and necessary pathway to releasing the stored energy of hurt and resentment, but do not direct your anger at others.
9. Empathy and compassion are essential to meaningful forgiveness.

When you do not forgive, it is a deliberate decision to carry the hurt with you every moment of every day. While forgiveness means grieving and probing the depths of our wounds, it also means gradually moving closer and closer to living in present time—the place where all healing really begins.

Two key factors that foster forgiveness are closeness and empathy. Researchers have recently found that people in relationships that are closer, more affectionate and more committed before a betrayal or hurt are more motivated to forgive. In addition, the ability to put oneself in the offending party's shoes, to experience empathy, is crucial to forgiveness.

THE PRACTICE OF TONGLEN

Tonglen is an ancient meditation practice that allows us to feel the connectedness of all things and not run from the suffering of another. It may be translated as "taking and sending." In the practice of forgiveness it allows us to recognize the suffering and the humanity in the person who has committed a hurtful act and to support him or her with our love. In short, you breathe the suffering of another into your heart and give back to them generosity, loving kindness and health. There is also a beautiful, hidden purpose behind tonglen that we will share following a note about this practice.

Visualize all the pain, suffering and hurt that is in the person with whom you are concerned. You may wish to begin this practice with someone more neutral rather than one who has hurt you badly. You might then graduate to a person who has hurt you badly when you feel ready. Inhale the person's pain and imagine it traveling down to the warmth of your heart. Since our hearts are much more abundant and vibrant than we think, this practice does no harm.

Hold the person's suffering in your heart. On exhaling, send your peace, freedom, love and goodness out to the other person, imagining that he or she is being bathed in this healing gift. Repeat the practice of inhaling the pain into your heart and exhaling the warmth of your heart. Repeat this "taking and sending" for five breaths, five minutes, or whatever you feel comfortable doing.

While it may seem contradictory to our feelings to send so much love and compassion to someone by whom we feel hurt, ask yourself this fundamental question. Would the world (or your life) be better if this person continued to act in hurtful ways or would it be better if the person were able to heal into wholeness, thus ceasing his or her hurtful actions?

The beauty of tonglen practice is that it begins to dull the illusion that we are separate from others. In addition, many of us spend our entire lives running from pain and toward pleasure. With the practice of tonglen, you actually move *toward* pain by breathing in the pain of another, and send out your most pleasant expression of kindness. This is, in essence, the reverse of what we usually do. This practice, therefore, can eventually break us from the endless cycle of avoiding pain and seeking pleasure. Once separated from this cycle, we cannot be easily hurt because we have developed a deeper sense of compassion and connectedness.

SUFFERING, GRATITUDE AND THE BREATH OF LIFE

Many hurts and betrayals seem beyond our capacity to cope with or understand, yet we rarely see what gifts lie beyond great suffering. One who is betrayed by a spouse may find that the truest, deepest love awaits them in a new relationship when the dust has settled. Or they may discover that their clinging and possessing has not allowed them to live life fully; that the betrayal has ripped them from a comfort and they can later be grateful for that. They may then rest more peacefully in their existing relationship.

Dr. Carolyn Myss has been quoted as saying, "Order is a human contrived phenomenon, chaos is divine. When chaos emerges, look for the hand of

God." She further notes that it is easy to find gratitude when the banquet table is full. Finding gratitude when the table is empty is much more difficult. In this light, one might begin to cultivate a *practice* of gratitude. No matter how severe the trial, you might attempt to find something for which to be grateful. Thich Nhat Han advocates a gratitude practice wherein he finds one new thing each day for which to be grateful.

John G. Bennet shares these poignant words on suffering:

You come to see ... that suffering is required; and you no more want to avoid it than you want to avoid putting your next foot on the ground when you are walking. In the spiritual path, joy and suffering follow one another like two feet, and you come to a point of not minding which "foot" is on the ground. You realize, on the contrary, that it is extremely uncomfortable hopping all the time on the joy foot.

There is a wise axiom that *suffering equals pain plus resistance*. It is our resistance that creates enduring suffering. We so often greet pain by holding our breath or breathing in shallow, contracted ways. It is one of the practiced (but harmful) ways of suppressing painful emotions.

Our adult lungs hold about 7 L of air, yet many of us breathe in an average of only 950 mL of air with every breath. The volume of air we take in with each breath dictates the amount of oxygen delivered to our tissues. Since oxygen is needed by every cell to generate energy, our shallow, oxygen-poor breaths deprive us of the vital fuel that drives our energy pathways. In short, when we do not breathe deeply and regularly we limit our ability to rebuild and repair.

The power of breath goes well beyond the biochemistry of cell energy. Many religious and spiritual traditions equate the breath with spirit. In the four canonical gospels, Jesus refers to "spirit" more than 100 times. In both Hebrew and Aramaic, the words *ruach* and *ruha* respectively stand for several English words: spirit, wind, air and breath. Christian, Jewish, Buddhist and other traditions suggest that the breath carries the spirit.

Rumi, the 12th-century mystic and poet, offers his thoughts on breath:

There is a way of breathing that is
a shame and a suffocation.
And there's another way of expiring a love breath,
that lets you open infinitely.

PRAYER AND MEDITATION

Members of the world's spiritual communities have long believed that prayer and meditation have the ability to heal and to deepen meaning in life. In the past two decades, the subject of prayer and healing has gained attention within the medical community as a serious, sensible means to improve health and quality of life. In a recent study of 4000 adults over 65, researchers at Duke University Medical Center studied health problems in those who prayed once a month, more than once a month or not at all. Those who never prayed ran a 50% greater risk of dying during the six-year study period. The risk of death held even after scientists controlled for risk factors such as drinking, smoking and social isolation.

Other studies have shown benefit to those who meditate. A study published in *Stroke: Journal of the American Heart Association* looked at the effect of meditation on the narrowing of blood vessels. Doctors began the study by taking ultrasound pictures of the carotid artery in the neck. All subjects tested had similar amounts of plaque buildup on the vessel walls, which narrowed the artery. Such narrowing can decrease blood supply to the brain and increase the risk of heart attack or stroke. It may also impair memory function as we age.

Test subjects then began a twice-a-day meditation program. After seven months, people who meditated showed a significant decrease in thickening of the carotid artery. Individuals who did not meditate experienced increased thickening over the same seven-month period.

Scientists learned some years ago that stress causes a buildup of substances called lipid peroxides in the brains of animals. Regardless of the type of stress, these nasty lipid peroxides appeared. More recent research with humans reveals that lipid peroxides increase in the blood after prolonged stress. For example, scientists in Russia discovered that the levels of MDA, a damaged fat molecule, correlated directly with the severity of the emotional stress.

What is so significant about lipid peroxides? Lipid means fat, while peroxide refers to a specific biochemical change that has occurred to damage the fat. In essence, lipid peroxides are rancid fats—not something you particularly want in the brain. The discovery that lipid peroxides may build up in the brain from stress is significant because the brain's *structure* is nearly 60% fat. In essence, the brain's structural fats may become rancid under stress, something that can affect brain performance and brain longevity.

Researchers showed that adults who were long-term practitioners of TM, or transcendental meditation, had lipid peroxides an average of 15% lower than those who did not meditate. Meditation was also found to lower the lipid peroxide levels in the elderly.

Even more interesting is a recent study suggesting that individuals who are prayed for without their knowledge also derive benefit. At St. Luke's Hospital in Kansas City, Missouri, doctors studied a group of patients, most of whom had suffered heart attacks. The patient's names were randomly assigned to a prayer group who prayed daily for the patients over a four-week period. The control group received standard medical care without prayer. Doctors discovered that patients who had been prayed for did about 10% better than those in the control group.

These studies and many like them raise interesting new questions about the potential for prayer and meditation to deepen one's healing journey. They suggest that prayer and meditation practices are health-building practices. We must say with some humility, however, that this is only logical to those who practise prayer and meditation. Yet more studies like this may be needed before medicine adopts these practices as a standard part of care.

A MINDFUL PATH TO WHOLENESS

On the journey of life, struggle, pain, suffering and illness are inevitable. Each of us has the choice to frame our circumstances in whatever way we choose, but the meaning we give our life experience bears strongly on whether struggle and pain is a growth experience or otherwise. As Mayo Clinic doctors found, those who explained their life in pessimistic ways had a 20% higher rate of death over a given period.

We have taken on the daunting task of describing mind-body-spirit influences on our health and longevity. We realize that we have omitted important features because of space. We also recognize that the mind-body-spirit language is an artificial separation.

We have tried to give some sense, through our own assembly of thought and research, that love, relationships, laughter, expression, forgiveness, prayer and meditation are components of a healthy life. Yet we also understand that a healthy life may not mean a life free of illness or disability. We believe that a healthy life is one that is full of meaning, purpose, richness, passion and above all, LOVE. We know of no hormone, vitamin or exercise that can replace the vibrancy that comes with love in all its forms.

Part III

Ten Steps to a Younger You

IT'S NEVER TOO LATE TO CHANGE YOUR BIO-AGE

Congratulations! You've made it through a complex journey through some of the most fascinating recent advances in anti-aging research. Now it's time to bring together all the steps you need to take to realize your quest for a younger you. So, how young do you want to be? These next pages will demonstrate that it really is up to you.

We hope that this book has now set the stage for a breakthrough approach in how you look, feel and perform. It is in your best interest not to put this task off any longer and change your old habits for these new ones, starting today. We all get caught up in our own comfort zones, and we tend to feel the least vulnerable while we remain in these zones, even when our actions are responsible for our failures. For many of us, in a sense our "failure" is that we're aging before our time. We've all heard the sayings "A leopard never changes its spots" and "The older you get, the more set in your ways and stubborn you become." While both of these statements can sometimes be true, they don't have to pertain to you. *You* are the only one who can make a difference in your Bio-Age.

This section will lay out a step-by-step Bio-Age life plan that you can put into effect immediately. We have amassed what we feel to be the top 10 steps that will allow you to reverse your own Bio-Age. We have tried our best to make these steps as short and straightforward as possible. Even though you have read through the information presented in *Bio-Age*, it is a lot to digest. These 10 steps contain some reminders of what you have already read and offer some new practical tips you can put into practice. If you follow them as closely as possible, you should notice results quickly.

These steps are not set out in any order of importance. Each of the steps is powerful in its own right. Make it a point to introduce them one at a time, a few at a time or all of them if you can for best results. Each step is followed by a few pages of elaboration The steps are easy to incorporate into your life; all you have to do is make a commitment to follow some or all of them every day. You can also choose the steps that you are most interested in. You don't have to incorporate all of them into your life at once; it's up to you.

After all, by following these guidelines you will most probably experience a profound difference in your life. You may actually *look*, *feel* and *perform* better than you had ever dreamed possible. You may be adding candles to your birthday cake each and every year, while all the time growing biologically younger. The newer, younger you is only 1 to 10 steps away. So let's get started.

BIO-AGE STEP #1: Increase Your Water Intake

You are mostly water! Even your bones are one quarter water. Your muscles are three quarters water and the wet matter of your brain is 85% water. Your blood and lungs are over 80% water. Next to oxygen, water is definitely our most important nutrient for sustaining life. Many people believe they get enough water from their juice, coffee, tea and sodas, but these do not satisfy the need for water. You may be suffering from dehydration and not even know it.

As you've read in Dr. Batmanghelidj's essay in Chapter 9, aging has been referred to as a process of drying up. Some medical experts, including Dr. Batmanghelidj, believe that at some point in human evolution our hunger and thirst signals got mixed up, so in a sense, when we are feeling hungry, we may in fact be thirsty.

Many other researchers now believe that water—not just fluid—is essential to our health and well-being and is therefore one of the keys to slowing down the aging process. A person weighing 68 kg contains approximately 37 L of water, which must be completely replaced every five to ten days. The average person loses almost eight cups of water a day just through normal metabolic processes. Intensive exercise increases this loss. Exercisers can easily lose 2–4 kg of fluid through perspiration, evaporation and exhalation. Studies show that for every kilogram of fluid lost, there is a significant drop in the efficiency with which the body produces energy. So if one of your goals is to increase your energy level (and who wouldn't want that?), then drink more water. After age 40 the kidneys begin to shrink and the bladder starts to lose elasticity.

Drinking at least eight glasses of water a day can help ward off these changes.

One more reason to consume lots of clean filtered water throughout the day is because of its positive effect on intracellular hydration. By increasing the water inside the cells of the body, the all-important process of anabolism is increased. Intracellular water causes the cell to expand, allowing for more amino acids to enter the cell for repair to take place. Remember, by increasing your anabolic metabolism, you slow down biological aging.

Some Water Is Better Than Others

As more than 60,000 different chemicals are known to contaminate our water supplies, it makes good sense to consume the cleanest water you can find. And since many of our water-treatment systems are underfunded and/or obsolete, it is becoming increasingly difficult to get rid of those contaminants. In 1993 the U.S. Environmental Protection Agency reported that 819 water systems throughout America had toxic levels of lead still remaining in fully treated water coming out of taps. Canadian concern about water safety was raised when E. coli bacteria seeped into the water system of one Ontario town, resulting in widespread illness and the deaths of at least 10 people. To avoid some of the possible hazards of drinking regular tap water, let's take a look at other alternatives.

Filters

Carbon filtration systems, such as the famous Brita® filters, are some of the most popular devices for cleaning our water, but how effective are these? Even though carbon filters have been shown to remove a significant portion of the chlorine content in water, they do very little for the thousands of other contaminants. Another downfall of these inexpensive systems is the problem with increased bacterial counts over time. In one recent study of the Brita® filter system, four out of six one-week-old filters tested had higher bacterial counts than those in regular tap water.

Reverse Osmosis Systems

These are a much better alternative than the carbon systems. The higher-quality ones use a four-step filtration method that can produce a very low contamination yield when completed. You can buy bottles of reverse osmosis water from health food stores.

Bottled Water/Home Distillation

Since most of the bottled water companies simply use regular tap water run through a filtration system, it is important to know the water company you are dealing with. If their starting supply is indeed regular tap water, the company should first be putting the water through the process of distillation to remove most contaminants. When purchasing bottled water, it is a good idea to contact the company that produced it to ask how many parts per million (ppm) contaminants are in their water. Good water companies test their water supply frequently and should have no problem giving out this information. Tap water typically has anywhere from 200 to 500 ppm of contaminants, while quality bottled water should contain no more than 40 ppm.

Water Tips
- Replace other liquids with clean filtered water and consume at least eight glasses throughout the day.
- Drink the water from a closed container and through a straw to avoid excess air and bloating.
- Consume the amount of water that your activity level and health profile require. The bare minimum should be eight to ten 250 mL glasses of water per day. If you are active, add at least another two 250 mL glasses to your intake. It's important to note that water is needed for detoxification and elimination of waste by-products through your metabolism. If you are consuming extra protein, then you should increase your water intake as well. Since you will be losing body fat and gaining muscle on the Bio-Age plan, you will need this extra water to safely eliminate the toxins that accumulate in the adipose tissue (fat cells) and that are then released as the fat is used as energy.
- Consume foods rich in water. Foods like watermelon contain large amounts of water per serving. In addition, the water in such foods is considered "structured" from a physics point of view, which makes it biologically more useful.

BIO-AGE STEP #2:

Sleep Deep
In order to perform at peak energy efficiency, one must get enough quality sleep. Before the advent of electric light in 1879, the average person slept 10 hours. Loss of sleep has been shown in research to have a cumulative negative effect on the overall outcome of energy production, glucose metabolism and aging.

As Dr. Daniel Crisafi suggested in the chapter "Waking Up Younger," the one third of our lives that we should spend sleeping will absolutely determine how we live the other two thirds of our lives in terms of overall health and productivity. Proper sleep is essential to replenish energy reserves, rebuild and repair muscle tissue, reenergize the immune system and cleanse the brain of excess cellular debris.

Tips for Restful Sleep

- Determine your sleep quota (i.e., the number of hours you need to feel refreshed and at your best), and try hard to reach it every night. The body repairs itself in the delta sleep phase, which occurs in the early hours of the morning, so the later you fall asleep, the less your body will repair itself for the morning.

- Do not eat (especially high-carbohydrate foods) too close to bedtime. Eating before sleep can alter your HGH production due to increased insulin levels. Not eating for two or three hours before bedtime allows for maximum HGH peaks. If you eat a high-carbohydrate source before sleeping, you run the risk of increasing your cortisol (stress hormone) levels in the middle of the night. Cortisol is also produced in response to low blood sugar (which usually follows a high-insulin response). This is one of the reasons people wake up in the middle of the night and can't get back to sleep.

- According to Dr. Edward Conley, author of the chapter "Running on Empty," approximately 58% of people tested in his clinic are deficient in the amino acid tryptophan, which is needed to produce melatonin (your sleep-inducing hormone). As we have mentioned, tryptophan can be found in soy protein, bananas, pineapples and milk products, and especially whey protein powders that contain high alpha-lactalbumin levels. (See Appendix II for recommendations.)

- For quality sleep, one must sleep in as complete darkness as possible. We all produce tiny, light-sensitive proteins in our skin called cryptochromes, which pick up the slightest light source and convey the message of light to our brains. These cryptochromes have the ability to lower our melatonin response. Cover or shut off all light sources during sleep, including light from clock radios, TVs, night-lights, room lights and hallway lights, and cover windows to shut out any street light source.

- Establish a regular daily schedule. Rise at the same time each morning. Go to bed at the same time each night, whether you feel sleepy or not, and whether you immediately go to sleep or not.

- Establish a regular eating schedule. Eat a light dinner, preferably three hours or more before bedtime. Don't eat anything after your evening meal, especially just before bedtime.

- Limit your intake of coffee, tea, cola drinks or chocolate.

- Avoid alcoholic beverages either as a nightcap or an "eye-opener." Remember that alcohol suppresses essential REM sleep. Very often the alcoholic beverage will help you fall asleep, but you will wake up earlier than warranted or you will notice a reduced quality of sleep.

- Develop a regular exercise program. This is especially important for sedentary individuals or where there is emotional or mental fatigue. A brisk walk for half an hour after supper may be all you need for a good night's sleep. Wait at least one hour after eating before vigorous exercise, but do not exercise vigorously within two hours of bedtime

- Apply gentle heat to your body, a very useful remedy for insomnia. Take a warm, non-alcoholic, non-caffeinated beverage such as camomile tea, or take a lukewarm bath with the essential oil of lavender.

- Try to sleep where it is quiet. Decrease noise pollution in your environment. Some people sleep soundly next to a busy railroad or in a factory, but most of us can't shut out the noise around us.

- Be sure the room you sleep in is well ventilated. Avoid drafts, but at least get indirect ventilation. Increased oxygen intake and cooler temperatures set the stage for sleeping soundly.

- Use a good-quality mattress. It surprises me how people can easily spend $20,000–$30,000 for a car and only a couple of hundred dollars on their bedding. You will spend as much as one third of your life in your bed, and a very good mattress will last 15 years or more. Investing in your sleep environment means investing in your life.

- Do not worry if you stay awake for a while. Don't let the anxiety of sleeplessness cause greater anxiety and greater sleeplessness. Practice relaxation techniques or meditation. Even if you just rest quietly for six or seven hours, you will get enough restorative rest to handle the next day. You will also be getting sleep you are not aware of. One consistent finding of sleep studies is that the subjects get more sleep than they think they do.

- Try to end your day on a low key. Avoid physical or mental high points near the end of the day (one of the reasons we don't recommend exercising late in the evening). Avoid exciting television programs or movies just before going to bed. Be wary of those stimulating computer videos. Try not to argue with others and do try to reconcile yourself with family members.

- In some cases, certain nutrient supplements and herbal formulas may be of value. Vitamin B3 is an activator of receptors for diazepam (a brain endorphin). Taking 50–100 mg at dinner may be helpful. Vitamin B3 in the form of niacinamide, the form that doesn't cause unpleasant flushing, is preferable. Griffonia, a source of hydroxy tryptophan, will help raise serotonin levels in the brain. Also, remember that calcium is required to trigger and maintain sleep. Calcium citrate can be a very valuable adjunct taken 30–60 minutes before bedtime. Magnesium glycinate can be another helpful sleep aid.

BIO-AGE STEP #3:

Nutrient Intervention

Your body's chemistry is an elaborate web of thousands of different molecules working beautifully in harmony. This web of interaction is entirely reliant upon the nutrients obtained through the diet. Because the body is absolutely dependent upon fundamental nutrients like vitamins and minerals, it is impossible to realistically name the "top" nutrients for optimal health.

However, if we assume that you are going to get the basic vitamins and minerals in adequate amounts, we can describe some of the important nutrients that we believe are essential to any program that will enhance your well-being. These are also the nutrients that are either usually deficient in modern diets or nutrients that help prevent some of the most common maladies in our society. Below is a brief description of the 10 nutrient categories that we think can be added to your support program. The basic list is accompanied by our reasons for suggesting the food or nutrient in question.

Fatty Acids
- borage oil (primrose oil, black currant seed oil)
- fish oil (or algae oil)
- flax seed oil
- krill oil

Fatty acids are the building blocks of all cells and are the key messenger molecules that govern the inflammatory system, immune system and hormonal system. They are the chief structural nutrients in the brain and are necessary to prevent brain degeneration as we age. Also, heart arrhythmia, one of the common causes of death from heart attack and stroke, can be prevented and, in some cases, eliminated by increasing our intake of fatty acids.

Western diets contain a ratio of omega-6 to omega-3 fatty acids of up to 20:1, when the ratio should be more like 2:1. In practice, this means that we are getting far too little of the important omega-3 fatty acid family. A combination of fish oil, flax seed oil and borage oil provides a very balanced fatty acid complex. Krill oil is another exceptional source of omega-3 fatty acids. In addition, krill oil is rich in carotenoids, vitamin E and phospholipids—all critical to any longevity program.

Proteins
- free essential amino acids
- whey protein
- soy protein

Protein is essential to maintain muscle mass, synthesize enzymes, make hormones and a vast array of other functions. These are made up of amino acids, which are the building blocks for these essential structural and functional roles. Branched-chain amino acids are critical to maintain muscle mass and are present in free-form amino acids as well as in whey protein. Whey protein also contains sulfur-based compounds that help build the very crucial glutathione molecule and aid in the detoxification processes. Recall that this molecule declines rapidly as we age. Proteins also contain the building blocks for the neurotransmitters that govern our mood, memory and behavior.

Antioxidants
- coenzyme Q10 (30–200 mg/day)
- glutathione (100 mg/day)
- lipoic acid (50–200 mg/day)
- mixed carotenoids (beta-carotene, lutein, zeaxanthin)
- N-acetyl carnitine (1000–1500 mg/day)
- N-acetylcysteine (50–200 mg/day)
- tocotrienols (30–60 mg/day)
- vitamin C (2000 mg/day)
- vitamin E (400 IU/day)

There are many, many antioxidant molecules in the body, but several have been identified as crucial substances that work in a network fashion to protect us from free radical injury, one of the hallmarks of aging. Taking one antioxidant in excess is no longer considered the wise form of supplementation. Combination antioxidants help ensure that balance will be maintained within the antioxidant system. Look for antioxidant formulas that contain the above network antioxidants, or purchase them separately; these should be included in your daily diet. For a complete formula containing all the essential network antioxidants refer to Appendix II.

One of the first changes that precedes illness or disease is a drop in energy efficiency. Mitochondria are the tiny structures within cells that produce energy from our dietary fuels. Decline in mitochondrial function in, for example, heart muscle, skeletal muscle and brain tissue is consistently associated with poor health outcomes. N-acetylcarnitine helps support mitochondrial energy production throughout the body and also supports acetylcholine synthesis in the brain. Coenzyme Q10 is a vital part of the electron transport so critical to energy production. Both nutrients have been studied and used in treatment of many adult disorders ranging from fatigue to brain disorders to heart conditions. These nutrients are known to improve cell energy at almost every level and can have extraordinary effects in supporting healthy longevity.

Our bodies are designed to make CoQ10 and carnitine, but frequently do not make enough. Moreover, making these two nutrients requires a number of other nutrients such as lysine, methionine, vitamin B6, vitamin C and others.

Plant Flavonoids

- apples
- blackberries
- blueberries
- cherries
- onions
- strawberries

Flavonoids are a family of molecules found widely in plants. Flavonoids have innumerable supportive functions in the human body. Their effects are wide-ranging and protect against conditions like diabetes, heart disease, memory impairment, cancer and many others. Flavonoids are also vital for regulating the inflammatory system as well as inhibiting formation of AGE proteins, as discussed in Chapter 16. Blueberries have among the richest flavonoid content of all and have been shown in animal studies to reverse the mental decline associated with aging. Some of the richest sources of flavonoids are listed above, though there are many others.

Methyl Donors

- betaine (10 mg/day)
- choline (10 mg/day)
- folic acid (1000 mcg/day)
- vitamin B6 (3 mg/day)
- vitamin B12 (1000 mcg/day)

In order to function properly, your body must become efficient at shuttling around tiny little molecules called methyl groups, which consist of one carbon and three hydrogens—CH_3. Methyl groups do tremendous things like help you synthesize DNA, but they also protect you from a toxic by-product of your own metabolism called homocysteine. The number one killer in North America is still heart disease, and elevated blood fat is only one cause. Elevated homocysteine is another important contributor. This toxic amino acid intermediate contributes to damage of blood vessels in the heart, brain and elsewhere. The key nutrient cofactors that prevent the buildup of the toxic homocysteine molecule are those listed above (though B6 is technically not a methyl donor). Note also that vitamin B12 deficiency can manifest as poor memory and concentration. Many people have been mistakenly diagnosed with Alzheimer's dementia when they actually had vitamin B12 deficiency.

Herbs and Spices
- garlic
- ginger
- green tea
- oregano
- rosemary
- thyme
- turmeric

Spices not only help food taste good, they are powerful substances that influence the aging process. Those mentioned above have multiple biochemical actions. Several are known to possess the ability to inhibit the COX-2 enzyme. This is an enzyme associated with inflammation and tissue damage. COX-2 levels have recently been found to be elevated in some cancers such as prostate cancer. COX-2–blocking substances may even protect against Alzheimer's disease. New drugs such as Vioxx™ and Celebrex™ are powerful COX-2–blocking drugs. Many of these spices listed above can perform most of the same metabolic functions as aspirin, but without the side effects.

Rosemary, thyme and turmeric influence glycation, the sugar–protein reaction that results in browning, stiffening and wrinkling in the body. We believe ginger will also be found to block glycation, but only further study will confirm this. Ginger, oregano, rosemary and turmeric are strong COX-2–inhibiting plants, so they can influence inflammation. Don't be concerned about dosage here. Just use the spices to taste as a regular part of your culinary habit. Fresh herbs are probably best, but dry herbs are fine as well.

Minerals
- chromium (200–400 mcg/day)
- magnesium (350 mg/day)
- selenium (50-100 mcg/day; up to 400 mcg under doctor's supervision)
- zinc (20 mg/day)

Minerals are essential components of body chemistry, so it is somewhat artificial to select only four for special mention, yet these four have been chosen because they are often found to be insufficient in adults and they influence some of the most common disorders of adulthood. Chromium has a powerful effect on blood sugar, diabetes and glycation (AGE). Selenium is one of the most widely documented trace elements with cancer-protecting activity. It also supports thyroid function and antioxidant enzyme protection. When magnesium levels decline, which is so very common in adults, over 100 enzyme systems suffer, including those responsible for energy production. Myelin, the covering around nerve cells that speeds nerve transmission, also requires magnesium for its production and maintenance.

Colostrum

Colostrum, as described in Chapter 13, has many important immunological benefits. It has also been shown to improve growth hormone synthesis, which is one of the most important means of retaining anabolic function as we mature. (Take 1000 mg twice daily on an empty stomach.)

Balancing Hormones with DIM
- DHEA (5 mg/day to support anabolic metabolism)
- DIM (150–200 mg/day for balancing hormones)
- DIM (200–400 mg/day for building lean muscle mass and increasing fat loss)

In Chapter 12, you learned about DIM (diindolylmethane) and its beneficial effects. DIM is *not* estrogen, but it helps the body produce more of the "good" 2-hydroxy estrogens while reducing the amount of "bad" 16-hydroxy estrogens. Also, DIM increases the amount of "free" or unbound testosterone. This is ideal for burning fat and increasing muscle mass in both men and women—vital steps toward attaining healthy longevity. As noted in Appendix I, a urine test is presently available should you wish to measure your existing ratio of 2-hydroxy to 16-hydroxy estrogens.

Supplements for Joint Support
- chondroitin sulfate (1500 mg/day)
- glucosamine sulfate (1500 mg/day)

As we move beyond age 35 our life activity, nutritional health, stress and trauma begin to show their effects on our joint tissue. Inflammatory changes in the joints grow more common with increasing years. Chondroitin sulfate and glucosamine sulfate have been shown to have very beneficial effects on reducing pain, inflammation and restoring cartilage integrity. There has been some debate over whether glucosamine sulfate is better or chondroitin sulfate is better. Our understanding of the medical literature and the chemistry of these two leads us to believe that both have considerable merit. Since glucosamine sulfate is much cheaper, many companies cast a negative shadow on chondroitin because they do not want to add this more expensive component and thus raise the cost of their product. The data support the value of chondroitin, however. If you have joint concerns, taking these two nutrients together can be invaluable. If you have no symptoms in your joints, there is probably no need for these supplements.

Bonus: A Glass of Wine

Red wine contains an abundant complement of flavonoids, including flavo-nols, anthocyanins, catechins and procyanins. Wine diluted by 1000 times had antioxidant protection greater than vitamin E and comparable to the flavonoid quercitin. New data suggest that red wine may protect against glycation. It has been estimated that if North Americans consumed two glasses of red wine a day, we could reduce our rate of heart disease by 40%. Two glasses per day may seem excessive to some and normal to others. We are not making a personal statement about the correct amount. However, the research is beginning to show that the flavonoids in grapes as delivered by red wine have considerable health benefits.

BIO-AGE STEP #4:

Raise Albumin Levels Through Optimum Hygiene

For more than 100 years, high concentrations of albumin in the serum have been regarded as the bellwether of health. More recent evidence from the British Regional Heart study, The National Institute on Aging (NIA), The National Health and Nutrition Examination Survey (NHANES) and many others, highlight a dramatic reduction in mortality and morbidity rates due to increasing concentrations of albumin. Medically speaking, the quality of life is influenced by the quantity of albumin.

Sound health, which basically means cell stability, can only be achieved in humans when albumin levels reach their highest levels. The higher the ratio of albumin to globulins (other serum proteins) the better. Anyone can figure out their albumin to globulin ratios by simply having your albumin and globulin level tested then dividing the amount of albumin by the amount globulin. For example, if your albumin ratio is 50 g/L and your globulin ratio is 25 g/L, then your A/G ratio would be 2.0 (50 divided by 25 = 2.0). Albumin should always be at least twice as high as the globulin for an adequate health profile, while three times the albumin to globulin would be optimum.

Steps to Achieving Optimal Albumin Profiles

For people over 65, those with cancer, diabetes, autoimmune diseases or chronic disease, it is essential to increase your albumin profiles by following the recommendations listed below. It is possible to maintain optimal albu-min profiles to at least 100 years of age.

- Use the Advanced Hygiene System consisting of a special soap that helps to wash away bacteria and viruses and a facial dip for the eyes and nose (see Appendix II for more information).

- For maximum efficacy, wash the fingernail area using the advanced hygiene tub of soap a minimum of five times per day. For best results, perform the facial dips, alternating between A, B and C every morning and night for best results. The dips should be performed at the first sign of headaches, congestion, sore throats, eye problems or allergies.
- Wash your hair a minimum of three times a week.
- Brush your teeth four times a day and floss at least once.
- Whenever possible visit the beach, swim and sunbathe without burning. Regular swimming in a clean pool is also beneficial.
- Maintain a clean environment. If you have pets, make sure they are kept clean.
- Get a sound night's sleep and get to bed as early as possible each night.
- Make sure your home and workplace are well ventilated.
- Biocize exercise will ensure that albumin leaves the bloodstream, surrounds cells and is returned via the lymphatic system.
- Supplement with high-quality proteins (see Appendix II for specific recommendations). Remember that albumin is a protein.
- Don't overeat. Overeating reduces albumin levels by stressing albumin cargo holds. When excess food breaks down into its smallest components and enters the bloodstream, albumin must transport the excess nutrients and fatty acids to the cells. This excess stress causes the albumin molecule to become overloaded and unable to clear excess toxins from the body.
- Drink plenty of clean filtered water each day.
- Many natural health experts believe that disease starts in the colon. To keep albumin levels high, cleanse the colon regularly with natural herbs such as Psyllium Seed Powder. Psyllium is an excellent colon and intestine cleanser that helps to remove excess toxins that accumulate in the intestinal tract. Always drink plenty of water when taking psyllium. Another great colon cleanser that has been around for centuries is actually a combination of three fruits called Triphala. Triphala is an Ayurvedic formula that has been used by billions of people around the world. Many health care experts believe it to be one of the most effective and safest laxative and colon tonic in existence today. The usual dose is one to three capsules before bed in a tea or with a glass of warm water.

BIO-AGE STEP #5:

Exercise Regularly Using the Biocize Exercise Philosophy

As we age we lose lean body mass and gain fat in its place. Weight-bearing activity (weight training) causes us to gain lean body mass and burn calories more efficiently, which helps reverse many of the biomarkers of aging.

After reading the "Biocize: Anti-aging Exercise" chapter you have a firm grasp on why proper exercise can help to reverse your Bio-Age. What we will provide for you here are some of the top resistance exercises that provide the greatest hormonal advantage for reducing your Bio-Age. Please consult a personal trainer if you have never trained with weights before. Also make sure to get medical clearance before performing any of the recommended exercises presented here.

Some Important Biocize Reminders

- Remember to perform your weight-bearing exercises first in the program, followed by cardio activity (such as walking). This will allow for optimum levels of fat to be burned while performing the cardio portion of Biocize.
- Try to consume a protein green drink approximately one half hour before exercising for optimal fat-burning hormonal response (see Appendix II for recommendations).
- Try to consume a high-quality whey protein, fresh fruit (berries) and organic flaxseed oil shake immediately after exercising for maximum anabolic activity (see pages 247–48 for suggested shake recipes).
- See Bio-Age shake recipes in Step #6 for a variety of delicious anabolic protein shakes. The ones listed are our personal favorites.
- As stated in the "Biocize: Anti-aging Exercise" chapter, your body will become accustomed to the resistance portion of any exercise routine in as little as a few weeks. Therefore, we recommend changing your routine every second month for best results.
- The resistance portion (weight training) of Biocize should never take you longer than 45 minutes to perform; any more than 45 minutes and you will most probably produce too many stress hormones.
- If you are a beginner, you can follow the highly successful routine outlined in *Fat Wars: 45 Days to Transform Your Body* published by CDG Books, Inc. You can also log onto *www.fatwars.com* for detailed descriptions and pictures of the various exercises.
- Don't get caught up in your weight. Remember that muscle weighs more than fat and gaining quality muscle is the name of the game, especially where fat loss is concerned.
- Men will experience results with the resistance portion of Biocize faster than most women due to their higher testosterone levels. Men usually experience a rapid increase in muscle mass and strength, as well as an increase in transport proteins, fat-burning enzymes and immune factors. Women will also experience an increase in strength and intracellular proteins, but without the bulk gains made by men. Levels of cortisol (the

muscle-wasting hormone) will begin to drop and levels of glucagon (the fat-releasing hormone) will begin to rise.

- Don't become discouraged in the first few weeks of your new Biocize routine. If you are like over two thirds of middle-aged North Americans, your body has become accustomed to the extra layers of fat that covers the "lean, younger you" underneath, so at first it may be reluctant to change. Just keep persisting and you will be amazed at your progress.
- Make a full commitment to yourself to complete your Biocize portion of the Bio-Age plan each and every day. It is one of the major keys in the success of the program. Stick to the recommendations as closely as possible.

Biocize: Before You Begin

- Always start with one or two warm-up sets when you begin to lift weights. The resistance should be light enough for you to handle 15–20 repetitions.
- Always use slow, controlled movements. Remember: You're in control of the weight—the weight isn't in control of you. Too many rush to lift the weight up and literally let it fall back down to the starting position. This will set you up for injuries as well as wasted effort. A good rule to follow is to count to three while lowering the weight.
- Never train the same muscle group two days in a row. Allow at least 48 hours between working each muscle group.
- Try working these muscle groups in the following manner: Day 1: Chest and back; Day 2: Legs; Day 3: Shoulders and arms. Day 1 could represent Monday, Day 2 Wednesday, and Day 3 Friday. On Tuesday, Thursday and the weekend, you would perform only the cardio portion of your Biocize plan, preferably first thing in the morning on an empty stomach.

The Top Biocize Exercises for Maximum Hormonal Release

As we have emphasized throughout this book, weight-resistant exercise is one of your most critical tools in achieving and maintaining a young Bio-Age. To obtain the most powerful anti-aging results follow the Biocize suggestions we have offered in this step and either get the help of a personal trainer, find a book on weight-training with detailed diagrams (one good resource is *Weight Training For Dummies* by Suzanne Schlosberg and Liz Neporent) or visit www.fatwars.com for more detailed Biocize exercise instructions. When you do consult with one of these exercise resources, you need to concentrate on the following Biocize exercises in order to elicit maximum anti-aging hormonal release. For each exercise, perform different sets of reps using both barbells and dumbbells. Select the weight appropriate to your size and fitness level:

- Incline Press (upper chest)
- Overhead Press (shoulder region)
- Lying Tricep Extension (triceps)
- Flat Bench Press (chest, shoulders, triceps)
- Squat (legs and buttocks)
- Stiffed-Legged Deadlift (hamstrings and lower back)
- Standing Curl (front of arms)

Cardio Portion of Biocize

Move Your Body Regularly

It is hard enough to deal with the day-to-day decline in lung function that seems to be a normal process of the aging cycle without also dealing with the excess burden of polluted air, less oxygen in our atmosphere and smoking (for those of us who are crazy enough to do so!). It has been proven that there are a few factors that can aid in the body's ability to improve its vital capacity. One of those factors happens to be a regular program of consistent and progressive aerobic exercise. In one recent study, it was shown that over a 20-week period of endurance training, there was an overall increase in vital capacity of 17.9%. That's a lot of extra oxygen that wasn't there to begin with. Can you imagine what you would achieve if you were to undertake a life-long commitment to exercise?

- Try walking 20–60 minutes a day, either first thing in the morning on non–weight-lifting days or right after the resistance portion of your workout.

Stretching and Flexibility

As we age our tissues often become more rigid and inflexible. This, in part, stems from the glycation process described in Chapter 16, which is a biochemical process of stiffening. We also become more rigid because we simply do not stretch enough and maintain our tissues in their most supple state. There is no escape. Flexibility is vital to a young Bio-Age.

BIO-AGE STEP #6:

Fuel Your Body on the Bio-Age Plan and Regulate Insulin

As Dr. Barry Sears mentions in his best-selling book, *Enter the Zone*, one famous British study demonstrated how detrimental a high-carbohydrate intake could be for fat loss even while on a calorie-restricted diet. The researchers studied a group of people on a 1000-calorie-per-day diet. One half of the group consumed the 1000 calories as 90% fat while the other half consumed the 1000 calories as 90% carbohydrates. The group on the high-fat diet lost an incredible amount of weight in a very short period of time, while the group consuming the high carbohydrates had *no* weight loss.

While we would never recommend a 1000-calorie-a-day diet of any kind, this study shows the powerful effect of insulin as a fat-storage hormone. Remember: When you are in a storage mode, you can't access fat as a fuel. The message is to not only watch the glycemic value (see pages 71–72 in Chapter 5) of carbohydrates but also to limit the total number of carbohydrates in your diet. In order to lower insulin levels and allow for greater insulin sensitivity, we recommend the following guidelines:

- If you are over 10% of your ideal lean body percentage (see Appendix I), it is our recommendation to limit carbohydrate consumption to no more than 50 g in any given day (weekends may be an exception). You can increase this number as the fat is lifted off your frame.
- For all of you who just want to stay healthy and keep insulin levels in check, we recommend limiting your carbohydrate consumption to approximately 100–150 g in any given day. If you wish, you may allow for a higher portion of carbohydrates one or two days during the week or on weekends. Again, use the glycemic index to guide you to the best carbohydrate choices.
- When it comes to safe and effective sweeteners there are two particular ones we recommend. Neither of these sweeteners will cause a drastic rise in blood sugar levels and therefore are good alternatives (especially for people with diabetes). Stevia extract comes from a plant originally from the rainforests of Brazil and Paraguay. Stevia is more than 100 times sweeter than table sugar (sucrose), but it does not appear to have any of the negative side effects associated with table sugar. It is very safe and widely used as a non-sugar sweetener in food and drink, and it is not broken down by heat, making it a great sweetener for cooking and baking. Another good choice is sorbitol powder: Sorbitol is a synthetically produced sweetener that naturally occurs in many fruits. It is 60% sweeter than table sugar (sucrose) with one-third fewer calories.

How to Eat on the Bio-Age Plan

As we get older, we tend to skip things more and more. Eating is no exception! We feel that if we skip breakfast, eat a small lunch and save the best for dinner, then by some biological miracle we will lose the extra winter coat we've been carrying around through all those summers since we turned 35.

We also tend to diet more as we reach middle age and beyond. Dieters are notorious for depriving themselves of essential nutrients and calories; one of the first things to go is snacks. But the right snacks at the right times can play a useful role in reversing your Bio-Age. Those of you who skip meals while dieting will notice that these lifestyle choices tend to work against your biochemistry, causing you to quickly pack on the fat. Healthy snacks fill the void between meals when blood sugar dips, which, if left unattended, leads to excess calorie consumption at the main meals and possibly binge eating.

Snacking can be good or bad, depending on what the snack is and how much of it you eat. On the *Bio-Age* plan, we recommend eating five or six small meals a day consisting of anywhere from 300 to 500 calories each (depending on your size). This is the optimum amount of calories to take in at each meal to increase the body's ability to burn fat. Any more than 500 calories and the body has a much easier time storing the excess as fat. Of course, as we've mentioned numerous times, the balance of protein, carbs and fat is also very important.

In *Bio-Age* we have focused on natural ways to increase the body's ability to burn fat and slow biological aging. With this in mind, we wouldn't be doing any justice to you if we didn't touch on the aspect of optimum caloric consumption throughout the day. It is through effective eating strategies along with all the other avenues we have laid out before you in *Bio-Age* that makes this plan so effective for overall success. The following are our recommendations for obtaining your optimum Bio-Age. Take stock of what you're eating now and how to change it. Make a commitment to assess your diet and start to buy and eat more healthy food five or six times a day. Take a step-by-step approach to making these new improved habits part of your life *today*.

In order to increase your energy levels, increase muscle and burn fat, you need the proper fuel for your body. Here's an easy equation to remember: Energy comes from calories and calories come from food; therefore, you absolutely need to eat (don't get overly excited yet) and you need to eat *frequently*. The key is to supply your body with the right fuel at the right intervals. Take the example of the sports car and the old clunker. A person with a slow metabolism is like an old clunker. The old clunker won't give you much performance; as a matter of fact, it's content just to make it from point A to point B. It doesn't require much fuel to "chug along." The person with a slow metabolism will take in any extra fuel and store it as a fuel reserve—body fat. Now a person with sufficient muscle and a fast metabolism is like a sports car. The sports car will give you all the performance you need, but it requires regular high-octane fuel to keep performing optimally.

Bio-Age Eating Tips

Metabolism influences the speed at which your body processes food into energy, and it is the major factor in restructuring your body composition. Here's where most diets fail: When you drastically limit the amount of food you take in without increasing the nutrient density of the available food, your metabolism will adjust by slowing down. The reverse is also true. If you supply your body with sufficient nutrient-dense foods, your metabolism will adjust by speeding up.

In order to take advantage of our natural circadian rhythms—the innate daily patterns of our bodies' various processes—we must realize that most of our fat will be burned during the waking hours when our metabolism is at its highest. Therefore, you should eat according to the rate at which your metabolism is able to utilize the fuel sources. And since your metabolism is at its highest in the daytime, with the morning being the most opportune time to burn fat, then your largest meal should be consumed at this time instead of at dinner. Don't skip breakfast! Many people operate under the assumption that skipping this important meal will limit their caloric intake and therefore help them avoid gaining fat—it won't!

- Avoid foods that are high in processed sugars, the wrong types of fat and that do not have enough quality protein. These foods are notorious for shutting off your fat-burning machinery for hours. And if you eat these foods at the end of the day, things get worse—soon afterwards it's bedtime, you usually still have a full tummy and guess what? Your body has a field day storing fat until the wee hours of the morning.

- The largest meals consumed should be in the morning, with the size of these meals decreasing throughout the day. The evening meal should be the smallest of all the meals of the day.

- You should try to eat every three to three-and-a-half hours. No one meal should be higher than 500 calories. The evening meal should be approximately 300–350 calories and should have very little to no carbohydrate source other than approved vegetables. The low insulin response to your last meal is the key to burning fat all night long.

- If you're unable to eat a nutritious, protein-rich breakfast, you should consider a Bio-Age shake that contains quality protein, fruit from the berry family (blueberries preferably) or the melon family. You might also consider adding 1 tbsp of organic flaxseed oil. One of the shakes should be consumed immediately after your Biocize routine (refer to the chapter on " Biocize" for details). Five Bio-Age shake recipes are listed below, including their macronutrient profiles.

- It is very important to your overall Bio-Age success to stick only with low-glycemic carbs like vegetables and certain fruits for your carbohydrate consumption. If you follow this rule in the Bio-Age plan, you can expect success. High-quality protein is also very important to consume at every meal.

Balancing Your Diet

The trick is to consume a balance of protein, carbs and essential fats every two-and-a-half to three-and-a-half hours (in your five or six small meals per day). The following is a simple overview of our bodies' nutritional requirements for proper energy metabolism, muscle gain and fat loss.

Carbohydrates

Consume your carbohydrates from low-glycemic foods such as vegetables, legumes, whole grains and fruits to provide fuel in the form of glucose (blood sugar) for both brain and muscle activity.

Fats

Consume your fats from unrefined oils, nuts and seeds to assist in the balance of blood sugar, provide raw materials for hormones, create fuel for long-term energy and strengthen cell walls and mucus membranes.

Proteins

Consume your proteins from both lean animal and plant sources (such as lean meat, chicken breast, fish, low-fat cottage cheese, soy and whey) to help stabilize blood sugar; promote cell growth and repair; assist hormone production; assist enzyme production (digestive and metabolic); assist neurotransmitter production, cell metabolism, body fluid balancing and maintenance of the immune system.

It is important to remember that all carbohydrates eventually break down into sugar in the body. It doesn't matter whether you consume 1/4 cup of pure sugar or eat a baked potato. They both are 1/4 cup of sugar to your body, and your body will take the appropriate steps to bring the sugar level back into balance.

In order to keep muscle tissue at optimum levels and assist the body in maintaining all of its other functions, the body must remain in a constant anabolic environment. Following this eating plan will ensure that maximum anabolic effects will take place.

Bio-Age Shakes

If you follow these shake recipes, you will enjoy the enormous anti-aging advantages of the phytochemical flavonoids that the skin of a fruit contains. Blended whole fruit, as opposed to drinking pure juice, is the key to reaping the benefits of great-tasting phytonutrition. For blending, we use the Vita-Mix® Total Nutrition Center/Whole Food Machine®, but if your blender is powerful enough to mix whole fruit, it will do just fine.

For a sweeter taste sensation, try using naturally flavored proteins. Avoid the many protein formulas on the market that contain unnatural flavoring agents such as aspartame, acesulfame potassium and sucralose. Even though there are no studies at this time showing any harm caused by ingredients like acesulfame potassium and sucralose, we urge caution when using these manufactured sweeteners. And don't be fooled by natural sweeteners such as fructose! As you'll remember from Chapter 5, fructose found in fruit is actually good for us; it's when you take it out of the fruit and use it as a sweetener that it begins to cause problems.

One final note before we outline the shake recipes. Remember: *Nothing takes the place of good clean water*. And whenever possible, use organic fruit and yogurt. The following is a list of five shakes that can help in lowering your Bio-Age. Before you make these, read over the following tips:

Shake Tip #1: When mixing specialized protein isolates, make sure to mix them up in a shaker cup first so as to not harm the delicate protein bonds. Then add them to the shake as the last ingredient and blend only for a few seconds on low speed (just enough to have them mixed in). This will ensure that the high-quality protein will reach your body undenatured.

Shake Tip #2: The macronutrient values listed below each shake give an approximate value of each nutrient, but use your own discretion when making these shakes. Depending on your individual protein needs, you may need to increase or decrease the amounts.

Shake Tip #3: Even though the consistency is liquid, always chew your shake for a few moments before swallowing. This will ensure maximum digestion potential since digestion starts in the mouth through saliva.

The base for these shakes is:
- 25–30 g/oz (dietary protein content) of unflavored whey, soy or mixed protein isolate powder, 350 mL/1 1/2 cups water.

Mix protein powder in shaker cup, blend other ingredients, then add protein powder and blend for a few seconds on low speed.

1. **Morning Energizer**
   250 mL/1 cup berries (your choice)
   1 apple (skin included)
   1 serving green food concentrate
   1 serving liquid or dry chlorophyll

15 mL/1 tbsp. flaxseed oil
Approx. Values: Calories: 400 Protein: 26 g Carbs: 36 g EFAs: 14 g

2. Memory Charge
250 mL/1 cup blueberries
125 mL/1/2 cup pineapples
1 capsule ginkgo biloba
15 mL/1 tbsp. dry lecithin
1 capsule full spectrum grape extract
15 mL/1 tbsp flax seed oil
Approx. Totals: Calories: 400 Protein: 25 g Carbs: 31 g EFAs: 20 g

3. Bio Body Fat Burner
100 g/4 oz. freshly squeezed grapefruit juice
250 mL/1 cup pineapples
1 capsule citrus aurantium (325 mg containing 6% synephrine)
1 capsule green tea extract
15 mL/1 tbsp. flaxseed oil
Approx. Totals: Calories: 360 Protein: 26 g Carbs: 30 g EFAs: 14 g

4. Immuno-Boost
100 g/4 oz. fresh squeezed orange juice
250 mL/1 cup blueberries
1000 mg vitamin C with quercetin
60 mg full spectrum grape extract
1 capsule echinacea
15 mL/1 tbsp. flaxseed oil
Approx. Totals: Calories: 365 Protein: 25 g Carbs: 33 g EFAs: 14 g

5. Post-Workout Maximizer:
1 cup mixed berries
1 small banana
5 g Creatine monohydrate
2 g pure L-glutamine
15 mL/1 tbsp. flaxseed oil
Approx. Values: Calories: 436 Protein: 35 g Carbs: 40 g EFAs: 14 g

Shake Ingredients: How They Contribute to Healthy Longevity

Protein Isolates will raise the levels of key neurotransmitters that revive the brain and help to stimulate the memory centers.

Berries are a very potent source of antioxidants that help to revitalize the energy-producing centers of our cells. They are also a slow trickling source of sugars for the body and brain that do not over-stimulate insulin production. In particular, blueberries are one of nature's richest natural brain protectors. Some studies show that the phytonutrients contained in blueberries are able to raise levels of very powerful antioxidants inside the brain. These special phytonutrients are also powerful immune boosters and modulators.

Apples are also a very good form of slow-releasing non-insulin stimulating sugars as long as they are blended with their skins. They are also a very good source of pyruvate, which is a key ingredient in our cells' energy production.

Green food concentrates supply the body with vital nutrients for energy production as well as key substances that act as potent antioxidants that help scavenge harmful free radicals.

L-glutamine is an amino acid essential for many of the body's functions, especially the immune system and gut function. Under normal conditions the glutamine level is kept in balance between release and use, but in situations that demand additional glutamine, such as stress or exercise, the available glutamine pool may not be enough to meet the protein-building demands.

Ginkgo biloba has been used in China for thousands of years to help treat memory loss, among other conditions. Many people in Europe and North America take it regularly to help stimulate brain function and boost memory. Ginkgo is also regarded as a cellular energizer that helps to slow the effects of aging. Use forms that have not been pressed into tablets.

Creatine monohydrate is an important part of the cells' energy system, as it combines with phosphates to make phosphocreatine (PC), an important energy-creating compound. Creatine has been shown to increase muscle power in speed-strength athletes such as football players, sprinters and weight lifters. Research also shows that creatine has a pronounced anabolic effect.

Vitamin C is a potent water-soluble vitamin. Its main job is to protect the watery interior of the cells. Since it belongs to the water-soluble family of nutrients, any excess is excreted in the urine.

Quercetin is a non-citrus bioflavonoid that helps increase the strength of the capillaries (blood vessels) and regulates their permeability. Bioflavonoids also act as cellular assistants to vitamin C by aiding its absorption. Quercetin has been shown to decrease many allergic reactions by helping to stabilize specific immune cells involved in the inflammatory process. Quercetin may be helpful in all kinds of inflammatory processes, including asthma, bursitis and rheumatoid arthritis. It has also shown great promise in inhibiting the development of certain viruses such as herpes, polio and Epstein-Barr.

Green tea extract is beneficial for the mind and body, and can speed up fat loss. Among the most impressive flavonoids in green tea are catechins, which are very effectively absorbed by the body. The catechins have powerful antioxidant activity and have been shown to inhibit certain cancers, improve blood flow in the cardiovascular system and reduce LDL (low density lipoprotein) cholesterol oxidation.

Full-spectrum grape extract contains all the protective chemicals of red wine that help diminish the signs of premature aging caused by pollution and other toxins. Research conducted by the University of Toronto found Biovin full-spectrum grape extract to provide strong protection against free radicals. It helps to protect your body against pollutants and free radicals, thereby slowing the rate of cellular damage. It can also improve age-related vision deterioration, reduce inflammation and restore elasticity to joints, skin and arteries.

Echinacea is one of the most trusted herbs for boosting immune function. It is one of the best-selling herbs for battling colds and the flu, and may also be a valuable weapon against bacterial and viral infections.

Citrus aurantium is a Chinese herb that helps to increase lipolysis (the breakdown of stored fat) by stimulating special metabolic receptors on cells called the beta-3 receptors. Once these beta-3 receptors are turned on, they cause an increase in the metabolic rate through thermogenesis (increased body heat).

Lecithin is the most common phospholipid (a type of fat synthesized by the liver) found in the body. Phospholipids serve as the structural framework that surround all cells. They also serve as insulation for the sheaths that surround nerve fibers. Lecithin is considered a memory-enhancer due to its high levels of choline, which can improve cognitive functions. Lecithin is taken predominantly for its choline content; however, it can also help break down both cholesterol and fats in the blood.

Chlorophyll is the green matter in plants. Through the chemical process photosynthesis, chlorophyll harnesses the sun's energy to perform various life-promoting functions. Combining carbon dioxide absorbed from the air with water, chlorophyll uses sunlight to make sugar. By using minerals from the soil, chlorophyll allows the plant to use the sun's energy to make vitamins, fats, proteins and starches. These elements can then be harvested for human consumption. Many people experience increased energy by taking this natural compound.

Flaxseed oil is one of nature's richest sources of the omega-3 fatty acids that help to manufacture powerful hormones in the body. These essential fatty acids are also important structural components of every one of our cells. For an in-depth explanation of essential fatty acids please refer to Chapter 7.

BIO-AGE STEP #7:

Increase Anabolic Metabolism Through High-Octane Protein

As we've emphasized throughout this book, aging is associated with a decline in anabolism that inevitably leads to disability and death. Huge amounts of research dollars have been spent investigating the role that protein synthesis plays in the development of disease and aging. As we saw in Chapter 6, administering a certain mixture of amino acids to elderly people resulted in a net gain in protein deposition and the restoration of youthful anabolic metabolism at the cellular level.

As we mentioned in the "Aging with Protein" chapter, *whey protein* isolates are excellent forms of protein for effective anabolism. They also offer many other benefits, such as increased antioxidant protection, hunger control, increased metabolism, cancer prevention, heart disease prevention and others. It is important to consume only the highest-quality whey protein supplements available (see Appendix II).

The alpha-lactalbumin levels in whey protein are key to anabolism as they are an ideal source of protein—instantly bioavailable. This means high alpha-lactalbumin (above 25%) whey protein goes immediately into use by the body in the repair process, slowing catabolism and cellular aging. When taking whey protein isolates, your increased anabolic rate means you will look, feel and perform better longer even as your chronological age increases. For an increased anabolic effect with whey protein, try incorporating products containing active ingredients such as Ekdisten, which helps increase the process of protein synthesis, boosting the effectiveness of the whey protein (see Appendix II for products containing Ekdisten).

In addition to whey protein, concentrate on incorporating into your diet moderate quantities of foods such as eggs, fish, poultry, low-fat milk and lean-cut beef, which are high in digestible protein. Though supplements are valuable, whole food remains one of our most important assets in achieving healthy longevity.

And a word of caution: As effective as, for example, whey protein is, it certainly does not mean that you should overconsume protein at any one sitting, because too much protein at one meal can cause excess stress to your liver and kidneys. The upper limit, depending on your size and activity level, seems to be 30–40 g at one sitting. Higher quantities seem to be better absorbed right after intense exercise.

Taken in the right quantities, one of the benefits of consuming a high-quality supplement containing protein isolates is that you are guaranteed to get the exact amount of protein that you need without the added fat and carbohydrates. From all the research on protein isolates combined with our own experience, we presently believe the supplemental protein source that stands out above all others when it comes to living a long, healthy, disease-free life is whey protein isolates.

Freeing Up Testosterone Naturally

As we have discussed, protein is a very important component of anabolism. But proteins without hormones are just building blocks with nowhere to go. Hormones are of paramount importance in the process of protein synthesis. In a sense they are the architects that give the orders on the construction site. Testosterone is one of the most important hormones in building new muscle. In Part I we discussed the importance of freeing up natural testosterone when it comes to maximizing our anabolic process and fat-burning potential.

One natural herb that will assist in this goal is *Urtica dioica*, but you may have heard of it before under a more common name: stinging nettle. In a paper published in 1995 in *Planta Medica*, a proprietary extract of stinging nettle plant was shown to inhibit SHBG from latching onto the cell membrane of the prostate gland. According to this and other studies, stinging nettle extract is not only a powerful booster of testosterone, but can also help to prevent and perhaps treat prostate disease.

There are many different forms of stinging nettle available on the market, but it is only the newer extracts of stinging nettle that are proving to be extremely powerful testosterone-helpers. Many of the stinging nettle products on the market today have been extracted from alcohol or ethanol. New studies have proven that ethanol extracts are inactive when it comes to inhibiting SHBG binding. But the research shows that both the aqueous (water) and methanolic extracts are capable of altering the SHBG activity. See Appendix II for specific recommendations.

Boosting Protein Synthesis Naturally

Muscle protein synthesis is a multistage process whose final outcome is protein assembly inside an area of the cell called the cytoplasm. This assembly is regulated to a great extent by the quantity and quality of ribonucleic acids (RNAs) along with cell energetics. In order to optimize the protein (muscle, enzyme and hormone) assembly process, a new class of natural anabolic activators may be incorporated into one's diet. When these anabolic activators are combined with an adequate hormonal environment and a diet rich in high-quality protein, a net increase in protein synthesis can be attained.

RNA and the cellular energy process can be effectively stimulated by taking a Brazilian rainforest herb called Ekdisten, a proprietary extract of the root of the plant *Pfaffia paniculata* (SUMA). This plant has been widely used in nutrition, especially by Russian athletes, due to its richness in various phytosterols.

For an enhanced anabolic effect, the oral dosage of Ekdisten should be in the range of 500–1000 mg daily taken along with 1000–2000 mg of water-extracted stinging nettle. Ekdisten has been shown to increase the synthesis of muscle proteins and other proteins, primarily albumin and hemoglobin. (See Appendix II.)

BIO-AGE STEP #8:

Consume High-octane Fat Fuels

As we better understand the body's critical dependence on specific fats and oils, we move beyond the commonly held view of fats and oils as mere sources of flavor or calories. Fats and oils now belong at the very top of our dietary and health considerations.

The knowledge that the brain is mostly fat should further compel us to place fats high on our list of vital foods. Selection of the appropriate fats, oils and supplements becomes one of the most important tasks we undertake in pursuit of optimal wellness. One of the first steps in this journey is to understand how to find and use quality oils.

Obtaining Quality Oils

As you've read in Chapter 7, techniques used in modern processing and preparation of oils for sale to the public result in damage to essential fatty acids, the presence of trans fatty acids and residue of solvent extraction. The food oil industry has a history of providing products to the marketplace based on ease of shipping and storage. Health considerations have often been secondary to shelf-life concerns. In order to derive the most benefit from consuming oils (and avoid making things worse), attention to quality is very important.

Below is a list of suggestions that will allow for selection of oil products of the highest quality and purity. Also included is a list of suggestions for storage that will maintain that quality once it's in your kitchen:

• Try to get your oils from whole foods whenever possible. This means consuming fish, walnuts, flaxseed meal, sesame seeds, brazil nuts or other products rather than just consuming the oil. Recall that foods such as flaxseed contain, in addition to fatty acids, compounds such as lignans with many significant health benefits.

- Use oils that are certified as organic. Many industrial and agricultural chemicals are fat-soluble and tend to concentrate in the oil portion of plants and animals. Organic products do not contain chemicals applied in the growing process and commonly have a nutrient density greater than non-organically grown products.
- Use oils that are stored in dark bottles. Essential fatty acids are likely to go rancid when exposed to light. Dark bottles prevent this from occurring. Grocery store shelves are filled with oils in clear glass or plastic bottles, which only invites light to further oxidize the fatty acids.
- Oils with a high content of unsaturated fatty acids spoil more easily with increasing air exposure. Oils should be kept covered.
- Oils with high unsaturated fatty acids spoil more easily when exposed to warm temperatures. Keep them refrigerated at all times. Those high in monounsaturates like olive oil need not be refrigerated. Oils rich in saturated fat, such as coconut oil or ghee, also need not be refrigerated.
- Use oils that are unrefined. Oils processed in this way are most closely related to the original product and are least likely to contain damaged fatty acids. Refined oils are commonly extracted with toxic solvents and processed at temperatures above 400° F/204°C.
- Oils should be cold processed, expeller pressed. Look for a statement on the label regarding the temperature at which the oil was processed. It should ideally be 86–110°F/30–43°C.
- If you taste an oil that seems bitter, it has probably become rancid. Consumption of these oils should be avoided.

Cooking with Oils

The Wet Sauté Method

Cooking with high temperatures is how many oils are damaged. One way to avoid this is to cook primarily with oils that contain mostly saturated fat, such as coconut oil, ghee or butter. Oils containing mostly monounsaturates such as olive oil are also fine for cooking. However, the taste of many other oils such as sesame are delightful. One way to preserve their integrity while still enjoying their taste is to "wet sauté." In this method, place a small amount of water in the pan or skillet and heat until just below boiling. Add the food you desire and sauté. As the food becomes cooked, add a small amount of oil. This shortens the time the oil is in contact with the heat, yet preserves the flavor in the food. Oils should not be heated to the point of smoking.

In Search of Omega-3

Since omega-3–containing foods are less common in our diets and more difficult to find, we've provided a brief separate guide to these foods. Following this discussion is an overview of the various oils used for consumption and their fatty acid content.

Choosing the Best Oils

In choosing oils, always remember to use organic oils or seeds. Seeds tend to concentrate pesticides and other undesirable substances. Moreover, many steps in the commercial processing of oils can add toxic residue and remove healthful components such as lignans. To maintain adequate levels of brain fats, we believe it is important to balance the intake of omega-6 and omega-3 fatty acids in an approximate 1:1 to 2:1 ratio. For most people living on modern diets, initially consuming more omega-3 oils may be necessary.

Foods Containing Omega-3 Alpha-Linolenic Acid

The following foods contain oil with their approximate percentage of alpha-linolenic acid (ALA) as a percentage of their total fat listed from highest to lowest. (Note: do not confuse *alpha-linolenic acid* with *linoleic acid*.)

- flax seed 58
- brazil nuts 40
- chia 30
- kukui (candlenut) 29
- hemp seed 25
- butternuts 16
- pumpkin seed 1–15
- canola 10
- soybean 7
- walnut 5
- wheat germ 5
- purslane (which is a leafy vegetable) 400 mg ALA/100 g
- green leafy vegetables (percentages vary)

Balancing Your Oils

The following oils are good oils, but they contain little or no omega-3 fatty acids. Therefore, they should always be balanced with an oil containing omega-3 fatty acids:

- black currant seed
- borage
- evening primrose
- rice bran
- sesame
- unrefined safflower
- unrefined sunflower

A Note on Sesame Oil and Red Palm Oil

Sesame oil is rich in omega-6 fatty acids—and we have said to reduce your intake of omega-6 fatty acids. However, sesame oil contains substances called sesamin, sesamol and sesaminol. As we discussed in Chapter 7, these substances are capable of benefiting the inflammatory system, and also have an antioxidant function in protecting some of the body's vital fatty acids against free radical injury. Thus, sesame oil, if organic, is considered a valued oil and can be used liberally.

Red palm oil is an ideal cooking oil because of its fatty acid profile. In addition, red palm oil is one of the richest sources of tocotrienols (in the vitamin E family) of any oil presently available. Red palm oil also contains a rich blend of carotenoids, another part of the antioxidant defense network. Red palm oil should not be confused with palm kernel oil, which has a notably different profile.

Foods Containing Omega-3 DHA

As you may recall from Chapter 7, cold-water fish are the richest sources of docosahexaenoic (DHA). Some species contain more than others and the content of an individual species varies somewhat from fish to fish. The DHA content of farmed versus wild fish can be considerably different depending upon the feed given to commercially raised fish. Consuming fish two or three times per week is an excellent way to increase the omega-3 fatty acid content in your diet. In general, the fish containing the highest amounts of DHA include:

- albacore tuna
- bluefin
- caviar
- herring
- krill
- mackerel
- plankton
- algae
- anchovies
- salmon
- sardines
- trout

Warm-water fish like orange roughy, red snapper and swordfish do not contain much DHA. EPA/DHA is also found (though in much smaller quantities) in freshwater fish such as:

- carp
- haddock
- lake trout
- northern pike
- walleye

Chicken and Eggs as Sources of DHA

Chicken meat may contain DHA if the bird has been raised on a high omega-3 fatty acid feed. Chicken eggs also naturally contain DHA. However, the amount is highly dependent upon what the chicken is fed. Dr. Artemis Simopoulos showed, for example, that Greek eggs (grown by feeding fish meal to laying hens) contained 6.6 mg of DHA for every gram of yolk, while regular supermarket eggs contained only 1.09 mg of DHA. High-DHA eggs should be labeled as such and are available in most grocery stores as well as at health food stores. Eggs contain as much as 20 times more omega-3 fatty acids than others. Since DHA is very susceptible to oxidation, cooking or overcooking chicken eggs may destroy some of this delicate fatty acid.

The Best Supplements

There are many supplement choices regarding fatty acids. We believe that a rich source of omega-3 fatty acids should be provided in the form of fish oil or algae oil. This will provide the brain with its needed fatty acids as well as those of the rest of the body. Flax seed oil provides crucial omega-3 fatty acids that are the parents of the brain's main omega-3. Borage oil provides yet another fatty acid helpful for the body's inflammatory balance.

As mentioned in Step #3, we suggest that a combined supplement of fish, flax and borage oil be considered. Krill oil (Neptune®) is a very rich source of omega-3 EPA and DHA. It also contains high amounts of phosphatidyl-choline, vitamin E and carotenoids. In some ways, krill oil is the ideal omega-3 source. The antioxidants in krill oil keep the oil safe from rancidity as well. Additions such as sesame oil (for sesamol or sesaminol) can be very useful as well. Red palm oil may be one of the best cooking oils because of its high carotenoid and tocotrienol content.

Check with the product's manufacturer that your fatty acid supplements have been tested for lipid peroxides, anisidine, volatiles and heavy metals.

Avoiding Foods High in Trans Fatty Acids

These altered fats are best left out of the diet. Common sources include:

- cake
- candy
- cookies
- corn chips
- deep-fried chicken nuggets
- deep-fried fish burgers
- deep-fried mushrooms, cheese curds, etc.
- doughnuts
- french fries
- margarine
- mayonnaise
- potato chips
- puffed cheese snacks
- salad dressing (other than olive oil–based)
- shortening
- tortilla chips

BIO-AGE STEP #9:

Stress Less

When describing ways to manage stress, there is a great tendency to over-simplify and to give little consideration to circumstances. For example, divorce is considered a very great stressor. But in a troubled marriage, immune function has been shown to decline. In such cases, divorce may actually be associated with diminished stress. Likewise, in examining the stress of divorce, those who wanted the divorce fared better physiologically than those who did not want the divorce. This shows the complexity of the stress response.

Our attempt to describe stress reduction should be taken with the understanding that there is no truly simple formula, no magic personality trait, no perfect coping strategy. Living in the world calls upon skills that we may be only slowly developing. Coping with a tragedy may call upon skills that we simply do not have because we have never been faced with the severity with which we are now faced. As you read our strategies for managing stress and enriching your life, consider that centuries' worth of wisdom-keepers have offered means to live in a complex world where things rarely go as we expect; where suffering seems as central to the human condition as food and water. What we offer, then, is given with a dose of humility and an understanding that there is more to healing from life's challenges than that mentioned below.

Acceptance

We're often told to accept that which we cannot change, yet we should honor the fact that acceptance may be a journey through time rather than an act that occurs quickly and easily. We should also consider that denial has temporary benefits to survival. Denial may allow us to cope initially when circumstances threaten to overwhelm.

Look for the Truth

While the facts of a situation can be painful, we often create undue suffering for ourselves as we imagine the worst scenarios. Avoid making assumptions. Once we have the facts, we can begin the process of healing, which may include acceptance, compassion, forgiveness, grieving or a new level of understanding. Recognizing the truth also allows us to take appropriate action.

Expression and Opening Up

Studies consistently show that expression of feelings is a time-honored path to healing. (On the other side, keep in mind that there may be circumstances when opening up is not appropriate. For example, when the environment for opening up is unsafe.) Gary Schwartz, Ph.D., of the University of Arizona, muses about whether aging is related to our inability to "release" old memories. He asks, "Are chronic diseases expressions of clogged systemic memories? Is 'old age' a side effect of being unable to release excessive information and energy that bogs us down? Have people who lived to be a hundred or more learned how to engage in a larger process of sharing and releasing information and energy?"

Forgiveness

Holding a grudge can sustain an ongoing stress response. Moreover, by constantly reliving a hurt that may be months or years in the past, we are kept from living in present time. Lack of forgiveness can also lead to a lack of joyfulness in life. An effort to forgive oneself and others from a place of deep empathy may be one vital path on the journey to renewal and freedom.

Don't Take Anything Personally

In reality, nothing other people do is because of you. They act out of their own beliefs, experiences and pain. Be careful not to "accept" the projection, blame and suffering that may be directed toward you by other people. It is not yours and it is not about you. Consider promising yourself, "I will no longer take anything personally." This includes criticism as well as accolades. This allows us to be free of the pain and motives of others. It also allows us to be more genuinely loving since our interactions will no longer be fueled by what we perceive others may think of us.

Laughter and Humor

While laughter and humor are among the most enjoyable of experiences, they are also associated with a reduced stress response. Recall that those who used humor to cope had lower levels of the stress hormones cortisol and adrenaline when faced with stressful circumstances.

Gratitude

Find something for which to be grateful in every difficult situation. During the Holocaust of World War II, a Jewish prisoner was found offering a prayer of gratitude in his barracks after witnessing horrible atrocities. A bunkmate reproached him harshly, saying that there was nothing for which to be grateful in this dark moment. But the man countered that he was grateful that he was incapable of carrying out the horrors that he had just witnessed.

Every circumstance contains something for which we can be grateful. When we practice gratitude in this way, we also begin to condition ourselves in a new way of seeing the world. We begin to realize that every difficulty contains hidden gifts.

Assertiveness

Assertiveness is needed to express the truth of our feelings, beliefs, responses and opinions. Without assertiveness, we are inclined to hold in feelings in order to achieve peace or for fear of rejection. Assertiveness allows us to speak in ways that honor what's inside us. Most people live their lives driven by the beliefs and expectations of other people. Make a commitment to speaking the truth that is inside your heart and to no longer acting a certain way merely because others expect this of you. Continue to treat others with honor and respect.

Touch

The average North American couple is said to touch about twice an hour, while those from some Caribbean cultures may touch well over 100 times per hour. Touch is a vital part of sustaining balance during stress. Consider more frequent touch with your children, your mate or your friends. Also consider massage.

A Helping Heart

The capacity to give joy to another is one of the highest human traits. So much personal suffering occurs when we constantly hold ourselves, our problems or our struggles in the center of our world. When we give to others, we essentially take ourselves out of the center of our world and realize that there is a greater cause than ourselves. Moreover, by helping we reinforce the sense that rather than being separate and isolated we are connected to others.

BIO-AGE STEP #10:

Pleasure and Play

Reread the "Mind over Aging" chapter and realize that life is about living! Take time for the things that really matter most in life, like family and friends. Find the child that still lives inside you. And remember that love, in the end, may be what matters most. Consider this: Yesterday is history, Tomorrow is a mystery, Today is a gift ... that's why we call it the present.

Conclusion

We are living in a time when the seemingly impossible can become the possible at any moment. Our biomedical knowledge is advancing at lightning speed; it's now easy to imagine that soon we will have the cures to many of the diseases that plague us today. And, as you've read, the future of anti-aging science is promising indeed! Scientists, like those who have contributed to *Bio-Age*, have already identified the mechanisms behind cellular aging and have isolated the factors that can slow or reverse those processes.

But, as we've also tried to emphasize, this purely technical advancement has its limits. Science can tell us much about the biology of life, health and longevity, yet it reveals little about the heart or the soul. Science is a clumsy poet; it shows us nothing about the longing to feel connected to others, or the feelings of awe and glory prompted by crimson sunsets or playful children.

We humans spend so little of life in present time; endless hours are spent looking back, in remembrance of past hurt or past joy. Likewise, we look forward, hopeful of better days or fearful of the next threat to our security. This living backward or forward in time is not living, for it makes the present time elusive. No one who lives in the past or future can live fully. No one caught in the trap that keeps him or her from this moment can heal fully, for this moment is all there truly is.

Life is a journey where everything that lies in our path is sacred, but are we not often blind to this abundance? How often do we really cherish all that surrounds us? Imagine a world where every person, every tree, every bird, every beating heart was honored as a special part of the web of creation. Imagine a world where you saw even your enemies as people who came bearing lessons, the gifts of which you cannot yet see.

There is a hidden mystery in all of this. One is tempted to view aging as something to be slowed, cut off or avoided. Yet the aging process, the time when our bodies begin to slow, our vision begins to dim, our movements are not so urgent, may be part of the call inward. This process may be what draws us deep into ourselves on our journey to true wisdom.

A long, fruitful life may be about maintaining our faculties at their highest possible functioning state, but a journey of good health without meaning, purpose or love is a journey few would likely embrace.

There are ages and stages that ask different things of us. Illness may teach us perseverance that is required for later. Struggle may be needed for the strength that is asked on the next step of the road to wholeness. A life of healthy longevity is not just about remaining disease-free or living longer; it is about living now, in the present moment—about accepting the gifts as they come. There is living long and there is living fully. They may coexist, but quite often they do not. We hope that in reading *Bio-Age* you have come away with an appreciation for an all-encompassing approach to healthy longevity—one that incorporates a respect for your body and what it requires in order to function at its ideal level, and for the importance of treating yourself gently and making rest, pleasure and those you love priorities in your life. In *Bio-Age* we have tried to present a cohesive picture of some of the factors behind your biological aging.

Yet, we realize that life is a great, complex mystery. Explorers have, for millennia, tried to tease out the answers to some of life's perplexing questions, only to find more questions. Perhaps we will one day find that aging is life's greatest gift, that freed from the ambition of youth we embark on the greatest possible journey to self-discovery. Perhaps the wisdom of our years allows us to ponder the deeper meaning hidden in life's story.

Bio-Age is a humble blueprint to a more vigorous, robust, long life. We invite you to take whatever steps may suit you and use them as you see fit. At the same time, we urge that you not resist the sweeping process of change that can open you to a life you never thought possible.

Appendix I:
Evaluating Your Bio-Age

The "you" that exists today is the sum of your many years of diet, stresses, loves, hopes, injuries and, of course, time. Imagine if you could actually ask your body chemistry, "What is my Bio-Age and what are the specific factors that are influencing—for better or worse—my quest for healthy longevity?"

Then imagine if you could use those answers to tell a story, a story that is unique to you. Out of this story would emerge a picture of the vitamins, minerals, amino acids, fatty acids and other building blocks necessary to propel you successfully into the next phase of your life.

As we've emphasized throughout this book, the biochemical processes that run the body have a powerful influence on how you feel, how you resist stress and how you age. If you could take a picture of your body's chemistry, you would be able to design a supplement program that is based entirely on your own biochemistry. It would be custom-tailored to your needs.

In the past 10 years, exciting advances in laboratory testing have made it possible to discover the unique biochemical patterns of an individual. From this profile, a nutritional support program can be developed that corrects deficiencies and improves metabolism long before disease or disharmony occurs. Health care professionals worldwide are now using such tests to tailor programs to individual patients in an effort to cure disease, but also to optimize health.

The following is a discussion of some of the new, innovative tests available in the area of nutritional medicine. Each of the building blocks will be discussed and followed by suggested tests that might comprehensively discover the story hidden in your body's chemistry.

It is important to keep in mind that there are many lab tests available beyond those described here. We have highlighted those we believe are the most valuable and that can be applied to anyone who wishes to improve his or her biological age. Additional tests may be needed for an individual with more specific concerns. You can ask your doctor about each test and if there is a charge involved. There are two labs in the United States—contact information is listed after the tests—that will perform all of these and can supply you with further information.

Nutritional Tests

Amino Acids
Amino acids are the building blocks of all protein in the human body. They are also key factors in the immune system, energy generation, brain neurotransmitters, enzymes and many other domains. For example, if you don't have enough of the amino acid tyrosine, your body cannot make enough thyroid hormone. If you lack the amino acid tryptophan, you cannot make enough of the neurotransmitter serotonin. (There is reason to believe that some doctors may prescribe Prozac™ to solve the serotonin problem when in fact it may be due to amino acid deficiency.) The amino acid leucine is essential to building muscle. Taurine is needed as a calming amino acid in the brain and heart.

The list of vital functions of amino acids is quite long. Performing an amino acid test on blood (or urine) allows you to discover the status of these vital structural and functional molecules. Once you've discovered possible deficiencies, you can take amino acid supplements to improve your health. Amino acid tests also reveal much about the combined activities of vitamins and minerals, which make your biochemistry work.

Test: Plasma amino acids or 24-hour urinary amino acids

Fatty Acids
As you've read, fatty acids are another family of important structural and functional molecules. We are accustomed to thinking of fat as bad, but the body simply cannot function without fat in the proper forms and amounts. Many conditions of the brain and nervous system, such as depression, multiple sclerosis and Alzheimer's disease, are related to fatty acids. Heart arrhythmia has also been found to be related to deficiency of omega-3 fatty acids. Even bone formation and conditions like osteoporosis are related to essential fatty acids. When fatty acids are out of balance, inflammation of the skin, cartilage, muscles, brain and many other tissues can occur.

Measurement of your red blood cell fatty acids can tell the story of over 30 fatty acids and set you on a path to correcting deficiencies in one of your body's most important nutrient families. Moreover, establishing proper fatty acid balance today may prevent disabling illness in the future. One such example is Alzheimer's disease. In one study, those with the lowest level of the fatty acid DHA in middle age were almost twice as likely to develop dementia (mental decline) in the following 10 years.

Test: red blood cell fatty acid profile, plasma fatty acids

Minerals

Mineral or trace elements have vital structural and functional roles in the body. In fact, a single mineral deficiency can disrupt hundreds of different body processes. For example, zinc and magnesium are each required for over 100 different enzymes in the human body. Zinc is critical for brain function and for the function of growth hormone. Recall that human growth hormone is one of the key anti-aging substances in the human body. Without adequate zinc, proper growth hormone binding does not occur. Magnesium is vital to energy production.

The trace element selenium is one of the most well-studied nutrients with regard to cancer protection. Chromium is vital to balancing blood sugar and to preventing diabetes. You'll remember from Chapter 16 that chromium is also crucial to preventing glycation, the harmful sugar–protein reaction that browns and stiffens most body tissues.

In the blood chemistries that we have assessed over the past 15 years, deficiencies are of zinc, magnesium, selenium and chromium are commonplace. Other nutrient deficiencies are common as well. The key to tailoring a program, we believe, is to assess your own trace element status and tailor your supplement program to fit your needs.

Test: red cell trace elements or a white blood cell element analysis

Organic Acids

Organic acids refers to a family of molecules that perform a wide array of functions in the body. Everything from energy production to the formation of key building blocks involves organic acids. Testing organic acids can tell us which key vitamins and other nutrients are deficient. For example, deficiency of vitamins B1, B2, B3, B5, B6, B12 and folic acid can be ascertained from an organic acid profile. In addition, the status of certain crucial nutrients like carnitine, coenzyme Q10 and glutathione can be determined.

Test: urinary organic acid profile

Free Radical Stress

The free radical model of aging was described in Part I. There are several tests available to indirectly measure the free radical stress on your body. One common test is called the serum lipid peroxide test. Lipids, or fats, are extremely susceptible to free radical damage. This basic test measures this biochemical marker. There is also a simple urine test available in which a dropperful of urine is placed in an ampoule that is observed for color change. Recall in Chapter 18 that those who practiced meditation had lipid peroxide levels 15% lower than those who did not meditate.

Test: Serum lipid peroxides
Home Test: Urine MDA (malondialdehyde), 4-hydroxy nonenal

Vitamin B12 and Folic Acid

Vitamin B12 and folic acid are highlighted separately here because they are crucial to a biochemical process in the body called methylation. Methylation is a critical part of ensuring that your genes do not start issuing false commands. It is also necessary for a vast array of other important functions. When B12 and folic acid are low, toxic homocysteine molecules may also build up.

An additional reason for assessing vitamin B12 is that B12 deficiency is often associated with two common conditions of aging: poor memory and poor energy. In fact, by some estimates, as many as 10% of those diagnosed with Alzheimer's disease may actually suffer from B12 deficiency. Serum tests for vitamin B12 and folic acid may not be as sensitive as the functional tests described below. Any decline in mental sharpness or energy should be followed up with a test for vitamin B12 and folic acid.

Test: Homocysteine and methylmalonic acid

Hormone Panels

Hormones are among the key signaling molecules in the human body. Many of the hormones decline with age or shift in balance with age, which contributes to the onset of poor health in many individuals. Hormone testing has become much more readily available with the advent of better urine and saliva tests. This makes discovering the level of your key hormones as simple as a urine collection or a salivary swab.

Male Hormone Panel

As men age, their production of testosterone falls significantly. It is estimated that a 20-year-old man has roughly 700 million testosterone-producing (Leydig) cells. An 80-year-old man may have only 200 million such cells. Low testosterone can result in lack of energy, low sex drive, difficulty obtaining an erection, decrease in strength, decrease in endurance, altered mood and decreased mental function.

Test: Testosterone (unbound)

Balancing Estrogens

As discussed in Chapter 12, imbalance between 2-hydroxy estrogen and 16-hydroxy estrogen appears to contribute to a range of problems, including PMS, breast disease, prostate disease, cancer, obesity and other common conditions of adulthood. As the levels of 2-hydroxy estrogen fall and 16-hydroxy estrogen levels increase, the tendency toward disease increases. This test measures the levels of both estrogen compounds and provides a ratio of the two. If the levels of 2-hydroxy are too low, one can begin a supplementation program with such things as DIM (diindolylmethane) to restore estrogen balance and improve health.

Test: Urinary 2-hydroxy estrogen; 16-hydroxy estrogen;
ratio of 2-hydroxy to 16-hydroxy (blood may also be used)

Female Hormone Panel

Test: Estradiol, progesterone and testosterone

Adrenal Stress Profile

Most people have heard of adrenal stress, but most are unaware that lab tests can pinpoint the biochemical status of some of the key stress hormones. Two of the key adrenal hormones are cortisol and DHEA.

Cortisol has important effects on muscle tissue and heart tissue and also influences how the body handles protein, fat and carbohydrate. Symptoms of cortisol imbalance can include anxiety, depression, obesity, fatigue and diabetes. Stress is a powerful contributor to increased cortisol. Excessive cortisol is one of the critical negative influences on shrinking and aging of the brain.

DHEA is a hormone produced in the adrenal gland. It provides raw material for making estrogen and testosterone. It has a powerful influence on the brain and immune system, as well as on the energy-producing functions of the body. DHEA is also important in decreasing body fat and maintaining muscle mass.

Test: Urinary and salivary or cortisol and DHEA

Special Profiles

ION Panel

The ION panel is a combination of several tests that gives a comprehensive picture of your body chemistry with regard to nutrition and metabolism. In all, roughly 150 chemical substances are measured. A professional trained in nutritional medicine can interpret this vast array of chemicals and begin to tell the story of your individual biochemical/nutritional profile. The tests included are: amino acids, organic acids, fatty acids, trace minerals, some vitamins and lipid peroxides. When these individual tests are ordered as part of the ION panel, the cost is roughly one third of what the individual tests would cost alone.

Cardiovascular Profile

In order for us to thrive as we age, we have to survive heart disease, which kills more people than the next eight leading causes of death combined. To truly discover our risk of heart disease, we have to measure more than just blood fats. A comprehensive profile would also include things such as blood homocysteine, a toxic amino acid by-product and silent killer of those who die despite *normal* blood fats. C-reactive protein is a marker for inflammation. Fibrinogen is a marker for blood coagulation, or clotting. The comprehensive profile might include:

Tests for the following fats: Triglycerides, total cholesterol, HDL cholesterol. In addition, test for special markers: Apo(a) and Apo(b), homocysteine, C-reactive protein and fibrinogen.

Blood Sugar Balance Profile

Changing blood sugar balance is one of the most powerful factors we know of that is associated with accelerated biological aging. Thus, a basic blood profile to measure how your body regulates blood sugar is one of the most valuable tests described here. Many doctors who assess blood sugar status merely measure fasting blood glucose. While helpful, this measure provides only the most elementary picture of blood sugar balance. A true, detailed picture can be obtained with a profile that might include testing glucose, insulin, hemoglobin A1C, IGF-1 plus the adrenal stress profile (cortisol and DHEA).

Bone Density Assessment

Beyond age 35, bone density tends to steadily decline. Recent estimates suggest that more than 50% of healthy women aged 30–40 will experience fractures of the vertebrae due to osteoporosis at some time during older age. By the time osteoporosis appears on an X-ray, far too much bone has already been lost. Today, urine tests that measure compounds called pyridinium and D-pyridinium can provide a picture of accelerated bone loss far in advance of any changes that could be seen on X-rays. This would allow a woman in her forties, for example, to discover her risk of osteoporosis and take early steps to strengthen her bones. This is a simple urine test that can be collected at home and sent off to a laboratory for analysis

Women should be aware that doctors often do not take osteoporosis prevention as seriously as they should. According to an article in *Journal of Bone and Joint Surgery*, only 23% of women who developed fractures after age 55 were given osteoporosis treatment. Fracture is a classic warning sign of osteoporosis.

Tests: Urinary pyridinium and deoxypyridinium.

Finding a Good Laboratory

There are many excellent laboratories that can provide the tests described above. In order to make the process simple, we list just two of the labs below. We have a great deal of experience with these labs and are also aware that they offer panels similar to those described above. You can discuss using these or other laboratories with your doctor.

MetaMetrix Clinical Laboratory
5000 Peachtree Ind. Blvd.
Norcross, GA 30071
770-446-5483

Great Smokies Diagnostic
  Laboratory
63 Zillicoa St.
Asheville, NC 28801–1974
800-522-4762

RECOMMENDED METHOD FOR MEASURING YOUR BODY FAT

There are a number of ways to measure your body fat and lean body mass. The following is a method that can measure your body fat content directly without calculating it from other body elements.

Near Infrared Technology (Futrex)

The technique is a method approved by the U.S. Department of Agriculture to measure the fat content of meat. It is based on the fact that near-infrared light is absorbed differently by the different organic materials constituting tissue. In other words, when such a light is shone on body tissue, body fat absorbs the light, whereas lean body mass reflects the light. The reflected light is measured by a special sensor and transmitted into a computer, which has already been given data on the subject's weight, height, body frame, etc. The computer interprets all the information to produce percentage of body fat. As the body fat is measured directly, changes in the other elements of the body (e.g., water) have no bearing on the accuracy of the measurement.

Futrex recommends measuring the body fat on a single site, the center of the biceps of the dominant arm. Independent studies show that the single-site measurement provides an accuracy of 2.8%, which is well within the range of accuracy of underwater weighing. The remarkable accuracy and ease of use has made this the most desirable method.

CALCULATING YOUR DAILY PROTEIN REQUIREMENTS

Once you have had your lean body mass measured, you can calculate your daily protein requirement using the following formula:
• If you are sedentary: 0.75 x lean body weight (lbs) = protein grams per day

- If you are moderately active (i.e., you exercise one or two times per week): 1.00 x lean body weight (lbs) = protein grams per day
- If you are active (i.e., you exercise three times per week): 1.15 x lean body weight (lbs) = protein grams per day
- If you are very active (i.e., you exercise five or more times per week): 1.25 x lean body weight (lbs) = protein grams per day

Appendix II:
Bio-Age Product Supplement Recommendations

Throughout the book there have been recommendations for supplements and other products. Below you will find some more specific suggestions. Some of these products are marketed by ehn Inc., the distributor of the award-wining greens+. Brad King has confidently recommended these products for a number of years, believing them to be among the best in the industry. In 1999 he agreed to come aboard the greens+ team and develop cutting-edge products for the company, some of which are transform+, proteins+, protect+, enact+ and lean+. Brad has no other affiliation with any other manufacturer.

Through many years in the health industry we have come to realize that there are a number of respectable and trustworthy product manufacturers. The recommendations presented here are, to the best of our knowledge, some of the top ones in the industry.

Whey Protein Isolate (proteins+ and transform+)

AlphaPure® is a patented isolation process for whey protein isolate, creating the highest biological value of any protein on the market today. It contains 2.5 times the cysteine levels present in other whey protein isolates, and provides an excellent and unsurpassed source of natural glutathione builders.

The levels of the amino acid tryptophan in AlphaPure® are on average triple that of other whey protein isolates. Tryptophan is needed by the body to produce the neurotransmitter serotonin. Through extensive research over the past 40 years it has been established that the activity level of serotonin has a material impact on levels of insomnia, pain sensitivity, anxiety and depression. Serotonin has also been demonstrated to have appetite-suppressant qualities.

AlphaPure® contains the highest levels of glycomacropeptides (GMPs) found in any whey protein product. GMPs are powerful stimulators of a hormone called cholecystokinin (CCK), which plays many essential roles in our gastrointestinal system. CCK stimulates the release of enzymes from the pancreas and increases gall bladder contraction and bowel motility. One of CCK's most incredible actions lies in its ability to regulate our food intake by sending satiation signals to the brain, making it a potential diet aid. In animal studies, a rise in CCK is always followed by a large reduction in food intake. In human studies, whey protein glycomacropeptides were shown to increase CCK production by 415% within 20 minutes after ingestion.

AlphaPure® is a registered trademark of:
Protein Fractionations Inc.
1146 Castlefield Ave., Toronto, ON, M6B 1E9
Tel: 416-783-8315 Fax: 416-783-7589

AlphaPure® is distributed exclusively in Canada by ehn Inc.
ehn Inc. (greens+ Canada)
317 Adelaide Street West, Suite 501 Toronto, ON, M5V 1P9
Tel: 416-977-3505 Toll-free: 877-500-7888 Fax: 416-977-4184
Web Site: www.greensplucanada.com

Soy Protein Isolate

Look for the Supro® non-GMO brand of soy protein isolate. The Supro® non-GMO brand of soy protein isolate contains the highest-quality water-extracted soy protein on the market today. Supro® non-GMO soy protein isolate has a biological value of 100, the same as egg when it comes to protein quality. The product transform+ only uses Supro® non-GMO soy protein isolate as its soy protein source.

NOTE: Soy protein is a very good source of natural high tryptophan levels (stated above), as well as the muscle-building branched-chain amino acids (BCAAs).

Supro® is a registered trademark of:
Protein Technologies International
P.O. Box 88940 St. Louis, MO, 63188
Toll-free: Consumer Inquiries: 877-SOY4HEALTH (877-769-4432)
Customer or Business Inquiries: 800-325-7108 Fax: 314-982-2461

Essential Fatty Acid (EFA) Manufacturers and Distributors

Omega Balance Oil and Flax Oil

IN CANADA:
Omega Nutrition Canada Inc.
1924 Franklin Street
Vancouver, B.C., V5L 1R2
Tel: 604-253-4677
Toll-free: 800-661-3529
Fax: 604-253-4893
Web Site: www.omegaflo.com

IN THE UNITED STATES:
Omega Nutrition U.S.A. Inc.
6515 Aldrich Road
Bellingham, Washington 98226
Tel: 360-384-1328
Toll-free: 800-661-3529
Fax: 360-384-0700
Web Site: www.omegaflo.com

Udo's Choice Oil and Flax Oil

IN CANADA:
Flora Distributors Ltd.
7400 Fraser Park Drive
Burnaby, B.C., V5J 5B9
Toll-free: 800-663-0617
Fax: 606-436-6060
Web Site: www.florahealth.com

IN THE UNITED STATES:
Flora Distributors Ltd.
P.O. Box 73
805 Badger Road East
Lynden, Washington, 98264
Toll-free: 800-446-2110
Fax: 360-354-5355
Web Site: www.florahealth.com

Bioriginal Oils

IN CANADA:
Bioriginal Food & Science Corp.
102 Melville Street
Saskatoon, SK, S7J 0R1
Tel: 306-975-9268
Fax: 306-242-3829

Fish Oils, EPA and DHA

IN CANADA:
Ocean Nutrition Canada Ltd.
747 Bedford Highway
Bedford, Nova Scotia, V4A 2Z7
Tel: 902-457-2399
Toll-free: 800-980-8889
Fax: 902-457-2357
Web Site: www.ocean-nutrition.com

Concentrated Green Foods

Not all concentrated green foods are the same quality. Look for powders that contain an array of natural organic greens and herbs. We highly recommend the multi–award-winning greens+ formula.

IN CANADA:
ehn Inc. (greens+ Canada)
317 Adelaide Street West, Suite 501
Toronto, ON, M5V 1P9
Tel: 416-977-3505
Toll-free: 877-500-7888
Fax: 416-977-4184
Web Site: www.greenspluscanada.com

IN THE UNITED STATES:
Orange Peel Enterprises, Inc.
2183 Ponce de Leon Circle
Vero Beach, Florida, 32960
Toll-free: 800-643-1210
Web Site: www.greensplus.com

Green Foods Corporation
320 North Graves Avenue
Oxnard, California, 93030
Tel: 805-983-7470
Toll-free: 800-777-4430
Web Site: www.greenfoods.com

Vitamins, Minerals, Antioxidants and Flavonoids

Look for formulas that contain as close a mix to the network antioxidants as possible: Vitamins C, E, lipoic acid, and CoQ10, along with grape seed extract and a mix of the carotenoids, such as protect+™. *Full-spectrum grape extract:* There are many various qualities on the market, so choose wisely. Quality full-spectrum grape seed extract formulas should contain 95% pro-cyanidolic values with resveratrol and ellagic acid. A favorite is a product called grapes+, which contains all the values mentioned here.

NOTE: The best way to boost glutathione levels in the body is to take lipoic acid (or Alpha Pure® protein found in proteins and transform+).

IN CANADA grapes+ and protect+™ are distributed by:
ehn Inc. (greens+ Canada)
317 Adelaide Street West, Suite 501
Toronto, ON, M5V 1P9
Tel: 416-977-3505 Toll-free: 877-500-7888 Fax: 416-977-4184
Web Site: www.greenspluscanada.com

Nature's Secret, Natrol, Twin Labs and other high-quality products: distributed by Purity Life
Purity Life
6 Commerce Crescent
Acton, ON, L7J 2X3
Tel: 519-853-3511 Toll-free: 800-265-2615 Fax: 519-853-4660
E-mail: info@puritylife.com

Purity Professionals (distributor of professional nutritional products)
Division of Purity Life Health products
2975 Lake City Way
Burnaby, B.C., V5A 2Z6
Toll-free: 888-443-3323
Fax: 888-223-6111
E-mail: professional@puritylife.com

Herbal Products and Preparations

Milk Thistle:

Generally, milk thistle extracts come standardized to contain a minimum of 75% silymarin. At this potency a dose of 50–100 mg two to three times daily will really boost liver cell activity and keep your fat-burning army marching along toward victory. One of the most effective formulas for liver function presently on the market is called liv-tone™, marketed in Canada by:

ehn Inc. (greens+ Canada)
317 Adelaide Street West, Suite 501
Toronto, ON, M5V 1P9
Tel: 416-977-3505 Toll-free: 877-500-7888 Fax: 416-977-4184
Web Site: www.greenspluscanada.com

Herbal Products & Preparations recommended in the UNITED STATES:
Nature's Herbs
600 East Quality Drive
American Fork, UT 84003
Toll-free: 1-800-437-2257 Fax: 801-763-0789
Web Site: www.twinlab.com

Carnitine

L-Carnitine is presently restricted in Canada, however it is concentrated in colostrum, and supplementing with bovine colostrum may be a great way to increase natural carnitine levels.
IN CANADA:
Symbiotics Colostrum™, distributed by:

Purity Life
6 Commerce Crescent
Acton, ON, L7J 2X3
Tel: 519-853-3511
Toll-free: 800-265-2615
Fax: 519-853-4660
E-mail: info@puritylife.com

Smarte Brand Laboratories Ltd.
610F – 70 Avenue SE
Calgary, AB, T2H 2J6
Tel: 403-252-7150
Fax: 403-258-0689
Email: smarte@smarte.ab.ca

IN THE UNITED STATES:
Symbiotics, Inc.
2301 W Hwy 89A, Suite 107
Sedona, AZ, 86336
Toll Free Phone: 800- 784-4355 Local Phone: 520-203-0277
FAX: 520-203-0279
Web Site: www.symbiotics.com

Pharmaceutical Grade L-Carnitine and Acetyl L-Carnitine
ONLY IN THE UNITED STATES:

Twin Laboratories Inc.
2120 Smithtown Avenue
Ronkonkoma, NY., 11779
Tel: 631-467-3140
Fax: 631-630-3486
Web Site: www.twinlab.com

Life Extension Foundation (mail
   order only)
995 South West 24th Street
Ft. Lauderdale, Florida, 33315
Tel: 954-766-8433
Toll-free: 800-841-5433
Fax: 954-921-2069
Web Site: www.lef.org
Bio-Age Nutrient Formulas

A.G.E. INHIBITORS

In our chapter "AGEing with Sugar" and in other parts of *Bio-Age* we talked about the destructive process of glycation. When we finished our research on the myriad disorders that Advanced Glycation Endproducts (AGE) have been shown to inflict upon our bodies, we realized that no single product on the market could adequately protect the body from effects of AGE. So we created A.G.E. Inhibitors to help combat this destructive process. A.G.E. Inhibitors is the first nutritional anti-A.G.E. formula in the line.

A.G.E. Inhibitors contains:

AlphaPure™
   (100% alpha lactalbumin)
Ginger
L-Taurine
Quercetin
Alpha lipoic acid (99% pure)
N-Acetyl Cysteine (NAC)
Full spectrum grape extract
   (Biovin™)

Stinging nettles
Inositol
Lactoferrin
Reduced glutathione
Turmeric
Rosemary extract
Thyme

enact+ (Anabolic Activator with Ekdisten™)

Throughout *Bio-Age* we have made reference to the importance of anabolic metabolism in lowering your Bio-Age. We have also pointed out the effectiveness of various phytosteroids in boosting this important anti-aging process. All these natural phytosteroids can now be found in one product that also incorporates the testosterone-enhancing effects of stinging nettle. enact+ makes use of safe natural phytosteroids found in plants to activate and accelerate the body's anabolic rate. Energy is processed more efficiently, stores of fat are converted to lean body mass, and the structure of the body is repaired and rebuilt at a faster rate.

enact+ combines a proprietary Suma extract (Ekdisten) and Samambaia—two plants very high in natural ecdysterones—with stinging nettles (aqueous extract) to create a unique formula that enhances your body's natural processes.

lean+

For maximum fat burning, you can find the most effective nutrients in a special cocktail available as lean+. Designed by co-author Brad King, it contains seven of the star players in the war on fat.

lean+ contains:

Cayenne

Citrus aurantium

Coleus forskohlii

Grapefruit juice powder

Green tea

Guggulipid (plant compounds)

Hydroxycitric acid (HCA) from
  Garcinia cambogia

meno

To restore hormonal balance and eliminate or reduce menopausal symptoms naturally, without the risks and side effects commonly associated with HRT.

meno contains:

Red clover

Black cohosh

Dong quai

Chaste tree berry

Dandelion

protect+

All the ingredients discussed in Chapter 16 can be conveniently found in one supplement, protect+. This product provides strong protection against all forms of free radicals.

protect+ contains:

N-Acetyl cysteine (to increase
  glutathione levels)

Lipoic acid (also increases
  glutathione levels)

Vitamin C

Vitamin E

CoQ10

Mixed carotenoids blend

Full-spectrum grape extract
  (Biovin™)

Selenium

Anthocyanins

IN CANADA:

enact+, protect+, lean+ are manufactured and distributed by:
ehn Inc. (Greens+ Canada)
317 Adelaide Street West, Suite 501
Toronto, ON, M5V 1P9
Tel: 416-977-3505 Toll-free: 877-500-7888 Fax: 416-977-4184
Web Site: www.greenspluscanada.com

NOTE: Look for updated information on products, exercises and research on
the Fat Wars Website: **www.fatwars.com**

Dr. Seaton's Advanced Hygiene System (see Chapter 15) is available from:

High Performance Hygiene
24000 Mercantile Road, Suite 7
Cleveland, Ohio, 44122
Tel/Toll-free: 888-262-5700 Fax/Toll-free: 888-247-8500
Web Site: www.advancedhealth.cc

References

CHAPTER 1: HOW YOUNG DO YOU WANT TO BE?

Clevenger, W. *The Human Body*. New York: Michael Friedman Publishing Group, Inc., 1993.

Evans, W.J., and D. Cyr Campbell. "Nutrition, Exercise, and Healthy Aging." *J Am Diet Assoc* 97, no. 6 (June 1997):632–638.

Friedan, B. *The Fountain of Age*. New York: Dell Publishing, 1999.

Golan, M.I., et al. "Role of Physical Activity in the Prevention of Obesity in Children." *Int J Obes Relat Metab Disord* 23, Supplement 3 (1999):S18–S33.

Graci, S. *The Power of Superfoods*. Scarborough: Prentice-Hall, 1997.

Hayflick, L., *How and Why We Age*, Ballantine Books. New York, NY. 1994.

Herman-Giddens, M.E., et al. "Secondary Sexual Characteristics and Menses in Young Girls Seen in Office Practice: A Study from the Pediatric Research in Office Settings Network." *Pediatrics* 99, no. 4 (April 1997):505–512.

Hitt, R., et al. "Centenarians: The Older You Get, the Healthier You Have Been." *Lancet* 354, no. 9179 (August 1999):652

King, B. *Fat Wars: 45 Days to Transform Your Body*. Toronto: CDG Books Canada Inc., 2000.

Maharam, L.G., et al. "Masters Athletes: Factors Affecting Performance." *Sports Medicine* 28, no. 4 (October 1999):273–285.

Proceedings of the Nutrition Society 51 (1992):353–365.

Rowe, J.W., and R.L. Kahn. *Successful Aging*. New York: Dell Publishing, 1998.

Shulman, P. "Design for Living." *Scientific American Presents* (Summer 2000):19.

Suzman, R.M. "Centenarians in the United States," National Institute of Health & The US Census Bureau, P23–199, 1999.

Walford, R.L. and R.H. Marantz. "The Quest to Beat Aging, the Battle Against Aging," *Scientific American* (September 6, 2000)

CHAPTER 2: ASSESSING THE DAMAGE

Jpn J Cancer Res no. 88 (October 1997):971–976.

Evans W.J., and D. Cyr Campbell. "Nutrition, Exercise, and Healthy Aging." *J Am Diet Assoc* 97, no. 6 (June 1997):632–638.

CHAPTER 3: THE THREE PAUSES

Bhasin, S., et al. "The Effects of Supraphysiologic Doses of Testosterone on Muscle Size and Strength in Normal Men." *New England Journal of Medicine* 335 (July 1996):1–7.

"BPH: The Other Side of the Coin." *Life Extension* 5, no. 2 (February 1999):13–17.

Campbell, D.R., and M.S. Kurzer. "Flavonoid Inhibition of Aromatase Enzyme Activity in Human Preadipocytes." *Journal of Steroid Biochemistry & Molecular Biology* 46, no. 3 (September 1993):381–388.

Cantrill, J.A., et al. "Which Testosterone Replacement Therapy?" *Clin Endocrinol* 21, no. 2 (August 1984):97–107.

Crist, D.M., et al. "Body Composition Response to Exogenous GH During Training in Highly Conditioned Adults." *Journal of Applied Physiology* 65, no. 2 (August 1988):579–84.

Curtis, H. *Biology*, 4th ed. New York: Worth Publishers, 1986.

Dilman, V.M. *The Grand Biological Clock*. Moscow: Mir, 1989.

Drafta, D., et al. "Age-Related Changes of Plasma Steroids in Normal Adult Males." *Journal of Steroid Biochemistry & Molecular Biology* 17, no. 6 (December 1982):683–687.

Goldwasser, P., and J. Feldman. "Association of Serum Albumin and Mortality Risk." *Journal of Clinical Epidemiology* 50 (1997):693–703.

Hryb, D.J., et al. "The Effect of Extracts of the Roots of the Stinging Nettle (*Urtica dioica*) on the Interaction of SHBG with Its Receptor on Human Prostatic Membranes." *Planta Medica* 61, no. 1 (February 1995):31–32.

Hsieh C., et al.; "Predictors of Sex Hormone Levels among the Elderly: A Study in Greece." *Journal of Clinical Epidemiology* 51, no. 10 (October 1998):837–841.

Hsieh, C., and J. Granstrom. "Staying Young Forever: Putting New Research Findings into Practice." *Life Extension* 5, no. 12 (December 1999):23–25.

Itoh, N., et al. "Therapeutic Efficacy of Testolactone (Aromatase Inhibitor) to Oligozoospermia with High Estradiol/Testosterone Ratio." *Nippon Hinyokika Gakkai Zasshi* 82, no. 2 (February 1991):204–209.

Kamen, B. and P. Kamen. "The Remarkable Healing Power of Velvet Antler." *Nutrition Encounter*, Novato, CA, 1999.

King, B. *Fat Wars: 45 Days to Transform Your Body*. Toronto: CDG Books Canada Inc., 2000.

Klatz, R., and C. Kahn. *Grow Young with HGH*. New York: HarperCollins Publishers, 1997.

Kley, H.K., et al. "Conversion of Androgens to Estrogens in Idiopathic Hemochromatosis: Comparison with Alcoholic Liver Cirrhosis." *Journal of Clinical Endocrinology and Metabolism* 61, no. 1 (July 1985):1–6.

MacDonald, P.C. "Origin of Estrogen in Normal Men and in Women with Testicular Feminization." *Journal of Clinical Endocrinology and Metabolism* 49, no. 6 (December 1979):905–916.

Meikel, A.W., et al. "Familial Effects on Plasma Sex-Steroid Content in Man: Testosterone, Estradiol and Sex Hormone-Binding Globulin." *Metabolism* 31, no. 1 (January 1982):6–9.

Patterson, C.R. *Essentials of Biochemistry*. London: Pittman Books, 1983.

Peters, T. *All About Albumin*. San Diego: Academic Press, 1996.

Pugeat, M., et al. "Clinical Utility of Sex Hormone-Binding Globulin Measurement." *Horm Res* 45, no. 3–5 (1996):148–155.

Rosmond, R., and P. Björntorp. "Endocrine and Metabolic Aberrations in Men with Abdominal Obesity in Relation to Anxio-depressive Infirmity." *Metabolism* 47, no. 10 (October 1998):1187–1193.

_____, and P. Björntorp. "The Interactions Between Hypothalamic-Pituitary-Adrenal Axis Activity, Testosterone, Insulin-like Growth Factor I and Abdominal Obesity with Metabolism and Blood Pressure in Men." *Int J Obes Relat Metab Disord* 22, no. 12 (December 1998):1184–1196.

Samra, J.S., et al. "Suppression of the Nocturnal Rise in Growth Hormone Reduces Subsequent Lipolysis in Subcutaneous Adipose Tissue." *Eur J Clin Invest* 29, no. 12 (1999):1045–1052.

Seaton, K. "Carrying Capacity of Blood in Aging." Presented at the Anti-Aging Conference, Las Vegas, 1999. Abstract available from Advanced Health Products, LLC, Beachwood, Ohio, 1-888-262-5700.

Sonntag, W.E., et al. "Pleiotropic Effects of Growth Hormone and Insuline-like Growth Factor (IGF)-1 on Biological Aging: Inferences from Moderate Caloric-Restricted Animals." *J Gerontol A Biol Sci Med Sci* 54, no. 12 (December 1999):B521—B538.

_____, et al. "Moderate Caloric Restriction Alters the Subcellular Distribution of Somatostatin mRNA and Increases Growth Hormone Pulse Amplitude in Aged Animals." *Neuroendocrinology* 61, no. 5 (May 1995):601–608.

Schöttner, M., et al. "Lignans from the Roots of *Urtica dioica* and Their Metabolites Bind to Human Sex Hormone Binding Globulin (SHBG)." *Planta Medica* 63, no. 6 (December 1997):529–532.

Sherins, R.J., et al. "Alteration in the Plasma Testosterone: Estradiol Ratio: An Alternative to the Inhibin Hypothesis." *Ann N Y Acad Sci* 393 (1982):295–306.

Shippen, E., and W. Fryer. *The Testosterone Syndrome: The Critical Factor for Energy, Health and Sexuality*. New York: M. Evans and Company, 1998.

Suzuki, K., et al. "Endocrine Environment of Benign Prostatic Hyperplasia: Relationships of Sex Steroid Hormone Levels with Age and the Size of the Prostate." *Nippon Hinyokika Gakkai Zasshi* 83, no. 5 (May 1992):664–671.

Swartz, C. "Low Serum Testosterone: A Cardiovascular Risk in Elderly Men." *Geriatric Medicine Today* 7, no. 12 (December 1988).

Tchernof, A., et al. "Relationships Between Endogenous Steroid Hormone, Sex Hormone-Binding Globulin and Lipoprotein Levels in Men: Contribution of Visceral Obesity, Insulin Levels and Other Metabolic Variables." *Atherosclerosis* 133, no. 2 (September 1997):235–244.

Tenover, Joyce S. "Effects of Testosterone Supplementation in the Aging Male." *Journal of Clinical Endocrinology and Metabolism* 75, no. 4 (1992):1092–1098.

Vermeulen, A., et al. "Testosterone, Body Composition and Aging." *J Endocrinol Invest* 22, no. 5 Supplement (1999):110–116.

Wright, J., and L. Lenard. *Maximize Your Vitality & Potency: For Men Over 40*. Smart Publications, 1999.

Xu, X., and W.E. Sonntag. "Moderate Caloric Restriction Prevents the Age-Related Decline in Growth Hormone Receptor Signal Transduction." *J Gerontol A Biol Sci Med Sci* 51, no. 2 (March 1996):B167–B174.

CHAPTER 4: STRESS: THE INVISIBLE SABOTEUR

Borghese, C.M., et al. "Cortisol, the Muscle Eater." *Brain Res Bull* 31 (1993):697–700.

Charlesworth, E.A., and R.G. Nathan. *Stress Management*. New York: Atheneum, 1984.

Dinan, T.G., et al. *Acta Physiol Scand* 151 (1994):413–416.

Liakakos, D., et al. *Clin Chemica Acta* 65 (1975):251–255.

Marin, P., et al. "Cortisol Secretion in Relation to Body Fat Distribution in Obese Premenopausal Women." *Metabolism* 41, no. 8 (August 1992):882–886.

Markus, R.C., et al. "The Bovine Protein Alpha-lactoalbumin Increases the Plasma Ratio of Tryptophan to the Other Large Neutral Amino Acids, and in Vulnerable Subjects Raises Brain Serotonin Activity, Reduces Cortisol Concentration, and Improves Mood under Stress." *Amer J Clin Nut* 71, no. 6: 1536–1544.

Murray, D.J. "Cortisol Binding to Plasma Proteins in Man in Health, Stress and at Death." *J Endocrinol* 39 (1967):571–591.

Pelletier, Kenneth. *Mind as Healer, Mind as Slayer*. New York: Delta, 1992.

Samson, J.C. *J Clin Trials* 24 (1987):1–8.

Schaur, R.J., et al. *J Cancer Res Clin Oncol* 93 (1979):287–292.

Shannon, H., et al. *Journal of Clinical Endocrinology and Metabolism* 52 (1981):1235–1241.

CHAPTER 5: INSULIN: A HORMONE OF AGING?

Acheson, K.J., et al. "Glycogen Storage Capacity and De Novo Lipogenesis During Massive Carbohydrate Overfeeding in Man." *Amer J Clin Nut* 48 (1988):240–247.

"Adult Diabetes Type on Rise in Young." *The New York Times* (July 8, 1997):C7.

Bao, Wehang, et al. "Persistent Elevation of Plasma Insulin Levels Is Associated with Increased Cardiovascular Risk in Children and Young Adults." 93, no. 1 (January 1, 1996):54–59.

Barceló, A. "Monograph Series on Aging-Related Diseases: VIII. Non-Insulin-Dependent Diabetes Mellitus (NIDDM)." *Chronic Dis Can* 17, no. 1 (Winter 1996):1–20.

Betteridge, D.J. "Diabetic Dyslipidaemia: What Does It Mean?" *Diabetes News* 18, no. 2 (1997):1–3.

Bray, G.A. "Health Hazards of Obesity." *Endocrinol Metab Clin North Am* 25, no. 40 (1996):907–919.

Cassidy, C.M. "Nutrition and Health in Agriculturists and Hunter-Gatherers: A Case Study of Two Prehistoric Populations." *Nutritional Anthropology*, Pleasantville, New York; 117–145.

Cohen, B., et al. "Genetics and Diet as Factors in Development of Diabetes Mellitus." *Metabolism* 21, no. 3 (March 1972):235–240.

Colman, E., et al. "Weight Loss Reduces Abdominal Fat and Improves Insulin Action in Middle-Aged and Older Men with Impaired Glucose Tolerance." *Metabolism* 44, no. 11 (November 1995):1502–1508.

Eaton, S.B. "Humans, Lipids and Evolution." *Lipids* 27, no. 10 (1992):814–820.

_____, et al. "An Evolutionary Perspective Enhances Understanding of Human Nutritional Requirements." *Journal of Nutrition* 126 (June 1996):1732–1740.

Evans, W.J., and D. Cyr Campbell. "Nutrition, Exercise, and Healthy Aging." *J Am Diet Assoc* 97, no. 6 (June 1997):632–638.

Forbes, A., et al. "Alterations in Non-Insulin-Mediated Glucose Uptake in the Elderly Patient with Diabetes." *Diabetes* 47, no. 12 (December 1998):1915–1919.

Guerre Millo, M. "Glucose Transporters in Obesity." *Proc Nutr Soc* 55, no. 1B (March 1996):237–244.

King, B. *Fat Wars: 45 Days to Transform Your Body*. Toronto: CDG Books Canada Inc., 2000.

Lane, M.A., et al. "Calorie Restriction in Nonhuman Primates: Effects on Diabetes and Cardiovascular Disease Risk." *Toxicol Sci* 52, no. 2 Supplement (December 1999):41–48.

Maegawa, H., et al. "Obesity as a Risk Factor for Developing Non-Insulin Dependent Diabetes Mellitus—Obesity and Insulin Resistance." *Nippon Naibunpi Gakkai Zasshi* 71, no. 2 (March 1995):97–104.

Matsuzawa, Y., et al. "Pathphysiology and Pathogenesis of Visceral Fat Obesity." *Obes Res* 3, Supplement 2 (September 1995):187S–194S.

Muller, D.C., et al. "The Effect of Age on Insulin Resistance and Secretion: A Review." *Semin Nephrol* 16, no. 4 (July 1996):289–298.

Must, A., et al. "The Disease Burden Associated with Overweight and Obesity." *JAMA* 282, no. 16 (1999):1523–1529.

Nilsson, J., et al. "Relation Between Plasma Tumor Necrosis Factor-Alpha and Insulin Sensitivity in Elderly Men with Non-Insulin-Dependent Diabetes Mellitus." *Arterioscler Thromb Vasc Biol* 18, no. 8 (August 1998):1199–1202.

Pi-Sunyer, F.X. "Comorbidities of Overweight and Obesity: Current Evidence and Research Issues. *Med Sci Sports Exerc* 31, Supplement 11 (1999):S602–S608.

Preuss, H.G. "Effects of Glucose/Insulin Perturbations on Aging and Chronic Disorders of Aging: The Evidence." *J Am Coll Nutr* 16, no. 5 (October 1997):397–403.

_____, and R.A. Anderson. "Chromium Update: Examining Recent Literature 1997–1998." *Curr Opin Clin Nutr Metab Care* 1, no. 6 (November 1998):509–512.

Rexrode, K.M., et al. "Abdominal Adiposity and Coronary Heart Disease in Women." *JAMA* 280, no. 210 (1998):1843–1848.

Shimizu, M., et al. "Age-Related Alteration of Pancreatic Beta-Cell Function. Increased Proinsulin and Proinsulin-to-Insulin Molar Ratio in Elderly, But Not in Obese, Subjects without Glucose Intolerance." *Diabetes Care* 19, no. 1 (January 1996):8–11.

Stewart, P.M., et al. "Cortisol Metabolism in Human Obesity: Impaired Cortisone/Cortisol Conversion in Subjects with Central Adiposity." *Journal of Clinical Endocrinology and Metabolism* 84, no. 3 (March 1999):1022–1027.

Vincent, J.B. "Mechanisms of Chromium Action: Low-Molecular-Weight Chromium-Binding Substance." *J Am Coll Nutr* 18, no. 1 (1999):6–12.

Willey, T.S., and B. Formby. *Lights Out: Sleep, Sugar, and Survival*. New York: Pocket Books, 2000.

Yudkin, J. "Evolutionary and Historical Changes in Dietary Carbohydrates." *Amer J Clin Nutr* 20, no. 2 (1967):108–115.

CHAPTER 6: AGING WITH PROTEIN

Barenys, M., et al. "Effect of Exercise and Protein Intake on Energy Expenditure in Adolescents." *Rev Esp Fisiol* 49, no. 4 (1993):209–217.

Biolo, G., et al. "An Abundant Supply of Amino-Acids Enhances the Metabolic Effect of Exercise on Muscle Protein." *Amer J Phys* 273 (1997):E122–E129.

Bounous, G., et al. "The Biological Activity of Undenatured Dietary Whey Proteins: Role of Glutathione." *Clin Invest Med* 14, no. 4 (August 1991):296–309.

_____, et al. "Evolutionary Traits in Human Milk Proteins." *Med Hypotheses* 27, no. 2 (October 1988):133–140.

_____, et al. "The Immunoenhancing Property of Dietary Whey Protein Concentrate." *Clin Invest Med* 11, no. 4 (August 1988):271–278.

_____, et al. "The Influence of Dietary Whey Protein on Tissue Glutathione and the Diseases of Aging." *Clin Invest Med* 12, no. 6 (December 1989):343–349.

_____, et al. "Whey Proteins in Cancer Prevention." *Cancer Lett* 57, no. 2 (May 1991):91–94.

Brink, W. "Whey Protein Power." *Life Extension Magazine*, 4, no. 3 (March 1998): 16–17.

Campbell, W.W., et al. "Effects of an Omnivorous Diet Compared with a Lactoovovegetarian Diet on Resistance-Training-Induced Changes in Body Composition and Skeletal Muscle in Older Men." *Am J Clin Nutr* 70 (1999):1032–1039.

Chaitow, L. *Amino Acids in Therapy.* Rochester, VT: Thorsons Publishers, Inc., 1985.

Champe, P., and R. Harvey. *Biochemistry*, 2nd ed. Philadelphia: Lippencott, 1994.

Conley, E. *America Exhausted.* Flint, MI: Vitality Press Inc., 1998.

Coring, T., et al. (Conference paper: International Whey Conference, Chicago, 1997).

Coyne, L.L. *Fat Won't Make You Fat.* Calgary, Alberta: Fish Creek Publishing, 1998.

Demonty, I., et al. "Dietary Proteins Modulate the Effects of Fish Oil on Triglycerides in the Rat." *Lipids* 33, no. 9 (1998):913–921.

Froyland, L., et al. "Mitochondrion Is the Principal Target for Nutritional and Pharmacological Control of Triglyceride Metabolism." *J Lipid Res* 38, no. 9 (1997):1851–1858.

Gadzhieva RM, Portugalov SN, Paniushkin VV, Kondrat'eva II [A comparative study of the anabolic action of ecdysten, leveton and Prime Plus, preparations of plant origin] Sravnitel'noe izuchenie anaboliziruiushchego deistviia preparatov rastitel'nogo proiskhozhdeniia ekdistena, levetona i "Praim Plas." *Eksp Klin Farmakol* 8, no. 5 (September–October 1995):46–48.

Heine, W., et al. "Alpha-lactalbumin-Enriched Low-Protein Infant Formulas: A Comparison to Breast Milk Feeding." *Acta Paediatr* 85, no. 9 (September 1996):1024–1028.

Knudsen, C. "Super Soy: Health Benefits of Soy Protein." *Energy Times* (February 1996):12.

Lemon, P.W., et al. "Moderate Physical Activity Can Increase Dietary Protein Needs." *Can J Appl Physiol* 22, no. 5 (1997):494–503.

Life Extension Foundation. "The Wonders of Whey Restoring Youthful Anabolic Metabolism at the Cellular Level," May 1999.

Markus, R.C., et al. "The Bovine Protein Alpha-lactalbumin Increases the Plasma Ratio of Tryptophan to the Other Large Neutral Amino Acids, and in Vulnerable Subjects Raises Brain Serotinin Activity, Reduces Cortisol Concentration, and Improves Mood under Stress." *Amer J Clin Nutr* 71, no. 6 (June 2000):1536–1544.

Mindell, E. *Earl Mindell's Soy Miracle*. New York: Simon & Schuster, 1995.

Morr, C.V., and E.Y. Ha. "Whey Protein Concentrates and Isolates: Processing and Functional Properties." *Crit Rev Food Sci Nutr* 33, no. 6 (1993):431–476.

Pressman, A.H. *Glutathione: The Ultimate Antioxidant*. New York: St. Martin's Press, 1997.

Recommended Dietary Allowances, 10th ed. Washington, D.C.: National Academy Press, 1989.

Renner, E. *Milk and Dairy Products in Human Nutrition*. Munich, 1983.

Robinson, S.M., et al. "Protein Turnover and Thermogenesis in Response to High-Protein and High-Carbohydrate Feeding in Men." *Am J Clin Nutr* 52, no. 1 (1990):72–80.

Sahelian, R. *5-HTP, Nature's Serotonin Solution*. New York: Avery Publishing Group, Inc., 1998.

Satterlee, L.D., et al. "In vitro Assay for Predicting Protein Efficiency Ratio as Measured by Rat Bioassay: Collaborative Study." *J Assoc Off Anal Chem* 65, no. 4 (July 1982):798–809.

Soucy, J., and J. Leblanc. "Protein Meals and Postprandial Thermogenesis." *Physiol Behav* 65, no. 4–5 (1999):705–709.

Stroescu, V., et al. "Effects of Supro Brand Isolated Soy Protein Supplement in Male and Female Elite Rowers." XXVth FIMS World Congress of Sports Medicine, Athens, Greece, 1994.

Vandewater, K., and Z. Vickers. "Higher-Protein Foods Produce Greater Sensory-Specific Satiety." *Physiol Behav* 59, no. 3 (1996):579–583.

Volpi, E., et al. "Exogenous Amino Acids Stimulate Net Muscle Protein Synthesis in the Elderly." *Clin Invest* 101 (1998):2000–2007.

Westerterp, K.R., et al. "Diet-Induced Thermogenesis Measured over 24 h in a Respiration Chamber: Effect of Diet Composition." *Int J Obes Relat Metab Disord* 23, no. 2 (1999):287–292.

Whitehead, J.M., et al. "The Effect of Protein Intake on 24-Hour Energy Expenditure During Energy Restriction." *Int J Obes Relat Metab Disord* 20, no. 8 (1996):727–732.

Wurtman, J.J., and S. Suffers. *The Serotonin Solution*. New York: Ballantine Books, 1997.

Zed, C., and W.P. James. "Dietary Thermogenesis in Obesity. Response to Carbohydrate and Protein Meals: The Effect of Beta-adrenergic Blockage and Semistarvation." *Int J Obes* 10, no. 5 (1986):391–405.

CHAPTER 7: FATTY ACIDS

Adams, P., et al. "Arachidonic Acid to Eicosapentaenoic Acid Ratio in Blood Correlates Positively with Clinical Symptoms of Depression." *Lipids* 31 (Supplement):S157–S161.

Al, M.D.M. "The Effect of Pregnancy on the Cervonic Acid (Docosahexaenoic Acid) Status of Mothers and Their Newborns." Department of Human Biology, University of Limberg, Maastricht, The Netherlands. Second International Congress of International Society for Study of Fatty Acids and Lipids, Washington, D.C., June 8–11, 1995.

Bazan, N.G. "Supply of n-3 Polyunsaturated Fatty Acids and Their Significance in the Central Nervous System." In *Nutrition and the Brain*, edited by R.J. Wurtman and J.J. Wurtman, 1–24. New York: Raven Press Ltd., 1990.

Burgess, J.R. "Essential Fatty Acid Metabolism in Boys with Attention Deficit-Hyperactivity Disorder." *A J Clin Nutr* 62 (1995):761–768.

Chen, C. "The Shatin Community Mental Health Survey in Hong Kong II: Major Findings." *Arch Gen Psychiatry* 50 (1993):125–133.

Cross National Collaborative Group. "The Changing Rate of Major Depression Across National Comparisons." *JAMA* 268 (1992):3098–3105.

Deber, C.M., and S.J. Reynolds. "Central Nervous System Myelin: Structure, Function, and Pathology." *Clin Chem* 24 (1991):113–134.

Glen, A.I.M. "A Red Cell Membrane Abnormality in a Subgroup of Schizophrenic Patients: Evidence for Two Diseases." *Schiz Res* 12 (1994):53–61.

Golomb, B.A. "Cholesterol and Violence: Is There a Connection?" *Ann Intl Med* 128 (1998):478–487.

Grandgirard, A. "Incorporation of Trans Long-Chain n-3 Polyunsaturated Fatty Acids in Rat Brain Structure and Retina." *Lipids* 29, no. 4 (1994):251–258.

Hamazaki, T. "The Effect of Decosahexaenoic Acid on Aggression in Young Adults." *J Clin Invest* 97 (1996):1129–1134.

Hibbeln, J.R., and N. Salem. "Dietary Polyunsaturated Fatty Acids and Depression: When Cholesterol Does Not Satisfy." *Am J Clin Nutr* 62 (1995):1–9.

Holman, R.T., et al. "Deficiency of Essential Fatty Acids and Membrane Fluidity During Pregnancy and Lactation." *Proc Nat Acad Sci* 88 (1991):4835–4839.

Hudgins, L.C. , et al. "Human Fatty Acid Synthesis Is Stimulated by a Eucaloric Low-Fat, High-Carbohydrate Diet." *J Clin Invest* 97 (1996):2081–2091.

Innis, S. "Essential Fatty Acid Requirements in Human Nutrition." *Can J Physiol Pharmacol* 71 (1993):699–706.

Innis, S., et al. "Development of Visual Acuity in Relation to Plasma and Erythrocyte Omega-6 and Omega-3 Fatty Acids in Healthy Term Gestation Infants." *Am J Clin Nutr* 60, no. 3 (1994):347–352.

Jamrozik, K., et al. "The Role of Lifestyle Factors in the Etiology of Stroke: A Population-Based Case-Control Study in Perth, Western Australia." *Stroke* 25 (1994):51–59.

Kalmijin, S.E., et al. "Polyunsaturated Fatty Acids, Antioxidants, and Cognitive Function in Very Old Men." *Amer J Epidemiol* 145, no. 1 (1997):33–41.

Kidd, P. *Phosphatidylserine: A Remarkable Brain Cell Nutrient*. Decatur: Lucase Meyer, Inc., 1995.

Laugharne, J.D.E. "Fatty Acids and Schizophrenia." *Lipids* 31 (1996):S163–S165.

Ledwozyw, A., and K. Lutnicki. "Phospholipids and Fatty Acids in Human Brain Tumors." *Acta Physiol Hungarica* 79 (1992):381–387.

Liu, X., et al. "The Effects of Omega-3 Fish Oil Enriched with DHA on Memory." Congress Programs and Abstracts, Fatty Acids and Lipids from Cell Biology to Human Disease: 2nd International Congress of the ISSFAL International Society for the Study of Fatty Acids and Lipids, June 7–10, 1995.

Lucas, A., et al. "Breast Milk and Subsequent Intelligence Quotient in Children Born Preterm." *Lancet* 339 (1992):261.

Mackie, B.S., et al. "Melanoma and Dietary Lipids." *Nutrition and Cancer* 9, no. 4 (1987):219–226.

Maes, M. "Fatty Acid Composition in Major Depression: Decreased n-3 Fractions in Cholesteryl Esters and Increased C20:4n-6/C20:5n-3 Ratio in Cholesteryl Esters and Phospholipids." *J Affect Dis* 38 (1996):35–46.

Manku, M.S., et al. "Fatty Acids in Plasma and Red Cell Membranes in Normal Humans." *Lipids* 12 (1983):906.

Martin, D.D., et al. "The Fatty Acid Composition of Human Gliomas Differs from That Found in Nonmalignant Brain Tissue." *Lipids* 31, no. 12 (1996):1283–1288.

Martinez, M., and E. Vasquez. "MRI Evidence That Docosahexaenoic Acid Ethyl Ester Improves Myelination in Generalized Peroxisomal Disorders." *Neurology* 51 (1998):26–32.

Mitchell, E.A., et al. "Clinical Characteristics and Serum Essential Fatty Acid Levels in Hyperactive Children." *Clin Pediatr* 26 (1987):406–411.

Nightingale, S. "Red Blood Cell and Adipose Tissue Fatty Acids in Active and Inactive Multiple Sclerosis." *Acta Neurol Scand* 82 (1990):43–50.

Nomura, A.M.Y., et al. "The Effect of Dietary Fat on Breast Cancer Survival Among Caucasian and Japanese Women in Hawaii." *Breast Cancer Research and Treatment* 18 (1991):S135–S144.

Peet, M. "Essential Fatty Acid Deficiency in Erythrocyte Membranes from Chronic Schizophrenic Patients and the Clinical Effects of Dietary Supplementation." *Prost Leukotr Ess Fat Acids* 51, no. 1 and 2 (1996):71–75.

Petersen, J., and J. Opstvedt. "Trans Fatty Acids: Fatty Acid Composition of Lipids of the Brain and Other Organs in Suckling Piglets." *Lipids* 27, no. 10 (1992):761–769.

Rouse, L.R., et al. "Effects of Isoenergetic, Low-Fat Diets on Energy Metabolism in Lean and Obese Women." *Am J Clin Nutr* 60 (1994):470–475.

Rudin, D.O. "Modernization Disease Syndrome as Substrate Pellagra-Beriberi." *J Orthomolecular Med* 2, no. 1 (1987):3–14.

Schlundt, D. "Randomized Evaluation of a Low-Fat Diet for Weight Reduction." *Int J Obesity* 17 (1993):623–629.

Sibley, W.A. "Therapeutic Claims Committee of the International Federation of Multiple Sclerosis Societies." *Therapeutic Claims in Multiple Sclerosis*. New York: Demos Publications, 1992.

Simopoulos, A.T. "Omega-3 Fatty Acids." In *Handbook of Lipids in Human Nutrition*, edited by G.E. Spiller, 68. Boca Raton, FL: CRC Press, 1996.

Stevens, L.J., and J. Burgess. "Omega-3 Fatty Acids in Boys with Behavior, Learning, and Health Problems." *Physiology Behavior* 59, no. 4–5 (1996):915–920.

Stordy, B.J. "Benefit of Docosahexaenoic Acid Supplements to Dark Adaptation in Dyslexics." *Lancet* 346 (1995):385.

Swank, R., and B.B. Dugan. *The Multiple Sclerosis Diet Book*. Garden City, NY: Doubleday & Co., 1987.

Yam, D., et al. "Diet and Disease: The Israeli Paradox: Possible Dangers of a High Omega-6 Polyunsaturated Fatty Acid Diet." *Is J Med Sci* 32 (1996):1134–1143.

Yokota, A. "Relationship of Polyunsaturated Fatty Acid Composition and Learning Ability in Rat" [in Japanese]. *Nippon Saniujinka Clakkadji* 45 (1993):15–22.

CHAPTER 8: THE METABOLIC MODEL OF AGING

Aleman, A., et al. "Insulin-like Growth Factor-I and Cognitive Function in Healthy Older Men." *Journal of Clinical Endocrinology and Metabolism* 84, no. 2 (February 1999):471–475.

Bastianetto, S., et al. "Dehydropiandrosterone (DHEA) Protects Hippocampal Cells from Oxidative Stress-Induced Damage." *Brain Res Mol Braom Res* 66, no. 1–2 (March 1999):35–41.

Baulieu, E.E., et al. "Dehydropiandrosterone (DHEA), DHEA sulfate, and Aging: Contribution of the DHEAge Study to a Sociobiomedical Issue." *Proc Natl Acad Sci USA* 97, no. 8 (April 2000):4279–4284.

Bloch, M., et al. "DHEA Treatment of Midlife Dysthymia." *Biological Psychiatry* 45, no. 12 (June 15, 1999):1533–1541.

Diamond, P., et al. "Metabolic Effects of 12-Month Percutaneous Dehydropiandrosterone Replacement Therapy in Postmenopausal Women." *J Endocrinol* 150 (1996):S43–S50.

Gordon, C.M., et al. "Changes in Bone Turnover Markers and Menstrual Function After Short-Term DHEA in Young Women with Anorexia Nervosa." *J Bone Miner Res* 14, no. 1 (January 1999):136–145.

Khorram, O.; L. Vu and S.S. Yen. "Activation of Immune Function by Dehydropiandrosterone (DHEA) in Age-Advanced Men." *J Gerontol* 52A, no. 1 (1997):M1–M7.

Landin-Wilhelmsen, K., et al. "Postmenopausal Osteoporosis Is More Related to Hormonal Aberrations Than to Lifestyle Factors." *Clinical Endocrinology* 51, no. 4 (October 1999):387–394.

Ravaglia, G., et al. "The Relationship of Dehydropiandrosterone Sulfate (DHEAS) to Endocrine-Metabolic Parameters and Functional Status in the Oldest-Old: Results from an Italian Study on Healthy Free-Living Over-Ninety-Year-Olds." *Journal of Clinical Endocrinology and Metabolism* 81, no. 3 (March 1996):1173–1178.

Reiter, W.J. "Dehydropiandrosterone in the Treatment of Erectile Dysfunction: A Prospective, Double-Blind, Randomized, Placebo-Controlled Study." *Urology* 53, no. 3 (March 1999):590–594.

Stomati, M., et al. "Endocrine, Neuroendocrine and Behavioral Effects of Oral Dehydropiandrosterone Sulfate Supplementation in Postmenopausal Women." *Gynecol Endocrinol* 13, no. 1 (February 1999):15–25.

Wolkowitz, O.M., et al. "Dehydropiandrosterone (DHEA) Treatment of Depression." *Biological Psychiatry* 41 (1997):311–318.

_____, et al. "Double-Blind Treatment of Major Depression with Dehydropiandrosterone." *American Journal of Psychiatry* 156, no. 4 (1999):646–649.

Yen, S.S., and G.A. Laughlin. "Aging and the Adrenal Cortex. *Exp Gerontol* 33, no. 7–8 (November–December 1998):897–910.

Yen, S.S., et al. "Replacement of DHEA in Aging Men and Women: Potential Remedial Effects." *Ann NY Acad Sci* 774 (December 1995):128–142.

Zwain, I.H., and S.S. Yen. "Dehydropiandrosterone: Biosynthesis and Metabolism in the Brain." *Endocrinology* 140, no. 2 (February 1999):880–887.

CHAPTER 9: CELLULAR INSURANCE

Abraham, S.K. et al. "Inhibitory Effects of Dietary Vegetables on the In Vivo Clastogenicity of Cyclophosphamide." *Mutation Res.*, 172 (1986):51–54.

Baggott, J.E., T. Ha., et al. "Effects of Miso and NaCl on DMBA-induced Rat Mammary Tumors." *Nutrition and Cancer*, 14 (1990).

Cassidy, A., et al. "Biological Effects of a Diet of Soy Protein Rich in Isoflavones on the Menstrual Cycle of Premenopausal Women." *Amer. Jr. of Clin. Nut.* 60 (1994):333–40.

Cody V. et al, eds. *Plant Bioflavonoids in Biology and Medicine* vol. 1 and 2. New York, NY: Alan Liss, 1986; 1988.

Deshpande, R.G., et al. "Inhibition of Mycobacterium Avium Complex Isolates from AIDS Patients by Garlic (Allium sativum)." *J. Antimicrob Chemistry*, 32 (1993):623–626.

Fahey, J.W., Y. Zhang, and P. Talalay. "Broccoli Sprouts: An Exceptionally Rich Source of Inducers of Enzymes that Protect Against Chemical Carcinogens." *Proc. Natl. Acad. Sci. USA* 94 (September 1997):10367–72.

Graf, E., et al. "Phytic Acid, A Natural Antioxidant." *J. Biol. Chem.*, 262 (1987):11647–50.

Jankun, J., St. H. Selman, and S.J. Swiercz. "Why Drinking Green Tea Could Prevent Cancer." *Nature* 387 (June 5, 1997):561.

Kajikawa, M., et al. "Lactoferrin Inhibits Cholesterol Accumulation in Macrophages Mediated by Acetylated or Oxidized Low-Density Lipoproteins." *Biochem. Biophys. Acta* 1213, no. 1:82–90.

Kennedy, A. "The Condition for the Modification of Radiation Transformation in Vitro by a Tumor Promoter and Protease Inhibitors." *Carcinogenesis* 6 (1985):1441–45.

Kennedy, R.S., G.P. Konok, et al. "The Use of Whey Protein Concentrate in the Treatment of Patients With Metastatic Carcinoma: A Phase 1-11 Clinical Study." *Anticancer Research.* 15 (1995):2643–50.

Majeed, M., and V. Badmaev. *Turmeric and the Healing Curcuminoids*. New Canaan, Conn: Keats Publishing, 1996.

Mautner, G.G., G.M. Gardner, and R. Pratt. "Antibiotic Activity of Seaweed Extracts." *J. Am. Pharm. Assn.* 42 (1953):294–296.

Mazzio, E.A. et al. "Food Constituents Attenuate Monoamine Oxidase Activity and Peroxide Levels in C6 Astrocyte Cells." *Planta Med* 64 (1998):603–606.

National Research Council. *Recommended Dietary Allowances*, 10th ed. Washington, D.C.: National Academy Press, 1989.

Packer, L., Colman, C. *The Antioxidant Miracle*, New York: John Wiley and Sons, 1999.

Serraino, M., and L.U. Thompson. "Flaxseed Supplementation and Early Markers of Colon Carcinogenesis." *Cancer Letters* 63 (1992):159–165.

Sundaram, S.G., and J.A. Milner. "Diallyl Disulfide Inhibits the Proliferation of Human Tumor Cells in Culture." *Biochem Biophys Acta*, 1315 (1996):15–20.

Teas, J., M.L. Harbison, and R.S. Gelman. "Dietary Seaweed and Mammary Carcinogenesis in Rats." *Cancer Research* 44 (1984):2758–2761.

Zi Xetal, "Anticarcinogenic Effect of a Flavonoid Antioxidant, Silymarin, in Human Breast Cancer Cells." *Clin Cancer Res* 4 (1998):1055–1064.

Ziegler, R. "Vegetables, Fruits and Carotenoids and the Risk of Cancer." *Amer Jr of Clin Nut* (1991):2515–2595.

CHAPTER 10: RUNNING ON EMPTY

For a full list of references, please see Dr. Edward Conley's book *America Exhausted: Breakthrough Treatments of Fatigue and Fibromyalgia*. Vitality Press, 1998.

CHAPTER 11: DRYING UP

For a full list of references, please see Dr. F. Batmanghelidg's book *Your Body's Many Cries For Water*. Global Health Solutions: Falls Church: VA, 1997.

CHAPTER 12: A NEW APPROACH TO FEMALE TRANSITION FROM PMS TO MENOPAUSE

Ackerman, G.E., et al. "Potentiation of Epinephrine-Induced Lipolysis by Catechol Estrogens and Their Methoxy Derivatives." *Endocrinology* 109 (1981):2084–2088.

Aldercreutz, H. "Western Diet and Western Diseases: Some Hormonal and Biochemical Mechanisms and Associations." *Scand J Clin Lab Invest* 50, Supplement 21 (1990):3–23.

Arneson, D.W., et al. "Presence of 3,3'/Diindolylmethane in Human Plasma After Oral Administration of Indole-3-Carbinol." *Proceedings of the American Association for Cancer Research* 40 (March 1999):2833.

Baker, B. "Pilot Study: Cruciferous Veggies May Induce Cervical Dysplasia Regression." *Ob Gyn News* 15, no. 13 (May 1999).

Barnard, N.D., et al. "Diet and Sex Hormone-Binding Globulin, Dysmenorrhea, and Premenstrual Symptoms." *Obstet Gynecol* 95, no. 2 (February 2000):245–250.

Bell, M.C., et al. "Placebo-Controlled Trial of Indole-3-Carbinol in the Treatment of CIN." *Gynecologic Oncology* 78 (2000):123–129.

Bland, J.S. "Phytonutrition, Phytotherapy, and Phytopharmacology." *Altern Ther Health Med* 2, no. 6 (November 1996):73–76.

Boehm, S., et al. "Estrogen Suppression as a Pharmacotherapeutic Strategy in the Medical Treatment of Benign Prostatic Hyperplasia: Evidence for Its Efficacy from Studies with Mepartricin." *Wein Klin Wochenschr* 110, no. 23 (1998):817–823.

Bradlow, H.L., et al. "Effects of Pesticides on the Ratio of 16/2-Hydroxyestrone: A Biologic Marker of Breast Cancer Risk." *Environmental Health Perspectives* 103, Supplement 7 (1995):147–150.

_____, et al. 16- Hydroxylation of Estradiol: A Possible Risk Marker for Breast Cancer." *Annals NY Acad Sci* 464 (1986):138–151.

_____, et al. 2-Hydroxyestrone: The 'Good' Estrogen." *Journal of Endocrinology* 150 Supplement (September 1996):S259–S265.

Calef, I., and J. Alsina. "Benefits of Hormone Replacement Therapy: Overview and Update." *International Journal of Fertility and Women's Medicine* 42, Supplement 2 (1997):329–346.

Cohen, J.H., A.R. Kristal, and J.L. Stanford. "Fruit and Vegetable Intakes and Prostate Cancer Risk." *J Natl Cancer Inst* 92, no. 1 (January 2000):61–68.

Doostzadeh, J. "Pregnenolone-7Beta-Hydroxylating Activity of Human Cytochrome P450-1A1." *Journal of Steroid Biochemistry & Molecular Biology* 60, no. 1–2 (1997):147–152.

Ettinger, B. "Overview of Estrogen Replacement Therapy: A Historical Perspective." *Proc Soc Esp Biol Med* 217 (1998):2–5.

Farnsworth, W.E. "Estrogen in the Etiopathogenesis of BPH." *Prostate* 41, no. 4 (1999):263–274.

_____. "Roles of Estrogen and SHBG in Prostate Physiology." *The Prostate* 28 (1996):17–23.

Fishman, J., H.L. Bradlow, et al. "Increased Estrogen-16-Hydroxylase Activity in Women with Breast and Endometrial Cancer." *Journal of Steroid Biochemistry and Molecular Biology* 20 (1984):1077–1081.

Ge, X., et al. "3,3'-Diindolylmethane Induces Apoptosis in Human Cancer Cells." *Biochem Biophys Res Commun* 228, no. 1 (November 1996):153–158.

Ginsberg, E.L., et al. "Effects of Alcohol Ingestion on Estrogens in Postmenopausal Women." *JAMA* 276 (1996):1747–1751.

Grady, D., et al. "Postmenopausal Hormone Therapy Increases Risk for Venous Thromboembolic Disease: The Heart and Estrogen/Progestin Replacement Study." *Ann Intern Med* 132, no. 9 (2000):689–696.

Grodstein, F., et al. "Postmenopausal Hormone Therapy and Mortality." *New England Journal of Medicine* 336 (1997):1769–1775.

_____, et al. "Postmenopausal Hormone Use and Risk for Colorectal Cancer and Adenoma." *Annals of Internal Medicine* 128 (1998):705–712.

Hammarback, S., et al. "Relationship Between Symptom Severity and Hormone Changes in Women with Premenstrual Syndrome." *Journal of Clinical Endocrinology and Metabolism* 68, no. 1 (January 1989):125–130.

Hershcopf, R.J., and H.L. Bradlow. "Obesity, Diet, Endogenous Estrogens, and the Risk of Hormone-Sensitive Cancer." *American Journal of Clinical Nutrition* 45, 1 Supplement (1987):283–289.

Inestrosa, N.C., et al. "Cellular and Molecular Basis of Estrogen's Neuroprotection: Potential Relevance for Alzheimer's Disease." *Molecular Neurobiology* 17 (1998):73–86.

Jacobs, I.C., and M.A. Zeligs. "Facilitated Absorption of a Hydrophobic Dietary Ingredient." Proceedings of Controlled Release Society, 1998.

Klaiber, E.L., et al. "Serum Estrogen Levels in Men with Acute Myocardial Infarction." *American Journal of Medicine* 73 (1982):872–881.

Komura, S., et al. "Catecholestrogen as a Natural Antioxidant." *Annals NY Acad Sci* 15, no. 786 (June 1996):419–429.

Labrie, F. "DHEA as Physiological Replacement Therapy at Menopause." *J Endocrinol Invest* 21 (1998):399–401.

_____, et al. "Effect of 12-Month Dehydroepiandrosterone Replacement Therapy on Bone, Vagina, and Endometrium in Postmenopausal Women." *Journal of Clinical Endocrinology and Metabolism* 82 (1997):3498–3505.

Loch, E.G., et al. "Treatment of Premenstrual Syndrome with a Phytopharmaceutical Formulation Containing *Vitex agnus castus*." *J Women's Health Gend Based Med* 9, no. 3 (April 2000):315–320.

Manson, J.E. "Postmenopausal Hormone Replacement and Atherosclerotic Disease." *American Heart Journal* 128 (1994):1337–1343.

Maxim, P., et al. "Fracture Protection Provided by Long-Term Estrogen Replacement Therapy." *Osteoporosis Int* 5 (1995):23–29.

Michnovicz, J.J., et al. "Altered Estrogen Metabolism and Excretion in Humans Following Consumption of Indole-3-Carbinol." *Nutr Cancer* 16, no. 1 (1991):59–66.

_____, et al. "Dietary and Pharmacological Control of Estradiol Metabolism in Humans." *Ann N Y Acad Sci* 595 (1990):291–299.

Musey, P.I., et al. "Effect of Diet on Oxidation of 17-Beta-Estradiol in vivo." *Journal of Clinical Endocrinology and Metabolism* 65 (1987):792–795.

Muti, P., et al. "Metabolism and Risk of Breast Cancer: A Prospective Analysis of 2:16 Hydroxyestrone Ratio in Premenopausal and Postmenopausal Women." *Cancer Epidemiology and Biomarkers* (2000), in press.

Philips, G.B., et al. "Association of Hyperestrogenemia and Coronary Heart Disease in Men in the Framingham Cohort." *American Journal of Medicine* 74 (1983):863–869.

Purohit, A., et al. "Inhibition of Tumor Necrosis Factor Alpha-Stimulated Aromatase Activity by Microtubule-Stabilizing Agents, Paclitaxel and 2-Methoxyestradiol." *Biochem Biophys Res Commun* 261, no. 1 (July 22, 1999):214–217.

Redei, E. "Daily Plasma Estradiol and Progesterone Levels Over the Menstrual Cycle and Their Relation to Premenstrual Symptoms." *Psychoneuroendocrinology* 20, no. 3 (1995):259–267.

Santoro, N. "Characteristics of Reproductive Hormonal Dynamics in the Perimenopause." *Journal of Clinical Endocrinology and Metabolism* 81 (1996):1495–1501.

Schairer, C., et al. "Menopausal Estrogen and Estrogen-Progestin Replacement Therapy and Breast Cancer Risk." *JAMA* 283, no. 4 (2000):485–491.

Schneider, J., et al. "Abnormal Oxidative Metabolism of Estradiol in Women with Breast Cancer." *Prc Natl Acad Sci USA* 79 (1982):3047–3051.

Seeger, H., et al. "The Effect of Estradiol Metabolites in the Susceptibility of Low Density Lipoprotein to Oxidation." *Life Sciences* 61 (1997):865–868.

Seippel, L., and T. Backstrom. "Luteal-Phase Estradiol Relates to Symptom Severity in Patients with Premenstrual Syndrome." *Journal of Clinical Endocrinology and Metabolism* 83, no. 6 (June 1998):1988–1992.

Sepkovic, D.W., et al. "Estrogen Metabolite Ratios and Risk Assessment of Hormone-Related Cancers: Assay Validation and Prediction of Cervical Cancer Risk." *Annals of the New York Academy of Science* 768 (1995):312–316.

Service, R.F. "New Role for Estrogen in Cancer?" *Science* 13, no. 279 (March 1998):1631–1633.

Shaughn O'Brien, P.M., et al. "Premenstrual Syndrome Is Real and Treatable." *The Practitioner* 244 (2000):185–195.

Spector, T.D., et al. "Is Hormone Replacement Therapy Protective for Hand and Knee Osteoarthritis in Women?" The Chingford Study. *Annals of the Rheumatic Diseases* 56 (1997):432–434.

Spicer, L.J., and J.M. Hammond. "Comparative Effects of Androgens and Catecholestrogens on Progesterone Production by Porcine Granulosa Cells." *Molecular and Cellular Endocrinology* 56 (1988):211–217.

Steinmetz, K.A. "Vegetables, Fruit, and Cancer Prevention: A Review." *Journal of the American Dietetic Association* 10 (1996):1027–1039.

Thrys-Jacobs, S. "Micronutrients and the Premenstrual Syndrome: The Case for Calcium." *J Am Coll Nutr* 19, no. 2 (April 2000):220–227.

Wang, M., et al. "Relationship Between Symptom Severity and Steroid Variation in Women with Premenstrual Syndrome: Study on Serum Pregnenolone, Pregnenolone Sulfate, 5 Alpha-Pregnane-3,20-Dione and 3 Alpha-Hydroxy-5 Alpha-Pregnan-20-one." *Journal of Clinical Endocrinology and Metabolism* 81, no. 3 (March 1996):1076–1082.

Wenger, N.K., et al. "Early Risk of Hormone Therapy in Patients with Coronary Heart Disease." *JAMA* 284, no. 1 (2000):41–43.

Wong, G.Y., et al. "Dose-Ranging Study of Indole-3-Carbinol for Breast Cancer Prevention." *J Cell Biochem Suppl* (1999):28–29, 111–116.

Zeligs, M.A. "Diet and Estrogen Status: The Cruciferous Connection." *Journal of Medicinal Food* 1 (1998):67–82.

_____. "Plant-Powered Weight Loss." *BioResponse*, LLC. Boulder, CO (2000).

_____. "Safer Estrogen with Phytonutrition." *Townsend Letter* 189 (1999):83–188.

Zhu, B.T., et al. "Is 2-Methoxyestradiol an Endogenous Estrogen Metabolite That Inhibits Mammary Carcinogenesis?" *Cancer Research* 1 (June 1998):2269–2277.

Zumoff, B., et al. "Estradiol Transformation in Men with Breast Cancer." *Journal of Clinical Endocrinology and Metabolism* 26 (1966):960–966.

CHAPTER 13: MOM'S BEST-KEPT SECRET, COLOSTRUM: THE PERFECT ANTI-AGING FOOD

AARP Poll. *Time* (June 7, 1999).

Bengtsson, G.H., et al. "Treatment of Adults with Growth Hormone (GH) Deficiency with Recombinant Human." *Journal of Clinical Endocrinology and Metabolism* 76 (February 1993):309–317.

Casswall, T.H., et al. "Treatment of *Helicobacter pylori* Infection in Infants in Rural Bangladesh with Oral Immunoglobulins from Hyperimmune Bovine Colostrum." *Aliment Pharmacol Ther* 12 (1998):563–568.

Davidson, G.P., et al. "Passive Immunization of Children with Bovine Colostrum Containing Antibodies to Human Rotavirus." *Lancet* 2 (1989):709–712.

Francis, G.L., et al. "Insulin-like Growth Factors-1 (IGF-1) and 2 (IGF-2) in Bovine Colostrum." *Biochem J* 251 (1988):95–103.

_____, et al. "Purification and Partial Sequence Analysis of Insulin-like Growth Factor-1 (IGF-1) from Bovine Colostrum." *Biochem J* 233 (1986):207–213.

Jackson, J.R., et al. "Effects of Induced or Delayed Parturition and Supplemental Dietary Fat on Colostrum and Milk Composition in Sows." *J Animal Sci* 73 1906–1913.

Keusch, G.T. "Effect of Protein-Energy Interaction with Reference to Immune Function and Response to Disease." In *Protein-Energy Interactions*, UN ACC-Subcommittee on Nutrition, the International Dietary Energy Consultancy Group. New York: UNY Press.

Khansari, D.N., and T. Gustad. "Effects of Long-Term, Low-Dose Growth Hormone Therapy on Immune Function and Life Expectancy of Mice." *Mech Ageing Dev* 57 (January 1991):87–100.

Mero, A., et al. "Effects of Bovine Colostrum Supplementation on Serum IGF-1, IgF, Hormone, and Saliva IgA During Training." *Journal of Applied Physiology* 83 (1997):1144–1151.

Mitra, A.K., et al. "Hyperimmune Cow Colostrum Reduces Diarrhea Due to Rotavirus: A Double-Blind Study, Controlled Clinical Trial." *Acta Paediatr* 84 (1995):996–1001.

Oda, S., et al. "Insulin-like Growth Factor-1 (IGF-1), Growth Hormone (GH), Insulin and Glucagon Concentrations in Bovine Colostrum and in Plasma of Dairy Cows and Neonatal Calves Around Parturition." *Comp Biochem Physiol* 94A, no. 4 (1989):805–808.

Pakkanen, R., and J. Aalto. "Growth Factors and Automicrobial Factors of Bovine Colostrum." *International Dairy Journal* (1997):285–297.

Palmer, E.L., et al. "Antiviral Activity of Colostrum and Serum Immunoglobulins A and G." *J Med Virol* 5 (1980):123–129.

Playford, R.J., et al. *Gut* 44 (May 1999):653–658.

Rouse, B.T., et al. "Antibody-Dependent Cell-Mediated Cytoxtoxicity in Cows: Comparison of Effector Cell Activity Against Heterologous Erthrocyte and Herpes-Virus-Infected Bovine Target Cells." *Infection and Immunity* 13 (1976):1428–1441.

Rudman, D., et al. "Effects of Human Growth Hormone in Men Over 60 Years Old." *New England Journal of Medicine* 323 (1990):1–6.

Rump, J.A., et al. "Treatment of Diarrhea in Human Immunodeficiency Virus-Infected Patients with Immunoglobulins from Bovine Colostrum." *Clin Investig* 70 (1992):588–594.

Sabin, A.B. "Antipoliomylitic Activity of Human and Bovine Colostrum and Milk." *Pediatrics* 29 (1962):105–115.

_____. "Antipoliomylitic Substance in Milk from Human Beings and Certain Cows." *Journal of Disease in Children* 80 (1950):866.

Shen, W.H., and R.J. Xu. "Stability of Insulin-like Growth Factor I in the Gastrointestinal Lumen in Neonatal Pigs." *J Pediatr Gastroenterol Nutr* 39 (March 2000):299–304.

Shomail, M.E., and R. Wolfsthal. "The Use of Anti-Aging Hormones." *Maryland Medical Journal* 46 (1997):181–186.

Tacket, C.O., et al. "Efficacy of Bovine Milk Immunoglobulin Concentrate in Preventing Illness After Shigella flexneri Challenge." *Am J Trop Med Hyg* 47 (1992):276–283.

Thompson, L.V. "Aging Muscle: Characteristics and Strength Training." Section on Geriatrics. American Physical Therapy Association.

Ungar, B.L. "Cessation of Cryptosporidium-Associated Diarrhea in an Acquired Immunodeficiency Syndrome Patient After Treatment with Hyperimmune Bovine Colostrum." *Gastroenterology* 98 (1990):486–489.

United States Census Bureau Statistical Brief by Economics and Statistics Administration, U.S. Department of Commerce, May 1995.

Watson, *Journal of Dairy Research* 59 (1992):369–380.

X.U.J. "Development of the Newborn Gastrointestinal Tract and Its Relationship to Colostrum, Reproduction, Fertility, Development." (1996).

CHAPTER 14: WAKING UP YOUNGER

Andreasen, Nancy M.C. *The Broken Brain*. Cambridge: Harper and Row, 1984.

Armitage, R., et al. "Slow-Wave Activity in NREM Sleep: Sex and Age Effects in Depressed Outpatients and Healthy Controls." *Psychiatry Res* 95, no. 3 (July 11, 2000):201–213.

Boyd, et al. "Stimulation of Human-Growth-Hormone Secretion by L-Dopa." *New England Journal of Medicine* 283, no. 26:1425–1429.

Edinger, J.D., et al. "Slow-Wave Sleep and Waking Cognitive Performance II: Findings Among Middle-Aged Adults with and without Insomnia Complaints." *Physiol Behav* 70, no. 1–2 (July 2000):127–134.

Guinness Book of World Records. New York: Stirling, 1984.

Hartman, Ernest. "How to Help Your Patients Sleep Better." *Medical Times* 100, no. 3 (March 1972).

Hauri, Peter. "Treatment of Sleep Disorders." *Basic Psychiatry for Primary Care Physicians*. Boston: Little, Brown and Co., 1976.

Kales, Anthony. "Treating Sleep Disorders." *American Family Physician* (November 1973).

Merritt, S.L. "Putting Sleep Disorders to Rest." *RN* 63, no. 7 (July 2000):77.

Miyamoto, Y., and A. Sancar. "A Circadian Regulation of Cryptochrome Genes in the Mouse." *Brain Res* 71, no. 2 (August 25, 1999):238–243.

Munson, B.L. "Myths & Facts About Sleep Deprivation." *Nursing* 30, no. 7 (July 2000):77.

Puig-Antrich, J., et al. "Growth Hormone Secretion in Pre-pubertal Children with Major Depression." *Arch Gen Psychiatry* 41, no. 5 (1984):463–466.

Restag, Richard. *The Brain*. Toronto: Bantam Books, 1984.

Saidel, W.E., et al. "Daytime Alertness in Relation to Mood, Performance, and Nocturnal Sleep in Chronic Insomniacs and Noncomplaining Sleepers." *Sleep* 7, no. 3 (1984):230–238.

Scheen, A.J., and E. Van Cauter. "The Roles of Time of Day and Sleep Quality in Modulating Glucose Regulation: Clinical Implications." *Horm Res* 49, no. 3–4 (1998):191–201.

Schneider, H. "DSIP in Insomnia." *Eur. Neurology* 23, no. 5 (1984):358–363.

Sei, H., et al. "Differential Effect of Short-Term REM Sleep Deprivation on NGF and BDNF Protein Levels in the Rat Brain." *Brain Res* 877, no. 2 (September 22, 2000):387–390.

Shahana, T.L., and C.A. Czeisler. "Physiological Effects of Light on the Human Circadian Pacemaker." *Semin Perinatol* 24, no. 4 (August 2000):299–320.

Sung, E.J., and Y. Tochihara. "Effects of Bathing and Hot Footbath on Sleep in Winter." *J Physiol Anthropol Appl Human Sci* 19, no. 1 (January 2000):21–27.

Van Cauter, E., and G. Copinschi. "Interrelationships Between Growth Hormone and Sleep." *Growth Hormone IGH Res* Supplement (April 2000):S57–S62.

_____, R. Leproult and L. Plat. "Age-Related Changes in Slow-Wave Sleep and REM Sleep and Relationship with Growth Hormone and Cortisol Levels in Healthy Men." *JAMA* 284, no. 7 (August 16, 2000):861–868.

Wasnes, K., and D. Harburton. "A Comparison of Temzepam and Flurazepam in Terms of Sleep Quality and Residual Changes in Performance." *Neuropsychobiology* 11, no. 4 (1984):244–246.

Williamson, A.M., and A.M. Feyer. "Moderate Sleep Deprivation Produces Impairments in Cognitive and Motor Performance Equivalent to Legally Prescribed Levels of Alcohol Intoxication." *Occup Environ Med* 57, no. 10 (October 2000):649–655.

Winget, C.M., et al. "A Review of Human Physiological Performance Changes Associated with Dysynchronosis of Biological Rhythms." *Aviation Space Environment Medicine* 55, no. 121 (1984):1085–1086.

CHAPTER 15: THE AGING PROCESS: HOW TO SLOW IT OR REVERSE IT WITH ALBUMIN

Bourlie F., and J. Vallery-Masson , *Epidemiology & Ecology of Aging*, Textbook of Geriatric Med Ed. Brocklehurst, Churchill Livingstone New York 1985:3–5.

Goldwasser P., Feldman J., "Association of Serum Albumin & Mortality," *J. Clin Epidemiol* 50 (1997): 693–703.

Masoro E. Hayflick, Lecture 1996 Annual Meeting of American Aging Association Age 19:141–145 1996 , Also *Age News*, 27 (Spring 1998):1–4.

Peters T., *All About Albumin*, San Diego: Academic Press, 1996.

Schmidt M., et al., "Markers of Inflammation & Prediction of Diabetes," *Lancet*; 353.

Seaton K. "Is Cortisol the Aging Hormone?," Report of The National Hygiene Foundation Washington DC 1997.

Seaton K., "Albumin & Alzheimer's," *Age* 18 (1995): 1–2.

Seaton K., "Carrying Capacity of Blood in Aging. Abstract Presented At Conference on Anti-Aging Medicine" Las Vegas 1999 American Academy of Anti-Aging Medicine Dec 1999.

Seaton K., "Health, Wealth & Hygiene," *JNMA* 86 (1994):327.

Seaton K., Micozzi M., "Is Cortisol the Aging Hormone?" *J Adv. Med*. 11 (1998): 73–94.

Steven, Richard, Blumberg Baruch, "Serum Albumin and the Risk of Cancer Macronutrietnts Investigating Their Role in Cancer."

Todaro G., and H. Green, "Albumin Supplemented Medium for Long-Term Cultivation of Cells," *Proc Soc Exp Bio* Med, 1964, 16, 688–692.

Walford R., "The Immunologic Theory of Aging," *Advances in Gerontological Research*, 2 (1967): 159–204.

Walford R., *Maximum Lifespan*, New York: W. Norton,1983.

CHAPTER 16: AGEING WITH SUGAR: BROWNING AND STIFFENING FROM THE INSIDE OUT

Anderson, R.A., et al. "Urinary Chromium Excretion and Insulinogenic Properties of Carbohydrates." *American Journal of Clinical Nutrition* 51 (1990):864–868.

Aoki, Y., et al. "Stiffening of Connective Tissue in Elderly Diabetic Patients: Relevance to Diabetic Nephropathy and Oxidative Stress." *Diabetabetologica* 36 (1993):79–83.

Artwerth, B.C., and P.R. Olesen. "Glutathione Inhibits the Glycation and Cross Linking of Lens Proteins by Ascorbic Acid." *Exp Eye Res* 47, no. 5 (1988):737–750.

Ashoor, S., and J.B. Zent. "Maillard Browning of Common Amino Acids and Sugars." *J Food Sci* 49 (1984):1206–1207.

Avendano, G.F., et al. "Effects of Glucose Intolerance on Myocardial Function and Collagen-Linked Glycation." *Diabetes* 48, no. 7 (July 1999):1443–1447.

Bailey, A.J., et al. "Chemistry of Collagen Cross-links: Glucose-Mediated Covalent Cross-linking of Type IV Collagen in Lens Capsules." *Biochem J* 296 (1993):489–496.

Beutler, E. "Nutritional and Metabolic Aspects of Glutathione." *Annu Rev Nutr* 9 (1989):287–302.

Bierhaus, A., et al. "Advance Glycation End Products-Induced Activation of NF-Kappa B Is Suppressed by Alpha-Lipoic Acid in Cultured Endothelial Cells." *Diabetes* 46, no. 9 (1997):1481–1490.

Blakytny, R., and J.J. Harding. "Glycation (Non-Enzymatic Glycosylation) Inactivates Glutathione Reductase." *Biochem J* 288 (1992):303–307.

Booth, A.A., et al. "Thiamine Pyrophosphate and Pyridoxamine Inhibit the Formation of Advance Glycation End-products: Comparison with Aminoguanidine." *Biochem Biophys Res Comm* 220, no. 1 (1996):113–119.

Colaco, C.A.L.S. *The Glycation Theory of Atherosclerosis*. New York: Chapman and Hall, 1997.

Davies, S., et al. "Age-Related Decrease in Chromium Levels in 51,665 Hair, Sweat, and Serum Samples from 40,872 Patients: Implications for the Prevention of Cardiovascular Disease and Type II Diabetes Mellitus." *Metabolism* 46, no. 5 (1997):469–473.

Devamnoharan, P.S., et al. "Attenuation of Sugar Cataract by Ethyl Pyruvate." *Mol Cell Biochem* 200, no. 1–2 (1999):103–109.

Dunn, J.A., et al. "Accumulation of Maillard Reaction Projects in Skin Collagen in Diabetes and Aging." *J Clin Invest* 91 (1993):2463–2469.

Durany, N. "Investigations on Oxidative Stress and Therapeutical Implications in Dementia." *Eur Arch Psych Clin Neurosci* 249, Supplement 3 (1999):68–73.

Dyer, D.G., et al. "Accumulation of Maillard Reaction Products in Skin Collagen in Diabetes and Aging." *J Clin Invest* 91, no. 6 (June 1993):2463–2469.

Fu, M.N., et al. "Role of Oxygen in Cross Linking and Chemical Modification of Collagen by Glucose." *Diabetes* 43 (1996):676–683.

Gerbityz, K.D., et al. "Mitochondrial and Diabetes: Genetic, Biochemical, and Clinical Implications of the Cellular Energy Circuit." *Diabetes* 45 (1996):113–126.

Gillery, P., et al. "Glycation of Proteins as a Source of Superoxide." *Diabetes and Metabolism* 14 (1996):25–30.

Glomb, M.A., and V.M. Monnier. "Mechanism of Protein Modification by Glyoxal and Glycoaldehyde, Reactive Intermediates of the Maillard Reaction." *J Biol Chem* 276 (1996):10017–10025.

Halliwel, B., and J.M. Gutteridge. *Free Radicals in Biology and Medicine.* Oxford: Clarendon Press, 1989.

Isenberg, D.A., and T.W. Rademacher. *Abnormalities of IgG Glycosylation and Immunologic Disorders.* New York: John Wiley & Sons, 1996.

Jacob, S., et al. "Enhancement of Glucose Disposal in Patients with Type 2 Diabetes by Alpha-Lipoic Acid." *Arxneimittelforschung* 45 (1994):872–874.

Koschinsky, T., et al. "Orally Absorbed Reactive Glycation Products (Glycotoxins): An Environmental Risk Factor in Diabetic Nephropathy." *Proc Natl Acad Sci USA* 94, no. 12 (1997):6474–6479.

Lyons, T.J. "Glycation and Oxidation: A Role in the Pathogenesis of Atherosclerosis." *Am J Cardiol* 71 (1993):26B–31B.

Makita, Z., et al. "Hemoglobin-AGE: A Circulating Marker of Advanced Glycosylation." *Science* 258 (1992):651–653.

Monnier, V.M., et al. "Maillard Reactions Involving Proteins and Carbohydrates *in vivo*: Relevance to Diabetes Mellitus and Aging." *Prog Food Nutri Sci* 5 (1981):315–327.

Morimitsu, Y., et al. "Protein Glycation Inhibitors from Thyme (*Thymus vulgaris*)." *Biosci Biotechnol Biochem* 59, no. 11 (1995):2018–2021.

O'Brien, Morrisey. "Metal Ion Complexation By-products of the Maillard Reaction." *Food Chem* 58 (1997):17–27.

Oya, T., et al. "Spice Constituents Scavenging Free Radicals and Inhibiting Pentosidine Formation in a Model System." *Biosci Biotechnol Biochem* 61, no. 2 (1997):263–266.

Ramakrishnan, S., et al. "Two New Functions of Inositol in the Eye Lens: Antioxidation and Possible Mechanisms." *Indian J Biochem Biophys* 36, no. 2 (1999):129–133.

Schmidt, A.M., et al. "Advanced Glycation Endproducts Interacting with Their Endothelial Receptors Induce Expression of Vascular Cell Adhesion Molecule-1 (VCAM-1) in Cultured Human Endothelial Cells and in Mice: A Potential Mechanism for the Accelerated Vasculopathy of Diabetes." *J Clin Invest* 96 (1995):1395–1403.

Sernau, T., "Thioctic Acid Prevents AGE-Mediated TF Induction by Blocking Translocation of NF-kappaB *in vitro* and *in vivo*." *Arch Pharmacol* S351 (1995):R91.

Stamler, J.S., and A. Silvka. "Biological Chemistry of Thiols in the Vasculature and in Vascular-Related Disease." *Nut Rev* 1 (1996):1–30.

Thornalley, P.J. "Glutathione-Dependent Detoxification of Alpha-Oxoaldehydes by the Glyoxalase System: Involvement in Disease Mechanisms and Antiproliferative Activity of Gloxalase I Inhibitors." *Chem Biol Interact* (1998):111–112.

_____. "The Glyoxalase System in Health and Disease." *Molec Aspects Med* 14 (1993):287–371.

Yan, S.D., et al. "Amyloi-B Peptide—Receptor for Advanced Glycation Endproduct Interaction Elicits Neuronal Expression of Macrophase-Colony Stimulating Factor: A Proinflammatory Pathway in Alzheimer Disease." Proceedings of the *National Acad Sci USA* 94 (1997):5296–5301.

CHAPTER 17: BIOCIZE: ANTI-AGING EXERCISE

Alessio, H.M.; Exercise-induced Oxidative Stress, *Med Sci Sports Exerc*, (Feb 1993), 25:2, 218–24.

Aniansson A., et al; Effect of a Training Program for Pensioners on Condition and Muscular Strength, *Arch Gerontol Geriatr*, 3 (Oct 1984):229–41.

Batmanghelidj, F.; *Your Body's Many Cries For Water*, Falls Church, VA: Global Health Solutions, 1998.

Blumenthal J.A., et al; Effects of Exercise Training on Older Patients with Major Depression, *Arch Intern Med*, 159 (Oct. 1999):2349–56.

Borst S.E., et al; "Growth Hormone, Exercise, and Aging: The Future of Therapy for the Frail Elderly," *J Am Geriatr Soc,*, 42:5 (May, 1998):528–35.

Burke, ER.; *Optimal Muscle Recovery*, Avery Publishing Group, 1999.

Buxton OM., et al; "Roles of Intensity and Duration of Nocturnal Exercise in Causing Phase Delays of Human Circadian Rhythms," *Am J Physiol*, (Sep 1997) 273:3 Pt 1, E536–42.

Buxton O.M. et al; "Acute and Delayed Effects of Exercise on Human Melatonin Secretion," *J Biol Rhythms*, 12 (Dec 1997):568–74.

Brsheim, E., et al; "Adrenergic Control of Post-exercise Metabolism," *Acta Physiol Scand*, 162 (Mar 1998):313–23.

Carlson, LA., et al; "Studies on Blood Lipids During Exercise," *J Lab Clin Med*, 61 (1963):724–729.

Cashmore A.R., et al; "Cryptochromes: Blue Light Receptors for Plants and Animals," 284 *Science*, (Apr 1999):760–5.

Coggan A.R. et al. "Fat Metabolism During High-Intensity Exercise in Endurance-Trained and Untrained Men," *Metabolism* 49 (2000):122–8.

Colgan, M; *The New Nutrition*, Vancouver: Apple Publishing, 1995.

Devlin P.F.; Kay SA; Cryptochromes—Bringing the Blues to Circadian Rhythms," *Trends Cell Biol*, 9 (Aug 1999):295–8.

Fernández Pastor V.J., et al; "Function of Growth Hormone in the Human Energy Continuum During Physical Exertion," *Rev Esp Fisiol*, 47 (Dec 1991):223–9.

Fiatarone, M.A., et al; "High-intensity Strength Training in Nonagenerians. Effects on Skeletal Muscle." *J of the American Medical Association*, 263 (1990):3029–3034.

Fryburg D.A., et al; "Short-Term Modulation of the Androgen Milieu Alters Pulsatile, But Not Exercise- Or Growth Hormone (GH)-Releasing Hormone-Stimulated GH Secretion In Healthy Men: Impact of Gonadal Steroid and GH Secretory Changes on Metabolic Outcomes," *J Clin Endocrinol Metab*, 82 (Nov 1997):3710–9.

Hagberg J.M., et al; "Metabolic Responses to Exercise in Young and Older Athletes and Sedentary Men", *J Appl Physiol*, 65 (Aug 1988):900–8.

Harro J., et al; "Association of Depressiveness with Blunted Growth Hormone Response to Maximal Physical Exercise in Young Healthy Men," *Psychoneuroendocrinology*, 24 (Jul 1999):505–17.

Karlsson J.; Metabolic Adaptations to Exercise: A Review of Potential Beta-adrenoceptor Antagonist Effects, *Am J Cardiol*, 55 (Apr 1985):48D–58D.

Kennaway D.J.; Van Dorp C.F.; "Free-running Rhythms of Melatonin, Cortisol, Electrolytes, and Sleep in Humans in Antarctica," *Am J Physiol*, (Jun 1991):1137–44.

Klatz, R. & Kahn, C. *Grow Young with HGH*. NewYork: Harper Collins, 1997.

Kostka T.; "Aging, Physical Activity and Free Radicals" *Pol Merkuriusz Lek*, 7 (Oct 1999):202–4.

Kraemer W.J. et al. "Effects of Heavy-Resistance Training on Hormonal Response Patterns in Younger and Older Men," *J Appl Physiol* 87(1999):982–92.

Kraemer W.J., et al; "Endogenous Anabolic Hormonal and Growth Factor Responses to Heavy Resistance Exercise in Males and Females," *Int J Sports Med*, 12 (Apr 1991):228–35.

Lucas R.J.; Foster R.G.; "Circadian Rhythms: Something to Cry About?" *Curr Biol*, 9 (Mar 1999):R214–7.

Luger A., et al; "Plasma Growth Hormone and Prolactin Responses to Graded Levels of Acute Exercise and to a Lactate Infusion," *Neuroendocrinology*, 56 (Jul 1992):112–7.

Maharam L.G., et al; "Masters Athletes: Factors Affecting Performance," *Sports Med*, 28 (Oct 1999):273–85.

McAuley E.; Talbot H.M.; Martinez S.; "Manipulating Self-efficacy in the Exercise Environment in Women: Influences on Affective Responses," *J Health Psychol*, 18 (May 1999):288–94.

McAuley E.; Mihalko SL; Bane SM; "Exercise and Self-Esteem in Middle-Aged Adults: Multidimensional Relationships and Physical Fitness and Self-Efficacy Influences," *J Behav Med*, 20 (Feb 1997):67–83.

McCartney, N.A., et al; "Usefulness of Weightlifting Training in Improving Strength and Maximal Power Output in Coronary Artery Disease," *Amer J Cardiol*, 67 (1991):939.

Morrow L.A., et al; "Effects of Epinephrine on Insulin Secretion and Action in Humans. Interaction with Aging," *Diabetes*, 42 (Feb 1993):307–15.

Nelson, M., *Stealing Time, The New Science of Aging*, PBS Video, Episode 2, 1998.

Noble E.G.., et al; "Differential Expression of Stress Proteins in Rat Myocardium After Free Wheel or Treadmill Run Training," 86 *J Appl Physiol*, (May 1999):1696–701.

Paffenbarger, R.S., et al; "Physical Activity, All-cause Mortality, and Longevity of College Alumni," *N Engl J Med*, 10 (Mar 1986):605–13

Poehlman, E.T.; "A Review: Exercise and its Influence on Resting Energy Metabolism in Man," *Med Sci Sports Exerc*, 21 (Oct 1989).

Rahim A., et al; "The Effect of Body Composition on Hexarelin-Induced Growth Hormone Release in Normal Elderly Subjects," *Clin Endocrinol* (Oxf), 49 (Nov 1998):659–64.

Rudolph D.L.; McAuley E.; "Cortisol and Affective Responses to Exercise," *J Sports Sci*, 16 (Feb 1998):121–8.

Scheen, A.J., et al; "Effects of Exercise on Neuroendocrine Secretions and Glucose Regulation at Different Times of Day," *Am J Physiol*, 274 (Jun 1998):1040–9.

Schneider J.K.; "Self-regulation and Exercise Behavior in Older Women," *J Gerontol B Psychol Sci Soc Sci*, 52 (Sep 1998): 235–41.

Seals D.R.., et al; Endurance Training in Older Men and Women: Cardio-vascular Responses to Exercise," *J Appl Physiol*, 57 (Oct 1984):1024–9.

Sears, B., *The Anti-Aging Zone*, Regan Books, 1999.

Seaton, K.; *Life Health and Longevity*, 1994.

Shephard, R.J. & Montelpare, W. "Geriatric Benefits of Exercise as an Adult." *J. Gerontology*, 43, (1998):M86–M90.

Shephard, R.J. Fitness and aging. In: Aging into the Twenty First Century. C. Blais (ed.). Downsview, Ont.: Captus University Publications, 1991, pp. 22–35.

Thuma J.R., et al; "Circadian Rhythm of Cortisol Confounds Cortisol Responses to Exercise: Implications for Future Research," *J Appl Physiol*, 78 (May 1995):1657–64.

Touitou Y., et al; "Effects of a Two-Hour Early Awakening and of Bright Light Exposure on Plasma Patterns of Cortisol, Melatonin, Prolactin and Testosterone in Man," *Acta Endocrinol* 126 (Mar 1992):201–5.

Ullis, K., & Ptacek, G.; *Age Right: Turn Back the Clock with a Proven, Personalized Anti-aging Program*, New York: Simon & Shuster, 1999.

Van, E.M., et al; "The Effect of Perceived Stress, Traits, Mood states, and Stressful Daily Events on Salivary Cortisol," *Psychosomatic Medicine* 58, no. 5 (Sept. 1996):447–458.

Woods J.A., et al; "Effects of 6 Months on Moderate Aerobic Exercise Training on Immune Function in the Elderly," *Mech Ageing Dev*, 109 (June 1999):1–19.

Woods J.A., et al; "Effects of Maximal Exercise on Natural Killer (NK) Cell Cytotoxicity and Responsiveness to Interferon-alpha in the Young and Old", *J Gerontol A Biol Sci Med Sci*, (Nov 1998) 53:6, B430–7.

CHAPTER 18: MIND OVER AGING

Aihara, M., et al. "A Case of Atopic Dermatitis Which Showed Correlation of Psychological State and Lesions—Change of Value of Psychological Test, Skin Lesion and NK Cell Activity." *Arerugi* 49, no. 6 (2000):487–494.

Aleksandrovskii, U., et al. "Lipid Peroxidation in Emotional Stress and Neurotic Disorders" [Russian]. *Zh Nevropatol Psikhiatr Im SS Korsakova* 88, no. 11 (1988):95–101.

Amen, D. *Change Your Brain, Change Your Life*. New York: Times Books, 1998.

Angier, N. "Chronic Anger Is Major Health Risk: Studies Find." *The New York Times* (December 13, 1990). Paper presented at a 1990 conference of the American Heart Association.

Barks, C., and M. Green. *The Illuminated Rumi*. New York: Broadway Books, 1997.

Buske-Kirschbaum, A., et al. "Conditioned Increase of Natural Killer Cell Activity (NKCA) in Humans." *Psychosomatic Medicine* 54 (1992):123–132.

Cohen, S., et al. "Social Ties and Susceptibility to the Common Cold." *JAMA* 277 (1997):1940–1944.

Glaser, R., et al. "Stress-Related Impairments in Cellular Immunity." *Psychiatric Research* 16 (1985):233–239.

Harro, J., et al. "Association of Depressiveness with Blunted Growth Hormone Response to Maximal Physical Exercise in Young Healthy Men." *Psychoneuroendocrinology* 24, no. 5 (1999):505–517.

Jackson, L. Personal communication, Boulder, Colorado, 2000.

Jemmot, J.B., et al. Secretory IgA as a Measure of Resistance to Infectious Disease: Comments on Stone, Cox, Valdimarsdottir, and Neale." *Behavioral Medicine* (Summer 1989):63–71.

Kiecolt-Glaser, J., et al. "Marital Quality, Marital Disruption, and Immune Function." *Psychosomatic Medicine* 49 (1987):13.

Lasler, K.A., et al. "Forgiveness: Physiological and Psychological Correlates." Annual Meeting of the American Psychosomatic Society, Abstract #1310, 2000.

Martin, R.A., and J.P. Dobbin. "Sense of Humor, Hassles, and Immunoglobulin A: Evidence for a Stress-Moderating Effect." *International Journal of Psychiatry in Medicine* 18 (1988):93–105.

Maruta, T., et al. "Optimists vs Pessimists: Survival Rate Among Medical Patients Over a 30-Year Period." *Mayo Clin Proc* 75, no. 2 (2000):140–143.

McClelland, D. "Motivational Factors in Health and Disease." *American Psychologist* 44, no. 4 (1989):675–683.

_____, and C. Kirschnit. "The Effect of Motivational Arousal through Films on Salivary Immunoglobulin." *Psychology and Health* 2 (1988):31–52.

McCullough, M.E., et al. "Interpersonal Forgiving in Close Relationships II: Theoretical Elaborate and Measurement." *Journal of Personality and Social Psychology* 75, no. 6 (1998):1586–1603.

McKay, J.R. "Assessing Aspects of Object Relations Associated with Immune Function: Development of the Affiliative Trust-Mistrust Coding System." *Psychological Assessment* 3, no. 4 (1991):1991.

Mind-Body Health Digest 2 (1990):5.

Pennebaker, J.W. "Telling Stories: The Health Benefits of Narrative." *Lit Med* 19, no. 1 (2000):3–18.

Petri, K.J., et al. "The Immunological Effects of Thought Suppression." *Journal of Personality and Social Psychology* 75, no. 5 (1998):1264–1272.

Russek, L.G., and G.E. Schwartz. "Narrative Descriptions of Parental Love and Caring Predict Health Status in Mid-life: A 35-Year Follow-up of the Harvard Mastery of Stress Study." *Alternative Therapies in Health and Medicine* 2 (1996):55–62.

Schneider, R.H., et al. "Effects of the Transcendental Meditation Program on Lipid Peroxide Levels in Community-Dwelling Older Adults." Presented at the Third International Congress of Behavioral Medicine, Amsterdam, The Netherlands, July 6–9, 1994.

_____, et al. "Lower Lipid Peroxide Levels in Practitioners of the Transcendental Meditation Program." *Psychosomatic Medicine* 60, no. 1 (1998):38–41.

Schwartz, G.E.R., and L.G.S. Russek. *The Living Energy Universe.* Charlottesville, VA: Hampton Roads Publishing Company, Inc., 1999.

Strasser, J.A. "The Relation of General Forgiveness and Forgiveness Type to Reported Health in the Elderly." Ph.D. dissertation, Catholic University of America, 1984.

Temoshok, L. 1985. "Biopsychosocial Studies on Cutaneous Malignant Melanoma: Psychosocial Factors Associated with Prognostic Indicators, Progression, Psychophysiology, and Tumor-Host Response." *Social Science and Medicine* 29 (1985):833–840.

_____, et al. "The Relationship of Psychosocial Factors to Prognostic Indicators in Cutaneous Malignant Melanoma." *Journal of Psychosomatic Research* 2 (1985):139–153.

Trainer, M. "Forgiveness: Intrinsic, Role-Expected, Expedient, in the Context of Divorce." Ph.D. dissertation, Boston University, 1981.

Wolf, S. "Predictors of Myocardial Infarction over a Span of 30 Years in Roseto, Pennsylvania." *Integrative Phys and Behav Sci* 27, no. 3 (1992):246–257.

PART III: TEN STEPS TO A YOUNGER YOU

Acheson, K.J., et al. "Glycogen Storage Capacity and De Novo Lipogenesis During Massive Carbohydrate Overfeeding in Man." *Amer J Clin Nut* 48 (1988):240–247.

"Adult Diabetes Type on Rise in Young." *The New York Times* (July 8, 1997):C7.

Bao, Wehang, et al. "Persistent Elevation of Plasma Insulin Levels Is Associated with Increased Cardiovascular Risk in Children and Young Adults." 93, no. 1 (January 1, 1996):54–59.

Barceló, A. "Monograph Series on Aging-Related Diseases: VIII. Non-Insulin-Dependent Diabetes Mellitus (NIDDM)." *Chronic Dis Can* 17, no. 1 (Winter 1996):1–20.

Betteridge, D.J. "Diabetic Dyslipidaemia: What Does It Mean?" *Diabetes News* 18, no. 2 (1997):1–3.

Bray, G.A. "Health Hazards of Obesity." *Endocrinol Metab Clin North Am* 25, no. 40 (1996):907–919.

Index